Recent Advance in Biomaterials, Clinical Dentistry and Dental Diseases 2.0

Recent Advance in Biomaterials, Clinical Dentistry and Dental Diseases 2.0

Editors

Naji Kharouf
Davide Mancino
Salvatore Sauro
Louis Hardan

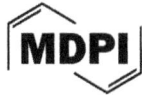

Basel • Beijing • Wuhan • Barcelona • Belgrade • Novi Sad • Cluj • Manchester

Editors

Naji Kharouf
Department of Biomaterials
and Bioengineering
University of Strasbourg
Strasbourg
France

Davide Mancino
Department of Biomaterials
and Bioengineering
University of Strasbourg
Strasbourg
France

Salvatore Sauro
Dental Biomaterials and
Minimally Invasive Dentistry
Universidad CEU-Cardenal
Herrera
Valencia
Spain

Louis Hardan
Department of Restorative
Dentistry
Saint-Joseph University
Beirut
Lebanon

Editorial Office
MDPI
St. Alban-Anlage 66
4052 Basel, Switzerland

This is a reprint of articles from the Special Issue published online in the open access journal *Bioengineering* (ISSN 2306-5354) (available at: www.mdpi.com/journal/bioengineering/special_issues/A4YZ96DJ8R).

For citation purposes, cite each article independently as indicated on the article page online and as indicated below:

Lastname, A.A.; Lastname, B.B. Article Title. *Journal Name* **Year**, *Volume Number*, Page Range.

ISBN 978-3-0365-9653-2 (Hbk)
ISBN 978-3-0365-9652-5 (PDF)
doi.org/10.3390/books978-3-0365-9652-5

© 2023 by the authors. Articles in this book are Open Access and distributed under the Creative Commons Attribution (CC BY) license. The book as a whole is distributed by MDPI under the terms and conditions of the Creative Commons Attribution-NonCommercial-NoDerivs (CC BY-NC-ND) license.

Contents

About the Editors vii

Preface ix

Antoun Farrayeh, Samar Akil, Ammar Eid, Valentina Macaluso, Davide Mancino and Youssef Haïkel et al.
Effectiveness of Two Endodontic Instruments in Calcium Silicate-Based Sealer Retreatment
Reprinted from: *Bioengineering* **2023**, *10*, 362, doi:10.3390/bioengineering10030362 1

Rami Zen Aldeen, Ossama Aljabban, Ahmad Almanadili, Saleh Alkurdi, Ammar Eid and Davide Mancino et al.
The Influence of Carious Lesion and Bleeding Time on the Success of Partial Pulpotomy in Permanent Molars with Irreversible Pulpitis: A Prospective Study
Reprinted from: *Bioengineering* **2023**, *10*, 700, doi:10.3390/bioengineering10060700 12

Tarek Ashi, Davide Mancino, Louis Hardan, Rim Bourgi, Jihed Zghal and Valentina Macaluso et al.
Physicochemical and Antibacterial Properties of Bioactive Retrograde Filling Materials
Reprinted from: *Bioengineering* **2022**, *9*, 624, doi:10.3390/bioengineering9110624 26

Louis Hardan, Jean Claude Abou Chedid, Rim Bourgi, Carlos Enrique Cuevas-Suárez, Monika Lukomska-Szymanska and Vincenzo Tosco et al.
Peptides in Dentistry: A Scoping Review
Reprinted from: *Bioengineering* **2023**, *10*, 214, doi:10.3390/bioengineering10020214 36

Claire El Hachem, Jean Claude Abou Chedid, Walid Nehme, Marc Krikor Kaloustian, Nabil Ghosn and Morgane Rabineau et al.
The Contribution of Various In Vitro Methodologies to Comprehending the Filling Ability of Root Canal Pastes in Primary Teeth
Reprinted from: *Bioengineering* **2023**, *10*, 818, doi:10.3390/bioengineering10070818 63

Maciej Zarow, Louis Hardan, Katarzyna Szczeklik, Rim Bourgi, Carlos Enrique Cuevas-Suárez and Natalia Jakubowicz et al.
Porcelain Veneers in Vital vs. Non-Vital Teeth: A Retrospective Clinical Evaluation
Reprinted from: *Bioengineering* **2023**, *10*, 168, doi:10.3390/bioengineering10020168 76

Mélanie Maillard, Octave Nadile Bandiaky, Suzanne Maunoury, Charles Alliot, Brigitte Alliot-Licht and Samuel Serisier et al.
The Effectiveness of Calcium Phosphates in the Treatment of Dentinal Hypersensitivity: A Systematic Review
Reprinted from: *Bioengineering* **2023**, *10*, 447, doi:10.3390/bioengineering10040447 88

Yi-Cheng Mao, Yen-Cheng Huang, Tsung-Yi Chen, Kuo-Chen Li, Yuan-Jin Lin and Yu-Lin Liu et al.
Deep Learning for Dental Diagnosis: A Novel Approach to Furcation Involvement Detection on Periapical Radiographs
Reprinted from: *Bioengineering* **2023**, *10*, 802, doi:10.3390/bioengineering10070802 106

Yi-Chieh Chen, Ming-Yi Chen, Tsung-Yi Chen, Mei-Ling Chan, Ya-Yun Huang and Yu-Lin Liu et al.
Improving Dental Implant Outcomes: CNN-Based System Accurately Measures Degree of Peri-Implantitis Damage on Periapical Film
Reprinted from: *Bioengineering* **2023**, *10*, 640, doi:10.3390/bioengineering10060640 124

Konstantin Johannes Scholz, Karl-Anton Hiller, Helga Ebensberger, Gerlinde Ferstl, Florian Pielnhofer and Tobias T. Tauböck et al.
Surface Accumulation of Cerium, Self-Assembling Peptide, and Fluoride on Sound Bovine Enamel
Reprinted from: *Bioengineering* **2022**, *9*, 760, doi:10.3390/bioengineering9120760 . . . . **143**

About the Editors

Naji Kharouf

Naji Kharouf is currently an Associate Professor in the Faculty of Dentistry and the department of Biomaterials and Bioengineering INSERM UMR_S 1121 at Strasbourg University, France. Prof Kharouf has been working in dental biomaterials, endodontic treatment, coronal restorative techniques, bioactive molecules, microsurgical skeels, and dental morphology since 2018 (H-Index: 14, 2024). He has been a speaker at several international conferences. He has published, in collaboration with international researchers, more than 68 scientific papers in international peer-review journals with a high impact factor in the dental and biomaterials field. He has a Certificate in Oral Implantology, a Master's degree in Biomaterials for Health, a Microsurgical Diploma, an Esthetic of Smile Diploma, a PhD in Endodontics, a post-doc in Dental materials, and finally an H.D.R. in dental materials modified with graphene. He is a lecturer and monitor in several dental courses at Strasbourg University, and he also supervises Master's, PhD, and post-doc students.

Davide Mancino

Professor Mancino graduated in Dentistry and Dental Prosthetics from the University of Palermo in 2001. In 2011, he successfully completed a Master's degree in Micro-Edodontics at the University of Turin. In 2019, he received a PhD in Biomaterials (chemistry and physics) from Strasbourg University. He is currently a Professor of Endodontics at the University of Strasbourg and has been a researcher at the Inserm Research Laboratory since 2014.

He is the director of the Diploma in Clinical and Surgical Microendodontics at the University of Strasbourg.

He is the author of several international publications in the field of endodontics, a speaker at national and international congresses, and a certified trainer in France, where he organizes several training courses in endodontics.

Salvatore Sauro

Dr Salvatore Sauro is currently a Professor in Dental Biomaterials and Minimally Invasive Dentistry at the "*Departamento de Odontología, Facultad de Ciencias de la Salud, Universidad CEU-Cardenal Herrera*", coordinator of "Dental Research", and Director (Principal Investigator) of the research group "In Situ Dental Tissues Engineering and Minimally Invasive Therapeutic Adhesive Rehabilitation". He is also a Visiting Senior Lecturer at the Faculty of Dentistry, King's College London Dental Institute (KCLDI), Visiting Professor at the School of Dentistry, Moscow, Sechenov University of Moscow (Russia), Visiting Professor at the School of Dentistry, University of Federico II of Napoli, as well as University Aldo Moro, Bari. He is also an Honorary Professor at the Dental School, University of Hong Kong. Dr. Sauro has been working in dental biomaterials and preventive and minimally invasive dentistry research for more than 15 years (H-Index: 46 2024) and he has published, in collaboration with internationally renowned researchers, more than 150 articles in international peer-review journals with a high impact factor in the dental and biomaterials field, along with more several research abstracts and lectures at international conferences.

Louis Hardan

Louis Hardan is a full professor at the Department of Esthetic and Restorative Dentistry, School of Dentistry, Saint-Joseph University, Beirut, Lebanon, and owns a private practice in his hometown of Byblos. He is the former Head of the Restorative and Esthetic Department at Saint-Joseph University, Beirut, Lebanon (2013–2019), has been a Director of a Master's program since 2019, and a Coordinator of the Prosthetic and Esthetic Master's program since 2021. He graduated in Dentistry in 1989 and continued his post-doctoral education at Saint-Joseph University; he obtained a certificate for Basic Science in 1993, completed his specialization in Restorative and Esthetic Dentistry in 1995, and completed his PhD in Oral Biology and Materials in 2009. He was an active member of the Lebanese Dental Association (LDA) board (2006–2009) and was assigned to be the General Secretary of the LDA in 2009. He has been the Country Chairperson for Lebanon of the European Society of Cosmetic Dentistry (ESCD) since 2020, is ESCD certified, an ESCD board member, and has been the International Affairs Chairperson since 2021. He was the winner of the Academic Award of the ESCD during the Oscar Night Ceremony of the 20th ESCD Anniversary in 2023. He is the inventor of Smile Lite MDP (Smile Line, Switzerland), a device which takes high-quality dental pictures with a mobile phone (winner of the best of class technology award for 2017 in the USA and winner of the CEDE 2022 in Poland), and Posterior Misura (LM instrument), an instrument for direct posterior composites. Prof. Hardan has many publications in many indexed and high-impact-factor international journals, chapters in international dental books, and is the author of a book entitled *Protocols for Mobile Dental Photography with Auxiliary Lighting* (Quintessence Publishing, 2020) and has given several international lectures and courses on dental adhesion, esthetic and restorative dentistry, and mobile dental photography.

Preface

The dental biomaterials field is developing very quickly. The dental market needs biomaterials which are biocompatible and bioactive. The bioactivity of dental material means that the material could ensure a biological effect or simulate this reaction. These bioactive biomaterials are used in all dental fields to enhance antibacterial activity and ameliorate the healing process.

Naji Kharouf, Davide Mancino, Salvatore Sauro, and Louis Hardan
Editors

Article

Effectiveness of Two Endodontic Instruments in Calcium Silicate-Based Sealer Retreatment

Antoun Farrayeh [1], Samar Akil [1], Ammar Eid [1], Valentina Macaluso [2], Davide Mancino [3,4,5], Youssef Haïkel [3,4,5] and Naji Kharouf [4,5,*]

1 Department of Endodontics, Faculty of Dental Medicine, Damascus University, Damascus 0100, Syria
2 ESTA, School of Business and Technology, 90000 Belfort, France
3 Pôle de Médecine et Chirurgie Bucco-Dentaire, Hôpital Civil, Hôpitaux Universitaire de Strasbourg, 67000 Strasbourg, France
4 Department of Biomaterials and Bioengineering, INSERM UMR_S, Strasbourg University, 67000 Strasbourg, France
5 Department of Endodontics, Faculty of Dental Medicine, Strasbourg University, 67000 Strasbourg, France
* Correspondence: dentistenajikharouf@gmail.com; Tel.: +33-(0)6-6752-2841

Abstract: The objective of the present in vitro work was to investigate the effectiveness and time required for the removal of calcium silicate-based sealer using two rotary retreatment systems. Sixty extracted, single-canal, lower premolars were used. After obturation using the single-cone technique with calcium silicate-based sealer, samples were divided into four groups according to the technique of desobturation: Group 1 (G1): D-Race; Group 2 (G2): D-Race followed by the use of XP–Endo Finisher R; Group 3 (G3): Protaper Universal Retreatment; and Group 4 (G4): Protaper Universal Retreatment followed by the use of XP–Endo Finisher R. Cone beam computed tomography (CBCT) images were used to calculate the remaining filling materials at the middle and apical thirds. Times required to perform each method were recorded. Scanning electron microscopy (SEM) and digital microscopy were used to evaluate the remaining filling materials. Data were statistically analyzed using the t-test and one way ANOVA on ranks tests. No statistically significant difference was found between G1 and G3 after CBCT observations ($p > 0.05$). Xp-Endo Finisher R significantly increased the ability to remove materials regardless of the initially used retreatment system ($p < 0.05$). Statistically significant longer time was found in G3 and G4 compared to G1 and G2, respectively ($p < 0.05$), to reach the full working length. No retreatment system was able to totally remove the calcium silicate-based sealer from the root canal at the middle and apical thirds ($p > 0.05$). Digital microscopy demonstrated that the residual materials were the remaining sealers on the canal walls. SEM showed the mineral depositions of calcium silicate materials onto the canal walls and into the dentinal tubules. However, that calcium silicate materials provide mineral deposition into the dentinal tubules might indicate that the traditional irrigants could not be sufficient to remove calcium silicate-based materials from the root canal, and other agents should be used to make retreatment considerably easier.

Keywords: root canal retreatment; calcium silicate-based cement; ProTaper Universal Retreatment; D-Race

1. Introduction

Non-surgical endodontic retreatment is the first option after the failure of conventional endodontic treatment [1]. It leads to elimination of the microorganisms that are responsible for persistent infections [2,3]. Bacteria such as *Enterococcus faecalis* remain after primary endodontic treatment in areas that were unreachable by instrumentation and irrigation [4,5]. It is impossible to totally remove the filling material from the root canal during retreatment using conventional instruments and techniques due to their anatomical complexity, especially in oval canals [6,7]. The residual microorganisms and filling materials could affect the final retreatment outcome [8]. In addition, the main purpose of endodontic retreatment is to retrieve healthy periapical tissue. It aims to regain access to the apical region through total removal of filling materials [9].

Removal of gutta-percha can be accomplished using hand files, rotary and reciprocating systems, ultrasonic methods, lasers, and chemical solvents [10–14]. Mechanized protocols were proposed to be supplementary steps after the initial removal of filling materials, including the use of Self-Adjusting File (SAF) instruments (ReDent, Ra'anana, Israel) [15], sonic and ultrasonic tips [7], the XP-endo Finisher (FKG Dentaire, La Chaux-de-Fonds, Switzerland), and the XP-endo Finisher R (FKG Dentaire, La Chaux-de-Fonds, Switzerland), with the main cause of removing the remaining materials from the root canal system.

The use of nickel-titanium (NiTi) rotary retreatment systems is an efficient and safe approach to remove filling materials during root canal retreatment [16]. In addition, several dental companies have introduced NiTi rotary retreatment systems on the dental market. The ProTaper Universal Retreatment system (Dentsply Maillefer, Ballaigues, Switzerland) includes three files—D1, D2 and D3—to remove filling materials from the root canal. These files have a convex triangular cross-section identical to the ProTaper shaping and finishing instruments [17].

The D-RaCe retreatment system (FKG Dentaire, La-Chaux-de Fonds, Switzerland) contains two instruments—DR1 (30/0.10) and DR2 (25/0.04)—for cleaning of the coronal third and to reach the working length (WL), respectively. Both instruments possess an active working tip to promote the initial penetration into the root canal filling material [18].

The XP-endo Finisher R (XPF-R) (FKG Dentaire, Switzerland) is a non-tapered file fabricated with NiTi MaxWire alloy (Martensite-Austenite Electropolish Flex). At temperatures less than 30 °C, this file is straight (martensitic phase "M-phase"), while the placement of this file inside the root canal at body temperature can transform it into an austenitic phase. In this phase, the file takes on a spoon shape in the last 10 mm, with a depth of roughly 1.5 mm. During entry of this file into the root canal, its austenite phase conversion and shape memory enhance its effectiveness in displacing and touching root-obturation materials. Therefore, this profile allows the instrument to attain irregular zones without modifying the original shape of the canal [1,8,19].

Various chemical compositions have been used in endodontic sealers to obturate the root canal with a gutta-percha point. These materials include zinc oxide-eugenol, gutta-percha flow, epoxy-resin, and calcium silicate cements [20]. Calcium silicate (CS) materials, called bioceramics, are considered a breakthrough in endodontic treatment due to their advantageous biocompatibility, antibacterial activity, appropriate filling ability, and good physicochemical properties. Their setting reaction could generate hydroxyapatite on their surfaces and cause tags in the dentinal tubules [21,22]. Different forms of calcium silicate sealers were introduced as powder-liquid and premixed products [23]. Premixed sealers demonstrated greater filling ability and easier application than conventional sealer. Ceraseal (Metabiomed, Korea) is a premixed calcium silicate sealer that demonstrated high obturation quality and appropriate biological, mechanical, and physicochemical properties [23]. The main disadvantage of calcium silicate materials is difficulty with their retreatment, especially at the apical third, and their removal requires both mechanical and chemical procedures [21].

Various dental companies have developed NiTi removal systems such as Mtwo retreatment (VDW, Munich, Germany), R-Endo, and Remover (Micro-Mega, Besançon, France). Hassan et al. studied the retreatment efficiency of R-endo and Xp-endo shaper files in root canals obturated using a bioceramic root canal sealer. The results showed that Xp-endo shaper files were significantly more effective in removing obturation materials. However, neither system totally removed the remaining materials from the coronal, middle, and apical thirds [24]. Donnermeyer et al. studied the retreatability of three calcium silicate sealers and one epoxy resin sealer with four different root canal instruments. They reported that engine-driven NiTi instruments were better suited to remove root canal fillings than stainless steel Hedström files [25].

Until now, there has been no validated protocol for the desobturation of calcium silicate material from the root canal in the literature; thus, research studies are still needed to enhance the efficacy of instruments and solvents in bioceramic retreatment.

The objective of this study was to evaluate the effectiveness of two retreatment instruments with or without a supplementary activation step in the removal of calcium silicate-based sealer. The null hypothesis was that there is no difference between the different instruments and the supplementary cleaning step regarding the quality of calcium silicate retreatment.

2. Materials and Methods

2.1. Teeth Preparation

After approval by the ethics committee of Damascus University, Damascus, Syria (protocol n. 3215-2020), 63 extracted single canal lower premolars without caries and previous endodontic treatment were selected for the present study. The exclusion criteria were teeth with resorption, incomplete apices, severe curvatures, and cracks. The canal curvature was measured as described in a previous study [26]; thus, teeth with a maximum canal curvature of 15° were selected. Root surfaces were cleaned, and all soft tissue and calculus were removed mechanically with periodontal curettes. Afterwards, the teeth were rinsed and then kept in 0.9% NaCl at 4 °C.

After preparation of the access cavity using diamond burs and ultrasonic tips, a size 10 stainless steel K-file (Mani, Takenzawa, Japan) was inserted to reach the apical foramen. All endodontic steps were performed under 4.5× magnification using Q-Optics Loupes (Q-Optics, Duncanville, TX, USA). To standardize the samples, all tooth crowns were sectioned to reach a root length of 17 mm and a working length (WL) of 16 mm. The same operator prepared all canals using ProTaper Next instruments (Dentsply Sirona, Konstanz, Germany) up to an X2 file at the WL with an electric motor (VDW, Munich, Germany) at a speed of 300 rpm and 3 Ncm of torque. After the use of each instrument, the canals were irrigated with 1 mL of 2.5% NaOCl using a 30-gauge needle. After shaping procedures, the smear layer was eliminated using 5 mL of 17% EDTA and 5 mL of 2.5% NaOCl for final irrigation, and then paper points were used to dry the canal. The single-cone technique was used to obturate the root canal with calcium silicate-based sealer (Ceraseal, Metabiomed, Cheongju, Republic of Korea). The intracanal tip was inserted into the coronal third of the canal, and the sealer was dispensed into the canal. The gutta-percha cone was then painted with the calcium silicate material and slowly inserted into the canal to the appropriate length. Finally, to remove the extra gutta-percha, a hot plugger was used to remove it. The access cavities were filled with a temporary filling material (MD-Temp, Metabiomed, Republic of Korea). The samples were then stored in phosphate-buffered saline (PBS10×, Dominique Dutscher, Bernolsheim, France) for 28 days to insure an appropriate setting of the filling material.

2.2. Non-surgical Root Canal Retreatment

After the storage period, coronal access was performed using size 3 and 2 files at 2000 rpm with Peeso drills (Mani, Takenzawa, Japan). The samples were randomly divided into four equal groups (n = 15) as follows:

- Group 1 (G1): D-Race files (Figure 1) were used with a speed of 600 rpm and torque of 1 Ncm. The coronal third of the obturation material was applied with a DR1 file (30/0.10) (Figure 1). Then, the DR2 file (25/0.4) was used for the two other thirds (middle and apical) to attain the working length.
- Group 2 (G2): the same procedure as in G1 was used with an additional step. The XP–Endo Finisher R file (XPF-R) (Figure 1) was used as a supplementary file following the initial retreatment procedures. The XPF-R file was used following the manufacturer's instructions at a torque of 1 Ncm and a speed of 800 rpm. A contra angle handpiece was used with the instrument. The XPF-R file was placed into the canal with no rotation. Subsequently, the instrument was activated for 1 min using slow and gentle

7- to 8-mm lengthwise movements up to the WL in a brushing action against the root canal walls.
- Group 3 (G3): ProTaper Universal Retreatment files (Figure 1) were used at a speed of 300 rpm with 3 Ncm of torque. A ProTaper D1 file (30/0.09) was used to prepare the coronal third of the canal. At the middle and apical thirds, D2 (25/0.08) and D3 (20/0.07) files were used to remove the filling materials.
- Group 4 (G4): the same procedure as in G3 was used with an additional step. The XP–Endo Finisher R file (XPF-E) (Figure 1) was applied as a supplementary file according the retreatment procedures.

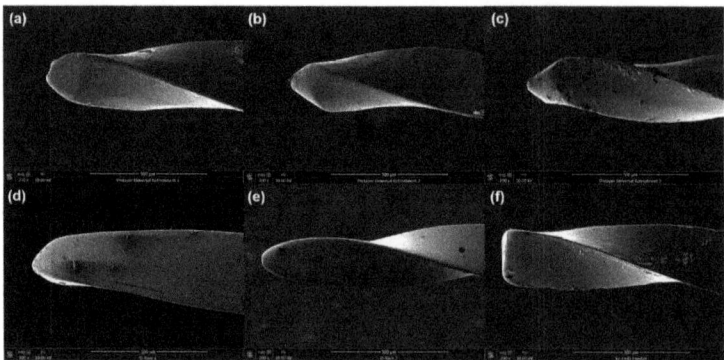

Figure 1. SEM images of the tips of (**a–c**) the ProTaper Universal Retreatment D1, D2 and D3, (**d,e**) the D-Race DR1 and DR2; and (**f**) the XP–Endo Finisher R file.

During instrumentation procedures, irrigation was performed with 2 mL of 2.5% NaOCl. All procedures were performed in an incubator at 37 °C. All steps were completed by the same operator. All errors during treatment, including instrument fracture, canal ledges, and blockages, were recorded. In case of a fractured instrument, the tooth was discarded and replaced with another one (three teeth were replaced due to procedural errors). Final irrigation was performed using 5 mL of 17% EDTA and 5 mL of 2.5% NaOCl. After the final irrigation step, the canals were dried with paper points. Two procedural times were recorded to obtain the total working time; including the time needed to attain the WL (T1) and the time needed to remove the gutta-percha (T2). The retreatment procedure was considered complete once the instrument flutes or the irrigation solution had no more residue from the calcium silicate-based sealer or gutta percha material [27].

2.3. Remaining Filling Materials Observations

2.3.1. Cone Beam Computed Tomography (CBCT) and Micro-computed Tomography (μCt)

CBCT scans were obtained using a PaX-i3D Green unit (Vatech, Hwaseong-si, Republic of Korea). The samples were exposed to 90 kV and 10.2 mA with an FOV of 5 × 5 cm and an isotropic resolution of 0.1 mm, with 12.57 s of exposure time. The artifacts created by the radiopaque root fillings were eliminated using inbuilt software. The images were evaluated in cross-sections plans, and the percentages of remaining materials at the apical and middle thirds were calculated using the inbuilt software. Finally, the CBCT cross-sections were analyzed, and scores were obtained for all CBCT images by two observers.

After the CBCT observations, the most meaningful sample from each group was analyzed using μCT (IRIS, Inviscan, http://www.inviscan.fr/product_iris_pet_ct.html accessed date: 15 December 2022) to show and evaluate the void percentages in them. The acquisition settings were 2000 projection (60 × 60 × 60 μm 3 voxel size) and 80 kVp. The images were visualized and manipulated using the Mimics Innovation Suite, version 24 (Materialise, Louvain, Belgium).

2.3.2. Digital Microscopy

After CBCT observations, the samples were prepared by creating two shallow longitudinal grooves in the buccolingual direction by a diamond bur. The grooves were created following the canal morphology and curvature. These grooves did not enter into the canal space. Each sample was split by a chisel and mallet to investigate the internal walls [28]. The internal walls of the root canal for each sample were investigated using a digital microscope (KEYENCE, Osaka, Japan) at 100× magnification to analyze the nature of the residual filling materials (gutta-percha and/or sealer), which could not be observed through CBCT analysis.

2.3.3. Scanning Electron Microscopy (SEM)

After digital macroscopy observations, the samples were dried in a graded series of ethanol (50, 70, 95, and 100%) for 10 min each. Finally, these samples were mounted on SEM stubs sputter-coated with gold–palladium (20/80) using a Hummer JR sputtering device (Technics, San Jose, California, USA). The samples were observed at different magnifications (100×–20.000×) with a working distance of 10 mm and a 10-kV acceleration voltage of the electrons through a scanning electron microscope (SEM, Quanta 250 FEG scanning electron microscope, FEI Company, Eindhoven, the Netherlands) [29].

2.4. Statistical Analysis

Statistical analysis was performed using SPSS software (version 17, SPSS, Chicago, IL, USA). The normality was verified with the Shapiro–Wilk test. However, when the normality test was not passed, an analysis of the variance on ranks, along with a multiple comparison procedure (Tukey's test), was performed to determine whether significant differences existed in the remaining material values between the different retreatments. The lapse to complete the retreatment of all groups was determined using the t-test, and the chi-square test was used to determine whether significant differences existed in the re-establishing of the working length. In all tests, a statistical significance level of $\alpha = 0.05$ was adopted.

3. Results

3.1. Ability to Reach WL and Required Time

The WL was re-established in 93.34%, 86.67%, 80%, and 86.67% of teeth for G1, G2, G3, and G4 respectively ($p > 0.05$) (Figure 2). Statistically longer time values were recorded for the groups in which Protaper Universal Retreatment was used compared to the groups in which D-Race was used regardless of the use of XP–Endo Finisher R (Table 1).

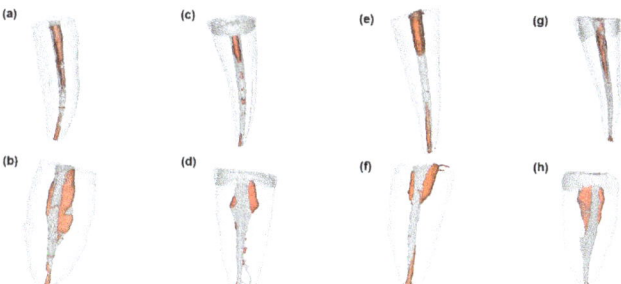

Figure 2. µCt images of the samples after retreatment procedures. (**a,b**) G1: D-Race files; (**c,d**) G2: D-Race and XP–Endo Finisher R; (**e,f**) G3: ProTaper Universal Retreatment; (**g,h**) G4: ProTaper Universal Retreatment and XP–Endo Finisher R file.

Table 1. Time required to re-establish the working length in the different groups. Different superscripted letters (a–d) indicate significant differences between the different groups ($p < 0.05$). Group 1 (G1): D-Race; Group 2 (G2): D-Race followed by the use of XP–Endo Finisher R; Group 3 (G3): Protaper Universal Retreatment; and Group 4 (G4): Protaper Universal Retreatment followed by the use of XP–Endo Finisher R.

	G1	G2	G3	G4	Statistical Analysis ($p < 0.05$)
Time (s)	214 ± 13 [a]	269 ± 28 [b]	304 ± 34 [c]	362 ± 35 [d]	a < c and b < d

3.2. CBCT and μCt Evaluations

No significant differences were found for the remaining material percentages between G1 and G3 ($p > 0.05$). The use of XP–Endo Finisher R (G2 and G4) demonstrated statistically greater efficacy in the removal of remaining materials than the other groups (G1 and G3) ($p < 0.05$) (Figure 2 and Table 2).

Table 2. Residual material percentages after all retreatment techniques. Different superscripted letters (a–d) indicate significant differences between the different groups ($p < 0.05$). Group 1 (G1): D-Race; Group 2 (G2): D-Race followed by the use of XP–Endo Finisher R; Group 3 (G3): Protaper Universal Retreatment; and Group 4 (G4) Protaper Universal Retreatment followed by the use of XP–Endo Finisher R.

	G1	G2	G3	G4	Statistical Analysis ($p < 0.05$)
Middle (%)	12 ± 6 [a]	8.4 ± 4.1 [b]	16.4 ± 11.1 [a]	8.8 ± 3.8 [b]	b < a
Apical (%)	14 ± 7 [a]	4.5 ± 0.6 [b]	15.4 ± 10.6 [a]	6.5 ± 6.4 [b]	b < a

3.3. Digital Microscope Observations

The use of CBCT did not reveal the nature of the remaining materials; thus, digital microscopy was used to investigate this finding. However, the most common residual materials were the calcium silicate sealers with small amounts of gutta-percha residue, as shown in Figure 3.

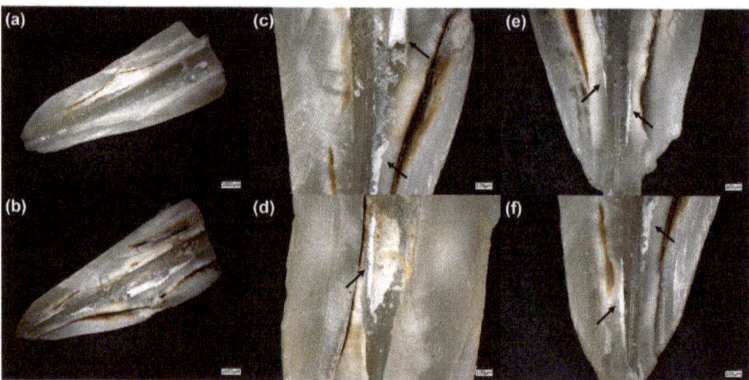

Figure 3. Digital microscope images demonstrate the effectiveness of the retreatment technique and the nature of the residual materials in (**a**,**b**) the root canal at (**c**,**d**) the middle and (**e**,**f**) apical thirds (black arrows).

3.4. SEM Observations

SEM was used to investigate the quality of smear layer and filling material removal after instrumentation and final irrigation using EDTA and NaOCl. Most dentinal tubules in all of the groups at the middle and apical thirds were not opened after the final irrigation (Figure 4a,b), while only a few zones in G2 and G4 demonstrated partially opened dentinal tubules (Figure 4c,d). Some zones were covered totally with sealer material, and this layer was not eliminated using the different protocols (Figure 4e). This layer covers the entrance of the dentinal tubules (Figure 4e) and prevented complete cleaning of the root canal system. After the immersion period, calcium silicate-based materials ensure the mineral deposition in the dentinal tubules, which could totally close them (Figure 4f). Therefore, the cleaning and opening of the dentinal tubules in root canals could be very difficult after the use of bioceramic material.

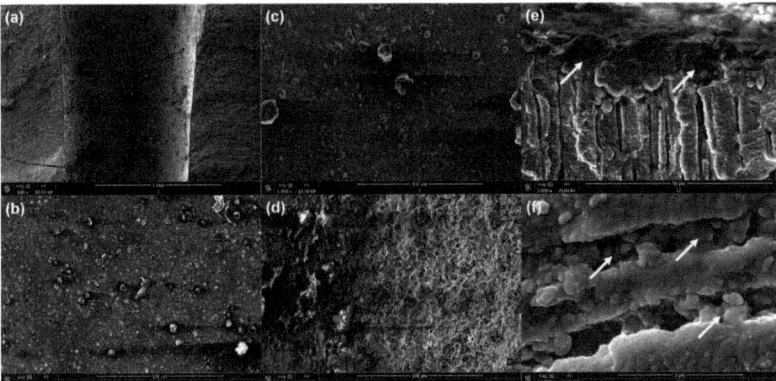

Figure 4. SEM images demonstrate (**a**,**b**) closed dentinal tubules; (**c**,**d**) partially opened dentinal tubules; (**e**) remaining calcium silicate sealer on the root canal walls; (**f**) dentinal tubules filled with mineral components (white arrows).

4. Discussion

Root canal treatments usually fail due to persistent periapical disorders after treatment [30]. Moreover, coronal leakage, periodical caries, necrotic tissue, tooth cracks and fractures, and bacterial biofilms could lead to treatment failure [31]. In addition, these etiological factors should be eliminated to establish adequate periapical recovery; thus, establishing patency and working length in retreatment cases could significantly provide for better periapical healing outcomes [32]. However, retreatment procedures are not always possible due to several factors, including root canal anatomy and resistant filling materials [21,27,33,34].

Currently, calcium silicate materials are used frequently in endodontic practice due to their great biological, mechanical, and physicochemical properties [35,36]. Ceraseal sealer, which was used in the present study, is one of these calcium silicate endodontic products that has demonstrated an alkaline pH and release of Ca^{2+} ions [23]. Therefore, these properties might enhance and provide for the mineralization process and the formation of hydroxyapatite tags in the dentinal tubules [21,23,29,35].

In the present in vitro study, SEM observations, digital analysis, and CBCT investigations demonstrated that there is no retreatment system that could totally eliminate the remaining filling materials and completely open the dentinal tubules. The results demonstrated that there are no statistically significant differences between the two rotary systems (G1 and G3) regarding the efficacy of filling material removal from the root canal at the middle and apical thirds ($p > 0.05$), while the supplementary cleaning step (XPF-R in G2 and G4) enhanced statistically the efficacy of retreatment ($p < 0.05$). These findings suggest that supplementary steps are able to decrease the amount of remaining filling materials. Moreover, the tested techniques in this study showed that they cannot provide for complete removal of the filling materials from the root canal system. Therefore the null hypothesis must be partially rejected.

The findings of the present work demonstrated that retreatment with the D-Race system required less time compared to ProTaper Universal Retreatment files, which might be attributed to the greater efficacy of D-Race files in removing gutta-percha, as well as two instruments being used in the D-Race system compared to three instruments being used in the ProTaper Universal Retreatment. Regarding the amount of remaining filling materials after retreatment, no statistically significant differences were found between the two systems: D-RaCe and ProTaper rotary instruments ($p > 0.05$). In contrast, the addition of a supplementary cleaning step using XPF-R (G2 and G4) demonstrated statistically higher cleaning efficiency results in all root segments compared to the two initial retreatment systems without this supplementary step ($p < 0.05$). This finding could be attributed to XPF-R metallurgy. The manufacture and improvement of these files depend on the shape-memory of its alloy. The file is straight in its M-phase, which is composed in cooled conditions. When the file is subjected to body temperature, its shape transforms into the A-phase. The shape in this phase permits the file to clean the zones that are otherwise inaccessible with regular instruments [37,38]. Therefore, novel instruments, systems, and supplementary steps and techniques are required for remaining filling material removal, especially in oval-shaped root canals, as well as in filled canals with bioceramic materials [28,39,40]. Removal of root filling materials during endodontic retreatment was previously evaluated using stereomicroscopy, scanning electron microscopy, digital microscopy, and x-ray radiography. Some studies used CBCT for the assessment of remaining filling materials. CBCT provides three-dimensional (3D) images on the axial, coronal, and axial planes, and it is capable of visualizing the root canal system and analyzing the quality of cleaning in extracted teeth [10,41].

Digital images demonstrated that most remaining materials in the root canals after retreatment procedures are the residues of calcium silicate sealers, which are stuck on the dentinal walls (Figure 3). Kaloustian et al. [28] used a digital microscope to investigate the amount of the remaining materials after different retreatment methods. Previous studies have reported that gutta-percha material could be eliminated mechanically using instruments and chemically by the application of different solvents [10–14]. In contrast, calcium silicate sealers and cements are very difficult in retreatment due to their high compressive strength, appropriate interactions with dental tissues, and mineralization reactions [20,21,23,29,35,36,42]. A previous study demonstrated that the use of special acids, such as formic acid, is the best route to retreat teeth filled with calcium silicate-based sealer [43].

Various studies have demonstrated that the use of EDTA and NaOCl as irrigants could provide for smear layer removal in permanent and primary teeth [44,45]. In contrast, SEM images in the present study rarely showed dentinal zones with opened dentinal tubules and an eliminated smear layer. Most observations showed debris in the root canal, closed dentinal tubules, remaining calcium silicate particles, and their mineralogical reactions in the dentinal tubules, which are near the principal root canal. In accordance, a previous study demonstrated that the use of calcium silicate-based material by orthograde obturation of the root canals could provide favorable conditions for bacterial entombment by intratubular mineralization [22]. Therefore, plugging the dentinal tubules with calcium silicate materials and/or their mineralogical reactions could close totally the dentinal tubules; thus, special solvent should be used to open them. In contrast, this plugging could enclose the remaining bacteria in the dentinal tubules and kill these microorganisms over time [22].

Finally, the findings of the present study are in accordance with previous studies reporting that retreatment with calcium silicate materials is considered a big challenge in endodontic treatment [21,34,46,47]. These materials could be considered to result in real blockage of the apical foramen, preventing patency of the root canal and the reestablishing of the WL, which are considered to be important outcomes. Further research is needed to evaluate the effects of different acids and solvents accompanying mechanical process and activation in retreatment with calcium silicate materials in straight and curved root canals. Moreover, the mineralization process of the different calcium silicate materials and the time needed to totally close the dentinal tubules will be further investigated. All the samples were observed using CBCT, while fewer samples were analyzed with μCt, which was used to obtain a higher resolution of data that were process using Mimics Innovation Suite software, version 24 (Materialise, Louvain, Belgium). This fact could be considered a limitation of the present work.

5. Conclusions

Within the limitations of the present in vitro study, none of the used systems was able to completely remove the CS material from the root canal. No significant difference was found between the two retreatment systems. Supplementary cleaning steps are effective tools to enhance the cleanliness of the root canal after a retreatment procedure. The traditional irrigants (EDTA and NaOCl) could not completely the open dentinal tubules after an obturation procedure using CS materials.

Author Contributions: Conceptualization, S.A.; methodology, A.F.; software, A.F.; validation, S.A.; formal analysis, A.F.; investigation, A.E.; resources, A.F.; data curation, A.F.; writing—original draft preparation, A.F.; writing—review and editing, N.K., D.M., V.M., A.E. and A.F.; visualization, N.K. and Y.H.; supervision, S.A.; project administration, S.A. All authors have read and agreed to the published version of the manuscript.

Funding: This research received no external funding.

Institutional Review Board Statement: This in vitro study was conducted according to the guidelines of the Declaration of Helsinki and approved by the ethics committee of Damascus University (protocol no. 3215-2020).

Informed Consent Statement: Each patient was informed of the study's procedure and objectives, and his or her non-opposition to the use of his or her tooth was recorded in his or her chart by the oral surgeon.

Data Availability Statement: The data presented in this study are available on request from the first author.

Conflicts of Interest: The authors declare no conflict of interest.

References

1. Volponi, A.; Pelegrine, R.A.; Kato, A.S.; Stringheta, C.P.; Lopes, R.T.; Silva, A.S.S.; Bueno, C.E.D.S. Micro-computed Tomographic Assessment of Supplementary Cleaning Techniques for Removing Bioceramic Sealer and Gutta-percha in Oval Canals. *J. Endod.* **2020**, *46*, 1901–1906. [CrossRef] [PubMed]
2. Nair, P.N. On the causes of persistent apical periodontitis: A review. *Int. Endod. J.* **2006**, *39*, 249–281. [CrossRef] [PubMed]
3. Siqueira, J.F., Jr.; Rôças, I.N. Clinical implications and microbiology of bacterial persistence after treatment procedures. *J. Endod.* **2008**, *34*, 1291–1301.e3. [CrossRef] [PubMed]
4. Berman, L.H.; Hargreaves, K.M. *Cohen's Pathways of the Pulp Expert Consult*, 12th ed.; Elsevier: Amsterdam, The Netherlands, 2020.
5. Nasiri, K.; Wrbas, K.T. Comparison of the efficacy of different Ni-Ti instruments in the removal of gutta-percha and sealer in root canal retreatment. *Indian J. Dent. Res.* **2020**, *31*, 579–584. [CrossRef]
6. Nguyen, T.A.; Kim, Y.; Kim, E.; Shin, S.J.; Kim, S. Comparison of the Efficacy of Different Techniques for the Removal of Root Canal Filling Material in Artificial Teeth: A Micro-Computed Tomography Study. *J. Clin. Med.* **2019**, *8*, 984. [CrossRef]
7. Martins, M.P.; Duarte, M.A.; Cavenago, B.C.; Kato, A.S.; da Silveira Bueno, C.E. Effectiveness of the ProTaper Next and Reciproc Systems in Removing Root Canal Filling Material with Sonic or Ultrasonic Irrigation: A Micro-computed Tomographic Study. *J. Endod.* **2017**, *43*, 467–471. [CrossRef]
8. Silva, E.J.N.L.; Belladonna, F.G.; Zuolo, A.S.; Rodrigues, E.; Ehrhardt, I.C.; Souza, E.M.; De-Deus, G. Effectiveness of XP-endo Finisher and XP-endo Finisher R in removing root filling remnants: A micro-CT study. *Int. Endod. J.* **2018**, *51*, 86–91. [CrossRef]
9. Kapasi, K.; Kesharani, P.; Kansara, P.; Patil, D.; Kansara, T.; Sheth, S. *In vitro* comparative evaluation of efficiency of XP-endo shaper, XP-endo finisher, and XP-endo finisher-R files in terms of residual root filling material, preservation of root dentin, and time during retreatment procedures in oval canals—A cone-beam computed tomography analysis. *J. Conserv. Dent.* **2020**, *23*, 145–151.
10. Madani, Z.S.; Simdar, N.; Moudi, E.; Bijani, A. CBCT Evaluation of the Root Canal Filling Removal Using D-RaCe, ProTaper Retreatment Kit and Hand Files in curved canals. *Iran. Endod. J.* **2015**, *10*, 69–74.
11. Fatima, K.; Nair, R.; Khasnis, S.; Vallabhaneni, S.; Patil, J.D. Efficacy of rotary and reciprocating single-file systems on different access outlines for gutta-percha removal in retreatment: An *in vitro* study. *J. Conserv. Dent.* **2018**, *21*, 354–358. [CrossRef]

12. Jiang, S.; Zou, T.; Li, D.; Chang, J.W.; Huang, X.; Zhang, C. Effectiveness of Sonic, Ultrasonic, and Photon-Induced Photoacoustic Streaming Activation of NaOCl on Filling Material Removal Following Retreatment in Oval Canal Anatomy. *Photomed. Laser Surg.* **2016**, *34*, 3–10. [CrossRef] [PubMed]
13. Bhagavaldas, M.C.; Diwan, A.; Kusumvalli, S.; Pasha, S.; Devale, M.; Chava, D.C. Efficacy of two rotary retreatment systems in removing Gutta-percha and sealer during endodontic retreatment with or without solvent: A comparative *in vitro* study. *J. Conserv. Dent.* **2017**, *20*, 12–16. [CrossRef] [PubMed]
14. Uzunoglu-Özyürek, E.; Küçükkaya Eren, S.; Karahan, S. Contribution of XP-Endo files to the root canal filling removal: A systematic review and meta-analysis of in vitro studies. *Aust. Endod. J.* **2021**, *47*, 703–714. [CrossRef] [PubMed]
15. Manker, A.; Solanki, M.; Tripathi, A.; Jain, M.L. Biomechanical preparation in primary molars using manual and three NiTi instruments: A cone-beam-computed tomographic in vitro study. *Eur. Arch. Paediatr. Dent.* **2020**, *21*, 203–213. [CrossRef]
16. Patil, A.; Mali, S.; Hegde, D.; Jaiswal, H.; Saoji, H.; Edake, D.N. Efficacy of Rotary and Hand Instrument in removing Gutta-percha and Sealer from Root Canals of Endodontically Treated Teeth. *J. Contemp. Dent. Pract.* **2018**, *19*, 964–968.
17. Dentsply. Available online: https://www.google.com/url?sa=t&rct=j&q=&esrc=s&source=web&cd=&cad=rja&uact=8&ved=2ahUKEwjmprL6vab9AhXYXaQEHaySCCkQFnoECAwQAQ&url=https%3A%2F%2Fwww.dentsplysirona.com%2Fcontent%2Fdam%2Fmaster%2Fregions-countries%2Fnorth-america%2Fproduct-procedure-brand%2Fendodontics%2Fproduct-categories%2Frestoration%2Fretreatment-files%2Fdocuments%2FEND-Step-By-Step-ProTaper-Universal-Retreatment-Files-EN.pdf&usg=AOvVaw1dITSqZuo2Of-2uH-bclhS (accessed on 12 January 2023).
18. FKG. Available online: https://www.fkg.ch/fr/produits/endodontie/retraitement/d-race (accessed on 12 January 2023).
19. De-Deus, G.; Belladonna, F.G.; Zuolo, A.S.; Cavalcante, D.M.; Carvalhal, J.C.A.; Simões-Carvalho, M.; Souza, E.M.; Lopes, R.T.; Silva, E.J.N.L. XP-endo Finisher R instrument optimizes the removal of root filling remnants in oval-shaped canals. *Int. Endod. J.* **2019**, *52*, 899–907. [CrossRef]
20. Kharouf, N.; Sauro, S.; Hardan, L.; Haikel, Y.; Mancino, D. Special Issue "Recent Advances in Biomaterials and Dental Disease" Part I. *Bioengineering* **2023**, *10*, 55. [CrossRef]
21. Kharouf, N.; Sauro, S.; Eid, A.; Zghal, J.; Jmal, H.; Seck, A.; Macaluso, V.; Addiego, F.; Inchingolo, F.; Affolter-Zbaraszczuk, C.; et al. Physicochemical and Mechanical Properties of Premixed Calcium Silicate and Resin Sealers. *J. Funct. Biomater.* **2023**, *14*, 9. [CrossRef]
22. Yoo, J.S.; Chang, S.W.; Oh, S.R.; Perinpanayagam, H.; Lim, S.M.; Yoo, Y.J.; Oh, Y.R.; Woo, S.B.; Han, S.H.; Zhu, Q.; et al. Bacterial entombment by intratubular mineralization following orthograde mineral trioxide aggregate obturation: A scanning electron microscopy study. *Int. J. Oral. Sci.* **2014**, *6*, 227–232. [CrossRef]
23. Kharouf, N.; Arntz, Y.; Eid, A.; Zghal, J.; Sauro, S.; Haikel, Y.; Mancino, D. Physicochemical and Antibacterial Properties of Novel, Premixed Calcium Silicate-Based Sealer Compared to Powder–Liquid Bioceramic Sealer. *J. Clin. Med.* **2020**, *9*, 3096. [CrossRef]
24. Hassan, H.Y.; Hadhoud, F.M.; Mandorah, A. Retreatment of XP-endo Shaper and R-Endo files in curved root canals. *BMC Oral. Health* **2023**, *23*, 38. [CrossRef] [PubMed]
25. Donnermeyer, D.; Bunne, C.; Schäfer, E.; Dammaschke, T. Retreatability of three calcium silicate-containing sealers and one epoxy resin-based root canal sealer with four different root canal instruments. *Clin. Oral. Investig.* **2018**, *22*, 811–817. [CrossRef] [PubMed]
26. Mancino, D.; Kharouf, N.; Cabiddu, M.; Bukiet, F.; Haïkel, Y. Microscopic and chemical evaluation of the filling quality of five obturation techniques in oval-shaped root canals. *Clin. Oral. Investig.* **2021**, *25*, 3757–3765. [CrossRef]
27. Baranwal, H.C.; Mittal, N.; Garg, R.; Yadav, J.; Rani, P. Comparative evaluation of retreatability of bioceramic sealer (BioRoot RCS) and epoxy resin (AH Plus) sealer with two different retreatment files: An *in vitro* study. *J. Conserv. Dent.* **2021**, *24*, 88–93. [PubMed]
28. Kaloustian, M.K.; Hachem, C.E.; Zogheib, C.; Nehme, W.; Hardan, L.; Rached, P.; Kharouf, N.; Haikel, Y.; Mancino, D. Effectiveness of the REvision System and Sonic Irrigation in the Removal of Root Canal Filling Material from Oval Canals: An In Vitro Study. *Bioengineering* **2022**, *9*, 260. [CrossRef]
29. Ashi, T.; Mancino, D.; Hardan, L.; Bourgi, R.; Zghal, J.; Macaluso, V.; Al-Ashkar, S.; Alkhouri, S.; Haikel, Y.; Kharouf, N. Physicochemical and Antibacterial Properties of Bioactive Retrograde Filling Materials. *Bioengineering* **2022**, *9*, 624. [CrossRef]
30. Siqueira, J.F., Jr. Aetiology of root canal treatment failure: Why well-treated teeth can fail. *Int. Endod. J.* **2001**, *34*, 1–10. [CrossRef]
31. Oltra, E.; Cox, T.C.; LaCourse, M.R.; Johnson, J.D.; Paranjpe, A. Retreatability of two endodontic sealers, EndoSequence BC Sealer and AH Plus: A micro-computed tomographic comparison. *Restor. Dent. Endod.* **2017**, *42*, 19–26. [CrossRef]
32. Arul, B.; Varghese, A.; Mishra, A.; Elango, S.; Padmanaban, N.; Natanasabapathy, V. Retrievability of bioceramic-based sealers in comparison with epoxy resin-based sealer assessed using microcomputed tomography: A systematic review of laboratory-based studies. *J. Conserv. Dent.* **2021**, *24*, 421–434.
33. Crozeta, B.M.; Lopes, F.C.; Menezes Silva, R.; Silva-Sousa, Y.T.C.; Moretti, L.F.; Sousa-Neto, M.D. Retreatability of BC Sealer and AH Plus root canal sealers using new supplementary instrumentation protocol during non-surgical endodontic retreatment. *Clin. Oral. Investig.* **2021**, *25*, 891–899. [CrossRef]
34. Zhekov, K.I.; Stefanova, V.P. Retreatability of Bioceramic Endodontic Sealers: A Review. *Folia Med.* **2020**, *62*, 258–264. [CrossRef] [PubMed]

35. Hachem, C.E.; Chedid, J.C.A.; Nehme, W.; Kaloustian, M.K.; Ghosn, N.; Sahnouni, H.; Mancino, D.; Haikel, Y.; Kharouf, N. Physicochemical and Antibacterial Properties of Conventional and Two Premixed Root Canal Filling Materials in Primary Teeth. *J. Funct. Biomater.* **2022**, *13*, 177. [CrossRef] [PubMed]
36. Kharouf, N.; Zghal, J.; Addiego, F.; Gabelout, M.; Jmal, H.; Haikel, Y.; Bahlouli, N.; Ball, V. Tannic acid speeds up the setting of mineral trioxide aggregate cements and improves its surface and bulk properties. *J. Colloid Interface Sci.* **2021**, *589*, 318–326. [CrossRef] [PubMed]
37. Hassan, R.; Elzahar, S. Cleaning Efficiency of XP Finisher, XP Finisher R and Passive Ultrasonic Irrigation Following Retreatment of Teeth Obturated with TotalFill HiFlow Bioceramic Sealer. *Eur. Endod. J.* **2022**, *7*, 143–149. [CrossRef] [PubMed]
38. Matoso, F.B.; Quintana, R.M.; Jardine, A.P.; Delai, D.; Fontanella, V.R.C.; Grazziotin-Soares, R.; Kopper, P.M.P. XP Endo Finisher-R and PUI as supplementary methods to remove root filling materials from curved canals. *Braz. Oral. Res.* **2022**, *36*, e053. [CrossRef] [PubMed]
39. Bernardes, R.A.; Duarte, M.A.H.; Vivan, R.R.; Alcalde, M.P.; Vasconcelos, B.C.; Bramante, C.M. Comparison of three retreatment techniques with ultrasonic activation in flattened canals using micro-computed tomography and scanning electron microscopy. *Int. Endod. J.* **2016**, *49*, 890–897. [CrossRef] [PubMed]
40. Keleş, A.; Arslan, H.; Kamalak, A.; Akçay, M.; Sousa-Neto, M.D.; Versiani, M.A. Removal of filling materials from oval-shaped canals using laser irradiation: A micro-computed tomographic study. *J. Endod.* **2015**, *41*, 219–224. [CrossRef]
41. Donyavi, Z.; Shokri, A.; Pakseresht, Z.; Tapak, L.; Falahi, A.; Abbaspourrokni, H. Comparative Evaluation of Retreatability of Endodontically Treated Teeth using AH 26, Fluoride Varnish and Mineral Trioxide Aggregate-based Endodontic Sealers. *Open. Dent. J.* **2019**, *13*, 183–189. [CrossRef]
42. López-García, S.; Myong-Hyun, B.; Lozano, A.; García-Bernal, D.; Forner, L.; Llena, C.; Guerrero-Gironés, J.; Murcia, L.; Rodríguez-Lozano, F.J. Cytocompatibility, bioactivity potential, and ion release of three premixed calcium silicate-based sealers. *Clin. Oral. Investig.* **2020**, *24*, 1749–1759. [CrossRef]
43. Garrib, M.; Camilleri, J. Retreatment efficacy of hydraulic calcium silicate sealers used in single cone obturation. *J. Dent.* **2020**, *98*, 103370. [CrossRef]
44. Kharouf, N.; Pedullà, E.; La Rosa, G.R.M.; Bukiet, F.; Sauro, S.; Haikel, Y.; Mancino, D. In Vitro Evaluation of Different Irrigation Protocols on Intracanal Smear Layer Removal in Teeth with or without Pre-Endodontic Proximal Wall Restoration. *J. Clin. Med.* **2020**, *9*, 3325. [CrossRef] [PubMed]
45. El-Hacham, C.; Nehme, W.; Kaloustian, M.K.; Ghosn, N.; Daou, M.; Zogheib, C.; Karam, M.; Mhana, R.; Macaluso, V.; Kharouf, N.; et al. The effectiveness of different irrigation techniques on debris and smear layer removal in primary mandibular second molars: An in-vitro study. *J. Contemp. Dent. Pract.* **2023**, in press.
46. Kontogiannis, T.; Kerezoudis, N.; Kozyrakis, K.; Farmakis, E. Removal ability of MTA-, bioceramic-, and resin-based sealers from obturated root canals, following XP-endo® Finisher R file: An ex vivo study. *Saudi Endod. J.* **2019**, *9*, 8–13.
47. Hess, D.; Solomon, E.; Spears, R.; He, J. Retreatability of a bioceramic root canal sealing material. *J. Endod.* **2011**, *37*, 1547–1549. [CrossRef] [PubMed]

Disclaimer/Publisher's Note: The statements, opinions and data contained in all publications are solely those of the individual author(s) and contributor(s) and not of MDPI and/or the editor(s). MDPI and/or the editor(s) disclaim responsibility for any injury to people or property resulting from any ideas, methods, instructions or products referred to in the content.

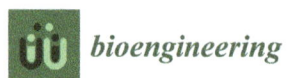

Article

The Influence of Carious Lesion and Bleeding Time on the Success of Partial Pulpotomy in Permanent Molars with Irreversible Pulpitis: A Prospective Study

Rami Zen Aldeen [1], Ossama Aljabban [1], Ahmad Almanadili [2], Saleh Alkurdi [3], Ammar Eid [1], Davide Mancino [4,5,6], Youssef Haikel [4,5,6,*] and Naji Kharouf [4,5,*]

[1] Department of Endodontics, Faculty of Dentistry, Damascus University, Damascus 0100, Syria; rami.zenaldeen@damascusuniversity.edu.sy (R.Z.A.); ossama.jabban@damascusuniversity.edu.sy (O.A.); ammarendo89@gmail.com (A.E.)
[2] Department of Oral Pathology, Faculty of Dentistry, Damascus University, Damascus 0100, Syria; dr.manadili@gmail.com
[3] Department of Pediatric Dentistry, Faculty of Dentistry, Damascus University, Damascus 0100, Syria; salekh1889@gmail.com
[4] Department of Biomaterials and Bioengineering, INSERM UMR_S 1121, Strasbourg University, 67000 Strasbourg, France; mancino@unistra.fr
[5] Department of Endodontics, Faculty of Dental Medicine, Strasbourg University, 67000 Strasbourg, France
[6] Pôle de Médecine et Chirurgie Bucco-Dentaire, Hôpital Civil, Hôpitaux Universitaire de Strasbourg, 67000 Strasbourg, France
* Correspondence: youssef.haikel@unistra.fr (Y.H.); dentistenajikharouf@gmail.com (N.K.); Tel.: +33-(0)6-6752-2841 (N.K.)

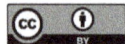

Citation: Aldeen, R.Z.; Aljabban, O.; Almanadili, A.; Alkurdi, S.; Eid, A.; Mancino, D.; Haikel, Y.; Kharouf, N. The Influence of Carious Lesion and Bleeding Time on the Success of Partial Pulpotomy in Permanent Molars with Irreversible Pulpitis: A Prospective Study. *Bioengineering* 2023, *10*, 700. https://doi.org/10.3390/bioengineering10060700

Academic Editors: Chengfei Zhang and Elena A. Jones

Received: 22 May 2023
Revised: 3 June 2023
Accepted: 6 June 2023
Published: 8 June 2023

Copyright: © 2023 by the authors. Licensee MDPI, Basel, Switzerland. This article is an open access article distributed under the terms and conditions of the Creative Commons Attribution (CC BY) license (https://creativecommons.org/licenses/by/4.0/).

Abstract: This prospective study aimed to evaluate the success rate of partial pulpotomy using mineral trioxide aggregate (MTA), in permanent molars with symptomatic irreversible pulpitis. Moreover, this study aimed to investigate the effect of carious lesion depth and activity and bleeding time on the outcome of partial pulpotomy. Forty permanent molars with deep and extremely deep carious lesions clinically diagnosed with symptomatic irreversible pulpitis were included. The status of the carious lesion was evaluated clinically and radiographically to determine its activity (rapidly or slowly progressing) and depth (deep or extremely deep). A partial pulpotomy was performed and MTA was used. Clinical and radiographic analysis were performed at 3, 6 and 12 months. Chi-square analysis and Fisher's exact test were used. Scanning electron microscope and energy dispersive X-rays were used to investigate the crystalline structures and their chemical composition onto MTA surfaces after immersion in several conditions. The partial pulpotomy was 88.9% successful, with no significant difference in outcome between deep and extremely deep carious lesions ($p = 0.22$) or between rapidly and slowly progressing lesions ($p = 0.18$). Nevertheless, all failed cases were associated with rapidly progressing lesions and extremely deep lesions. All failures occurred when the bleeding time was more than 3 min ($p = 0.10$). Different crystalline structures were detected on MTA surfaces, with higher calcium percentages in PBS conditions. Within the limitations of the present study, favorable results demonstrated that MTA might be recommended as a suitable agent for partial pulpotomy in permanent molars with irreversible pulpitis. The depth and activity of the carious lesion as well as the bleeding time are important factors in the success of partial pulpotomy treatment. The prolonged bleeding time and the extremely deep rapidly progressing caries could be related with the failure cases in partial pulpotomy treatment of irreversible pulpitis.

Keywords: carious lesion activity; irreversible pulpitis; partial pulpotomy; vital pulp therapy; mineral trioxide aggregate

1. Introduction

Numerous chemical, thermal, microbiological and traumatic factors can cause inflammation in the dental pulp [1]. Traditionally, in the reversible stage, the tooth could be healed by the elimination of the stimulus whilst, in the irreversible stage, the pulp tissue is so damaged that it is impossible to be recovered, and thus, root canal treatment (RCT) is recommended [2].

Several clinical signs could be considered as indicators of irreversible pulpits, such as severe pre-operative pain that is spontaneous or long-lasting and is accompanied by a deep carious lesion [2]. However, several histological studies demonstrated that inflammatory changes in pulp tissues are limited to the coronal region adjacent to the carious lesion, while the residual parts of the coronal pulp tissue remain normal and uninflamed [3,4]. These histological findings, along with recent improvements in the understanding of the pulp reparative processes [5], as well as developments in the field of bioactive materials, such as calcium silicate-based materials and their biological effects [6–8], have made it possible to change the concept of root canal treatment and to adopt more conservative treatment strategies such as vital pulp therapy (VPT) for the management of pulpitis in mature permanent teeth [9,10].

VPT is a minimally invasive, biologically based treatment aimed at preserving the vitality of the entire dental pulp or a portion of it by sealing the pulp wound with bioactive material after removing the infected tissue [11,12]. VPT represents a group of therapeutic strategies, including indirect pulp capping, direct pulp capping, partial pulpotomy, and full pulpotomy [13]. Several clinical studies over the last two decades have demonstrated that full and partial pulpotomy could be a promising biologically based treatment alternative to RCT for the management of carious mature teeth, even with symptoms of irreversible pulpitis [14–16]. Nevertheless, the medical literature is divided over whether or not a partial pulpotomy could be an indication for irreversible pulpitis management in mature permanent teeth, and more clinical studies are still required [17,18].

The success of the VPT is dependent upon an accurate assessment of the inflammatory status of the dental pulp. Due to the limited link between clinical signs and symptoms and the histological state of the pulp, this assessment is, unfortunately, more predictive than accurate in clinical practice [4,19]. Therefore, to limit the predictive diagnosis in teeth presenting with a carious lesion, it may be essential to pay attention to additional criteria such as the depth of penetration and activity state of the carious lesion [20]. It has suggested that the depth and activity of the carious lesion may be an important clinical measure for the regenerative potential of the pulp tissue and the degree of pulp inflammation and may influence the outcome of pulp exposure treatment [21]. Interestingly, data on carious lesion penetration and activity concerning VPT, including partial or full pulpotomy, are seldom described in the literature. In addition, the relation between depth and activity of carious lesion, and bleeding time with the success of partial pulpotomy treatment should be clarified. Furthermore, the appearance of the pulp tissues under the amputation level after partial or full pulpotomy, as well as the time needed to control bleeding, can ensure valuable information about the degree and extent of inflammation within the pulp tissues and determine the most appropriate treatment type and prognosis [9].

Calcium silicate materials, called bioceramics, are used in dentistry, especially in endodontic treatment due to their physicochemical, mechanical and biological effects [22–24]. PD-MTA White (Produits dentaires, Vevey, Switzerland) is one of the calcium silicate cements which is used in dental practice due to its thin hydrophilic particles, biological activities and short setting time (15 min) [25]. However, there is no previous study in the literature which investigates the effectiveness of PD-MTA on the dental pulp in term of VPT. Moreover, the crystallographic reactions of this material after contact with saliva, blood and phosphate-buffered solution have never been analyzed.

The aim of the present prospective study was to investigate the influence of the carious lesion depth and activity as well as the bleeding time on the partial pulpotomy using PD-MTA in permanent molars with irreversible pulpitis after one year of follow-up. The null hypothesis was that there is no impact of the carious lesion depth, activity and the bleeding time on the partial pulpotomy success in permanent molars with irreversible pulpitis after one year. Moreover, it aimed to evaluate the crystallographic reaction of MTA after exposure to artificial saliva, blood and phosphate-buffered solution (PBS) by using scanning electron microscope and energy-dispersive X-rays.

2. Materials and Methods

2.1. Ethical Considerations

The study protocol was approved by the Scientific Research and Postgraduate Board of Damascus University Ethics Committee, Syria (UDDS-1819-07052018/SRC-1450). The patients signed assent and informed consent forms. Patients were offered a full pulpotomy or root canal treatment in case of treatment failure.

2.2. Study Design and Sample Size Calculation

The study was a prospective longitudinal single-arm clinical investigation of the predictability of partial pulpotomy with MTA in permanent molars exhibiting symptoms and signs of irreversible pulpitis. The sample size was determined using a sample-size calculation program, based on the teeth numbers included in previous studies which investigated both the outcome of full and partial pulpotomy in teeth which have reversible and irreversible pulpitis [15,26,27]. Sample size was calculated using G*Power 3.1.9.2 software (Heinrich-Heine-Universität Düsseldorf, Düsseldorf, Germany) based on a previous study [15] in order to have 95% power, an alpha error probability of 0.05 and degree of freedom at 1 which has been concluded from a total sample size of 51 teeth.

2.3. Participants

Sixty-four patients aged from 18 to 65 years old attending the Restorative and Endodontic Dentistry Department, Faculty of Dentistry, Damascus University were enrolled. One permanent molar per patient was included.

2.4. Inclusion and Exclusion Criteria

Inclusion and exclusion criteria were summarized in Table 1.

Table 1. Inclusion and exclusion criteria.

Inclusion Criteria	Exclusion Criteria

o The patient should be ≥18 years old.
o Mature first/second (upper/lower) molar tooth.
o Clinical examination shows:
  • Tooth with a history of signs of irreversible pulpitis such as spontaneous pain or pain exacerbated by cold stimuli and lasting for a few seconds to several hours (interpreted as lingering pain) compared to control teeth, and which could be reproduced using cold testing.
  • Positive response to cold with no signs of pulpal necrosis including swelling or sinus tract.
  • The tooth is restorable with no need for crown or post-retained restoration.
  • Normal probing pocket depth and tooth mobility
o Radiographic examination shows:
  • Mature molar with deep or extremely deep carious lesion.
  • A pulp chamber of relatively normal dimensions without calcified forms (e.g., pulp stone, diffuse calcification, disk-like chamber)
  • No prominent radiolucency at the furcation or zones. No evidence of internal or external resorption.
	o Immature molar with open apex.
	o Radiolucency at the periapical zones or furcation
	o Existence of calcification and internal or external resorption
	o Existence of swelling of sinus tract and the negative response to cold indicator
	o Uncontrolled bleeding after partial pulpotomy (> 6 min)
	o Bleeding is not sufficient after pulp exposure; the pulp is judged partially necrotic.
	o Non-restorable teeth.

2.5. Patient Assessment and Operative Procedure

Before the operation, a medical/dental history and chief complaint were recorded as part of the clinical assessment. Afterward, the periodontal tissues, tooth mobility, and possibility for restoration were evaluated. In addition, the pulp response was assessed using the Endo Ice cold sensibility test (Coltene, Altstätten, Switzerland), and the pre-apical tissues were evaluated using the percussion and papulation tests. A preoperative periapical radiograph was performed using a digital sensor (Vatech, Ezsensor HD, Saul, Republic of Korea) with a film holder (Dentsply, Elgin, IL, USA) to evaluate the condition of the periapical and furcation areas. In addition, a bitewing radiograph was taken to assess the depth of penetration of the carious lesion (Figure 1a,b). The carious lesions were later divided, according to the depth of penetration within the dentine as shown radiographically, into deep (Figure 1a) (caries reaching the inner quarter of dentine but with a zone of hard or firm dentine between caries and the pulp) or extremely deep (Figure 1b) (caries penetrating the entire thickness of the dentine with certain pulp exposure) [13,28]. Later, radiographs were evaluated independently by the endodontist and a second examiner, for the depth of the lesion as a deep or extremely deep case. After that, a local anesthesia was applied using 2% lidocaine with epinephrine 1/80,000 (Scandonest; Septodont, Saint-Maur-des-fosses Cedex, France) and a rubber dam was applied. The cavity was prepared, under a dental operating microscope (Labomed, Los Angeles, CA, USA), by using a diamond bur (EX-41, Dia burs-Mani, Tochigi, Japan) with a water-cooled high-speed handpiece. Caries at the lateral walls of the cavity and only the superficial part of the demineralized dentin was removed with a sharp excavator, followed by rinsing of the cavity with saline. After drying the cavity using a sterile cotton pellet, the carious lesion was carefully examined to determine its activity. The operator assessed the level of caries activity based on the color and surface texture (moisture and consistency) of the carious dentine. The operator determined the demineralized dentine color by comparing the clinical situation with photographs of the five typical dentine color classes, which are light yellow, yellow, light brown, dark brown, or black [29]. The consistency of the dentine was categorized as soft dentine (when it can be excavated with minimum resistance using hand instruments), firm dentine (when it was resistant to excavation using manual instruments), and hard dentine (when it was resistant to probe penetration) [13]. Surface humidity was determined by inserting a probe into the carious tissue; if the tissue oozed moisture, it was categorized as wet, and if it did not, it was classified as dry [30]. Accordingly, demineralized dentin with a light yellow/yellow color and a soft/moist surface texture was classified as a rapidly progressing lesion (Figure 1c), while demineralized dentin with a light brown/brown color and a firm/dry surface texture was classified as a slowly progressing lesion (Figure 1d).

After that, the gross caries was removed in a non-selective manner with a round bur and a slow handpiece (Figure 2d). After the pulp was exposed (Figure 2d), a carbide bur on a high-speed handpiece was used to eliminate around 2 to 3 mm of coronal pulp tissues under water-cooling (Figure 2e). Following the rinsing of the pulp with 2.5% NaOCl [31] for one minute, the state of the pulp tissues below the amputation level was thoroughly evaluated under magnification. If the pulp tissues' appearance was normal with no sign of infection or degradation, hemostasis was attained by applying a cotton pellet drenched in 2.5% NaOCl to the wound pulp. Hemostasis was controlled every minute for up to 6 min [26]. The time to control bleeding was recorded and subsequently divided into two categories as follows: bleeding time between 1 and 3 min, and bleeding time between 4 and 6 min. Finally, mineral trioxide aggregate (MTA) (PD-MTA, Produits Dentaires SA, Verey, Switzerland) was prepared following the manufacturer's instructions and added gradually over the fresh pulp wound and surrounding dentine to a thickness of 2–3 mm using the MapOne carrier (MapOne system, Produits Dentaires SA, Verey, Switzerland) (Figure 2f). The MTA was coated with a sterile, moist cotton pellet immersed in saline for 15 min to provide primary hydration. After that, a layer of resin-modified glass-ionomer cement "RMGIC" (Fuji II LC; GC Corp, Tokyo, Japan) was placed on the MTA (Figure 2g) [32]. An universal adhesive system (Tetric-N Bond, Ivoclar Vivadent) was applied and covered by direct composite restorative resin (Tetric-Ceram, Ivoclar Vivadent) (Figure 2h) [33]. All the clinical steps are summarized in Figure 3.

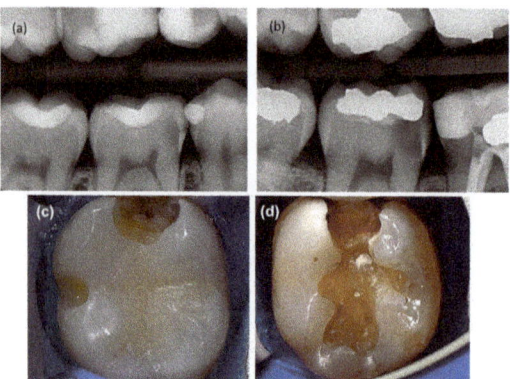

Figure 1. (**a**) Bitewing preoperative radiograph for first mandibular molar with deep carious lesion shows that the lesion involves the inner quarter of dentine with a radio-dense zone (hard or firm dentine) between caries and the pulp. (**b**) Bitewing preoperative radiograph for second mandibular molar with extremely deep carious lesion shows the lesion penetrating the entire thickness of the dentine with a radio-dense zone located within the pulp chamber indicative of tertiary dentine. (**c**) Intraoral image shows a rapidly progressing lesion and the yellow color of the demineralized dentine with soft and wet appearance of the surface texture. (**d**) Intraoral image shows a slowly progressing lesion and the brown color of the demineralized dentine with firm/dry appearance of the surface texture.

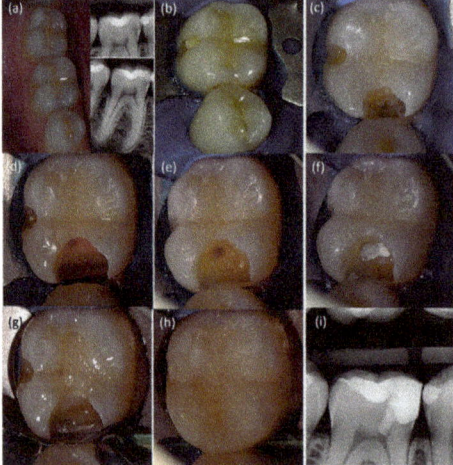

Figure 2. Mandibular right first molar presented with symptomatic irreversible pulpitis treated with partial pulpotomy using PD-MTA. (**a**) Clinical and radiographic examinations revealed deep carious lesion confined at a proximal surface with no evidence of dentine exposure, reflecting a close lesion environment. (**b**) Rubber dam application. (**c**) After removal of the undermined enamel and the exposition of the demineralized dentine. (**d**) Pulp exposure after non-selective caries removal. (**e**) Partial pulpotomy by removing of 2–3 mm of pulp tissues under exposure and hemostasis achieved. Note that the pulp tissues under level of amputation showed a normal appearance, texture, and color. (**f**) PD-MTA application as capping material. (**g**) Base of resin-modified glass–ionomer cement placed above MTA material. (**h**) Composite resin restoration. (**i**) Postoperative bitewing radiograph.

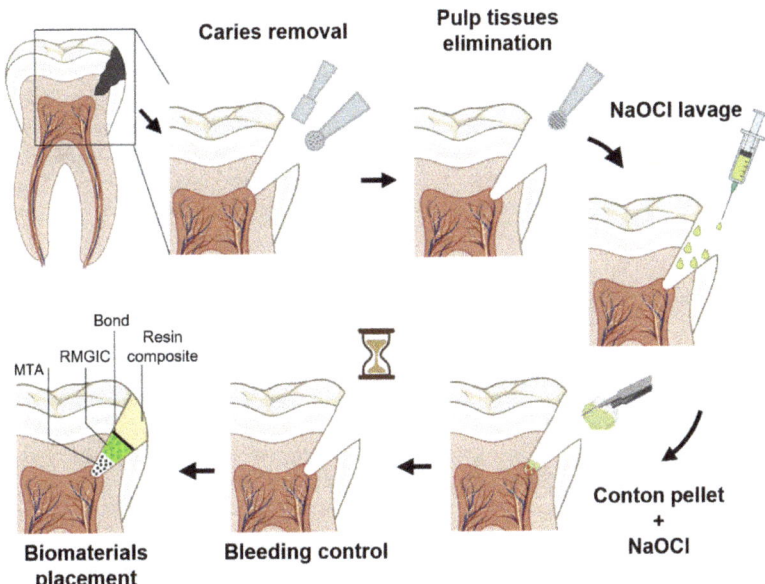

Figure 3. Schematic graph presents the different steps of clinical procedure in partial pulpotomy.

2.6. Outcome Evaluation

Three follow-up appointments (3, 6, and 12 months) were determined. At each time point, participants were clinically and radiographically examined by an endodontist who was blinded about the depth and activity of caries and the bleeding time. Different clinical parameters including the absence and presence of clinical signs, a vitality pulp test, a periodontal examination, and a percussion test were recorded. Periapical and bitewing radiographs were taken to evaluate any pathological changes at the periapical or furcal area and to detect dentinal bridge formation. The radiographs were later evaluated independently by two blinded examiners; the accuracy between the examiners was investigated by repeating the evaluation of the images after one week [34]. After one year, the teeth were classified as successful or failed treatments. To be classified as retaining overall success, the tested tooth should have both clinical and radiographic success. Treatment was considered successful when the tooth responded positively to a cold test within normal limits, there were no signs of pulpitis, there was no abnormal mobility or fistula, and there was no evidence of an apical radiolucency or internal and/or external root resorption.

2.7. Scanning Electron Microscope (SEM) and Energy Dispersive X-ray Analysis (EDX)

After the end of the follow-up (12 months), 9 samples of the same MTA material were prepared using Teflon molds (height: 3.8 mm/diameter: 3 mm). The samples were put at 37 °C for 48 h to achieve a good setting time [12]. Each of the three samples were stored in 50 mL of human blood, phosphate-buffered saline (PBS10x, Dominique Dutscher, Bernolsheim, France) or artificial saliva (Serlabo Technologies, Entraigues-sur-la-Sorgue, France) at 37 °C for 7 days. After the immersion time, the samples were gently rinsed with distilled water for 3 min and were sputter-coated with gold–palladium (20/80) using a Hummer JR sputtering device (Technics, San Jose, CA, USA). After that, the surface of each sample was investigated using SEM (Quanta 250 FEG scanning electron microscope "FEI Company, Eindhoven, The Netherlands"; 10 kV acceleration voltage of the electrons) and studied at a magnification of 1000× and 4000× for morphological evaluations and mineralization changes through SEM. Moreover, EDX analyses were performed for 30 s at 10 mm of distance in order to investigate the chemical composition.

2.8. Statistical Analyses

The SPSS 24.0 software (SPSS Science, Chicago, IL, USA) was used to perform the statistical analyses. The level of significant difference was at $\alpha = 0.05$. Fisher's exact test and the Chi-square test were used to assess the influence of the depth and activity of a carious lesion and the bleeding time on the outcome of treatment. The preoperative caries depth assessment inter-observer agreement and the postoperative intra-observer reproducibility and inter-observer agreement in terms of any pathological changes in the periapical or furcal area were assessed using Cohen's Kappa coefficient.

3. Results

Sixty-four patients were assessed for eligibility, having presented with signs symptomatic of irreversible pulpitis in molar teeth. Fourteen participants were excluded from the study due to refusal to participate (five patients) or not meeting inclusion criteria (nine patients). Fifty patients (50 teeth, one tooth per patient) were enrolled to be treated by partial pulpotomy treatment. Ten patients were subsequently excluded intraoperatively, three cases due to uncontrolled bleeding and seven cases due to extension of infected tissue to the root canal orifices or beyond. These patients were treated either with full pulpotomy or with RCT. Finally, forty teeth were included and treated in this study. Four participants could not attend the follow-ups, resulting in an overall recall rate of 90% (36/40) (Figure 4).

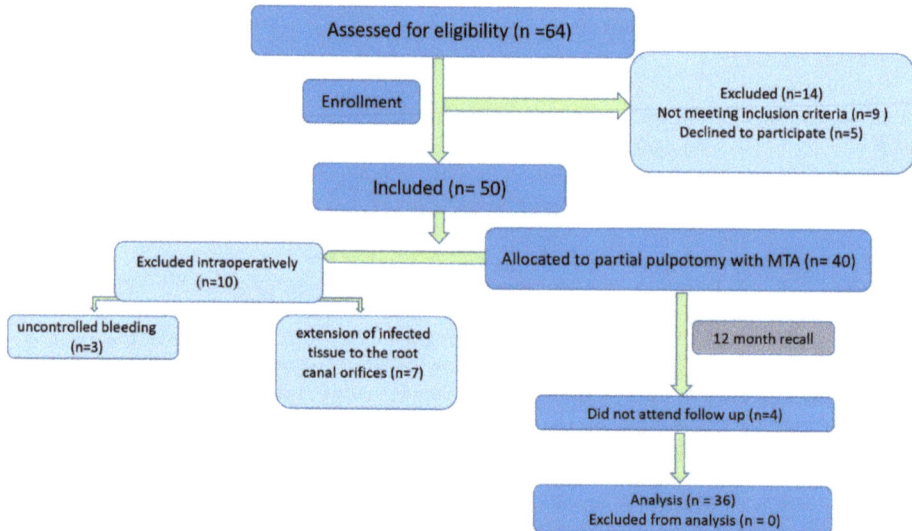

Figure 4. Study flow diagram.

The patients consisted of 13 males and 23 females, aged 18–65 years old (32.75 ± 10.7 years old). The included cases consisted of twenty teeth (55.5%) and sixteen teeth (44.5%) with deep and extremely deep caries, respectively. The carious lesion was actively progressing in twenty-four cases (66.7%) compared to twelve slowly progressing lesions (33.3%).

The mean bleeding time was 3.80 ± 1.47 min; fifteen teeth (41.7%) needed time between 1–3 min to achieve hemostasis, while twenty-one teeth (53.3%) needed time between 4–6 min to control the bleeding.

The success rate for partial pulpotomy managing irreversible pulpitis was 88.9% after one year of follow-up, and failure was observed in four cases. Early failure occurred within three months in three cases, while late failure was observed after 12 months in one case. For carious lesion activity, all failure cases were associated with actively progressing lesions, while no failure occurred in slowly progressing lesions. However, no statistically significant difference was observed ($p > 0.05$). Regarding caries depth, only one failure case was related to a deep lesion, whilst the other three failure cases were associated with extremely deep carious lesions ($p > 0.05$).

As for bleeding time, it was noted that all failure cases were associated with a bleeding time ranging between 4 and 6 min, whilst no failure was detected for cases with 1–3 min bleeding time ($p > 0.05$) (Table 2).

Table 2. Fisher's exact test results to compare the outcome according to the activity of carious lesion, carious lesion depth, and bleeding time.

Variables		n (%)	Overall Outcome		p-Value
			Success (%)	Failure (%)	
Activity of carious lesion	Rapid progression	24 (66.7)	20 (83.3)	4 (16.7)	0.18
	Slow progression	12 (33.3)	12 (100)	0 (0)	
Carious lesion depth	Deep	20 (55.5)	19 (95)	1 (5)	0.221
	Extremely deep	16 (44.5)	13 (81.3)	3 (18.7)	
Bleeding time	1–3 min	15 (41.7)	15 (100)	0 (0)	0.102
	4–6 min	21 (58.3)	17 (81)	4 (19)	

The results were subdivided by both depth and activity of carious lesions into four categories: rapidly progressing deep ($n = 14$), rapidly progressing extremely deep ($n = 10$), slowly progressing deep ($n = 6$), and slowly progressing extremely deep ($n = 6$). Three cases of rapidly progressing extremely deep lesions and one case of rapidly progressing deep lesions failed, whereas neither slowly progressing deep lesions nor slowly progressing extremely deep lesions failed ($p > 0.05$) (Table 3).

Table 3. Chi-Square test results to compare the outcome according to depth/activity of carious lesion.

State of Carious Lesion	n (%)	Overall Outcome		p-Value
		Success (%)	Failure (%)	
Rapidly progressing deep	14 (38.88)	13 (92.9)	1 (7.1)	
Rapidly progressing, extremely deep	10 (27.8)	7 (70)	3 (30)	0.149
Slowly progressing, deep	6 (16.66)	6 (100)	0 (0)	
Slowly progressing, extremely deep	6 (16.66)	6 (100)	0 (0)	

The two examinations showed a good level of accordance in investigating caries depth ($\kappa = 0.8$). When assessing the periapical and furcal areas, the Kappa value for the inter-observer accordance was 0.89, and for the intra observer reproducibility, the Kappa values were 0.95 and 0.92 for the 1st and 2nd observers, respectively.

SEM micrographs showed the reaction of MTA surfaces after 7 days of immersion in blood, PBS and artificial saliva at 37 °C. The crystalline textures of the MTA in the three conditions are demonstrated in Figure 5. Different crystalline appearances were detected. SEM images of MTA exposed to PBS demonstrated cubical crystalline, whilst MTA surfaces exposed to blood demonstrated small globular crystalline. MTA surfaces exposed to saliva did not show any crystalline structures. EDX analysis for MTA surfaces after 7 days presented different % of Ca, Si and P among the three conditions. Higher Ca mass percentages were detected on MTA surfaces in PBS condition compared to blood and saliva.

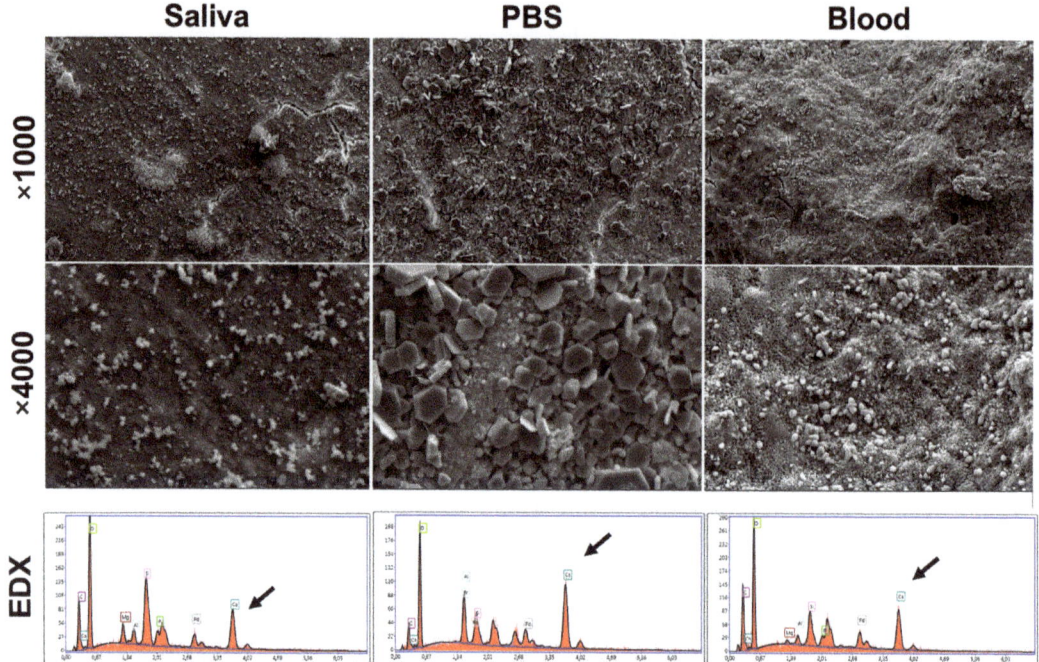

Figure 5. Scanning electron micrographs and Energy dispersive x-ray for Mineral Trioxide Aggregate surfaces in contact with saliva, PBS and blood at ×1000 and ×4000 magnifications. Different calcium percentages were detected by using EDX analysis (Black arrows).

4. Discussion

Partial pulpotomy is described as the removal of 2–3 mm of pulp tissue at the exposure site, followed by sealing of the pulp wound with bioactive material [13]. This procedure differs from pulp capping in that it removes the superficial layer of infected or inflammatory tissue and the accompanying biofilms [26]. In addition, it preserves a significant portion of the coronal pulp compared to a full pulpotomy, which removes the entire coronal tissue up to the canal orifices [12]. Therefore, partial pulpotomy could be the most conservative and predictable treatment for carious pulp exposure.

The success rate in the present study was 88.9% after one year of follow-up. Several clinical studies over the last 10 years have shown success for the partial pulpotomy procedure in treating carious pulp exposure in adult and young permanent teeth, even when there are symptoms and signs of irreversible pulpitis [15,16,26]. In accordance with the results of the present study, Uesrichai et al. noted a 90% success rate for partial pulpotomy in the management of irreversible pulpitis in mature and young teeth in children aged 6 to 18 years [16]. Another study showed a success rate of 90% after 12 months partial pulpotomy procedure on complete developed permanent teeth within a sample of reversible and irreversible pulpitis [26]. A longer follow-up study (2 years) performed on partial pulpotomy in complete developed adult teeth with symptomatic irreversible pulpitis showed a slightly decrease in the success rate to 80% [15]. In accordance with the previous study of Taha and Khazali [15], the current study relied on standardizing the initial diagnosis of the dental pulp and limiting it to irreversible pulpitis in adult mature permanent molars to analyze the partial pulpotomy procedure in such cases more precisely. In addition, the originality of the current study was to associate the effect of carious lesion activity and depth, as well as the use of PD-MTA on the success of a partial pulpotomy procedure, which was never previously investigated.

No statistically significant relation was found between the failure with deep or extremely deep lesions ($p > 0.05$). Therefore, the null hypothesis must be accepted. Only one failure case was related to a deep lesion, whilst three failure cases were associated with extremely deep carious lesions. This results could be explained by the fact that pulpitis will be present at the early stage of the carious process, and the severe inflammatory response and the significant levels of inflammatory cells are not identified in the pulp until caries have progressed to within around 0.5 mm near the pulp [35]. It was found that bacteria were mainly present in the primary dentine in deep carious lesions. Extremely deep lesions, on the other hand, were linked to pulp-reaching microorganisms, as well as inflammatory infiltration and subsequent partial necrosis [20]. Therefore, the majority of failure cases in the current study were associated with extremely deep lesions rather than deep ones. In accordance, Careddu and Duncan [26] noted that all failure cases in their study, which were treated with a partial pulpotomy using Biodentine as capping material, were in the extremely-deep caries group.

Ten patients were excluded intraoperatively due to either the extension of infected tissue to the root canal orifices or beyond, as confirmed by careful examination under magnification and illumination, or uncontrolled bleeding that may indicate advanced pulpal inflammation [36]. In addition, these patients had extremely deep caries. In accordance, a previous histological study [20] revealed that more than half of extremely deep caries were associated with inflammatory infiltrates that affected the complete coronal pulp and the most coronal part of the radicular pulp, which renders partial pulpotomy inappropriate in such cases. As there was no significant difference between deep and extremely deep lesions, extremely deep carious lesions can still be treated with partial pulpotomy if a magnified examination of the underlying tissues is performed to determine the extent of inflamed and infected tissues within the dental pulp.

No failure cases were detected after one year for slowly progressing lesions, whilst all failure cases were associated with actively progressing lesions. In addition, all cases presented with slowly progressing lesions were successful even if they had extremely deep penetration, while 30% of extremely deep lesions and 7.1% of deep lesions failed if they rapidly progressed. These findings could be due to rapidly progressing lesions being associated with the presence of heavily cariogenic biofilm, while the cariogenic biofilms are significantly diminished in slowly progressing lesions [20,30]. Moreover, a slowly progressing lesion with limited cariogenic biofilms is less likely to transmit stimuli into the pulp, which is associated with a low-intensity inflammatory response favorable for healing and repair [37]. Therefore, we can conclude that the rapidly progressing and extremely deep caries associated with clinically diagnosed irreversible pulpitis have less chance of being treated with a partial pulpotomy, even though no statistically significant difference was observed in treatment outcomes according to both depth and activity of the carious lesion.

It is commonly agreed that avoiding pulpal exposure and selectively removing carious tissue is the optimal strategy for the management of a deep carious lesion [38]. In the current study, all teeth were clinically judged to have irreversible pulpitis, necessitating the total or partial removal of coronal pulp tissue [14,15]. Therefore, regardless of the depth of caries, they were chosen to have the carious tissues removed non-selectively rather than selectively. Notably, the majority of included deep lesions were proximal caries, in which the undermined enamel maintains a closed ecosystem and a rapid progression rate. These carious lesion characteristics may be associated with no or less prominent tertiary dentine formation, and bacterial invasion of the pulp may be evident even before caries reaches the pulp radiographically [39]. Moreover, pulpitis may be induced by a highly acidogenic environment in such lesions even before the pulp is exposed [28,40]. This may explain the occurrence of irreversible pulpitis in a significant part of cases included in this study despite their presenting with deep lesions without reaching the pulp radiographically, and it highlights once again the importance of evaluating the activity of the carious lesion in addition to its depth to determine the most appropriate treatment.

All failed cases in the present study occurred when the bleeding time was more than 3 min. Consistently, the present results showed no significant difference in the success rates of partial pulpotomy with the difference in the time needed for hemostasis ($p > 0.05$). In accordance, several recent studies demonstrated that there was no marked association between bleeding time and the outcome of pulpotomy treatments [18,26]. The control of bleeding is essential for the success of VPT, as the profuse, difficult-to-stop pulp bleeding could be an indicator of advanced pulp inflammation [36]. However, the mechanical and chemical elimination of the infectious challenge at the pulp wound by partial pulpotomy and NaOCl lavage may make the bleeding time a less significant factor in the treatment outcome [31]. Moreover, the local anesthesia which was applied using 2% lidocaine with epinephrine 1/80,000 in the present study could play an important role on the bleeding time. Chu et al. demonstrated that the use of local anesthesia based on lidocaine and epinephrine decreases the pulpal blood flow and may protect the dental pulp by attenuating the increase in pulpal blood flow caused by tooth preparation [41]. Moreover, it is known that the infiltration anesthesia is used successfully in the maxillary teeth but is less effective in the mandibular molar regions due to the density of bone [42]; therefore, block anesthesia was used in the present study for the mandibular molar regions.

In order to clarify the outcomes of the use of MTA in partial pulpotomy, when this biomaterial is in direct contact with pulpal tissue, blood and dentinal fluids, SEM analyses were performed on a MTA surface after immersion in PBS, blood and artificial saliva at 37 °C for 7 days. PBS was utilized to simulate the in vivo dental tissue fluids [43] to assess the mineral development that could take place on the material surfaces. SEM images showed crystallite formation on the material surfaces in the cases of PBS and blood conditions, whilst no mineralization process and no notable changes were demonstrated for MTA surfaces after immersion for 7 days in artificial saliva. Therefore, MTA is a bioactive material which could promote the remineralization process. In addition, calcium silicate-based materials are capable of making calcium hydroxide and calcium silicate hydrate when it is in a humid medium [22,24,44]. Lower calcium peaks were found for the MTA surfaces immersed in blood and artificial saliva, whilst higher calcium peeks were detected for MTA surfaces exposed to PBS. These findings could be related to the different environmental conditions and the dissolution of calcium hydroxide because of hydration [45]. These outcomes are similar to the results of a previous study which was conducted on MTA ProRoot [45]. Moreover, in the present study, RMGIC was used on MTA in order to have the optimal bond strength with the final restoration (composite) as described previously [46,47]. In addition, several studies have also shown that the MTA's physical properties might be affected by the acidic environment that existed before composite buildup [48,49]. Therefore, RMDIC was used to have an optimal coronal sealing ability, which is related to the long success of VPT.

Some limitations were detected in the present study. For example, because the study was designed to investigate the effect of the depth and activity of the carious lesion, there was no control group to which the patients could be assigned randomly. Moreover, PD-MTA as a powder–liquid bioceramic material should be carefully mixed following the manufacturer's instructions in order to avoid errors during manual mixing, which could alter the physicochemical properties of this material [22]. Moreover, the irrigant which was used, NaOCl, is known for its high cytoxicity, which could lead to severe tissue damage if it is used in high concentrations [50,51]; in contrast, 2.5% NaOCl has a high efficacia as a lavage solution due to the unique capability of NaOCl to selectively dissolve necrotic soft tissue, thus reducing the necessity to mechanically remove infected tissues [31]. In addition, radiographic monitoring was crucial to follow the treatment results; however, the indication to take radiographs in clinical practice is limited to reasonable requests in order to decrease patients' exposure to ionizing radiation [52]. Further studies with higher numbers of included cases and longer follow-up periods should be performed to investigate the relation between the activity of a carious lesion and the success of partial pulpotomy treatment. In addition, the carious lesion depth was estimated on a bitewing radiograph.

Although there was a good inter-observer agreement (0.8), it was still challenging to identify the exact depth of caries on a two-dimensional radiograph. Finally, future studies should consider using cone-beam computed tomography (CBCT) as a more precise technique for this purpose. The color, moisture, and surface texture of the carious tissues were also used as indications of carious lesion activity. These indicators, however, are somewhat subjective, and a more reliable method is required.

5. Conclusions

Within the limitations of the present study, favorable results demonstrated that MTA might be recommended as suitable agent for partial pulpotomy in permanent molars with irreversible pulpitis, with an 88.9% success rate after one year. It could be concluded that the depth and activity of the carious lesion as well as the bleeding time are important factors in the success of partial pulpotomy treatment. The prolonged bleeding time and the rapidly progressing extremely deep lesions could be related to the failure cases in partial pulpotomy treatment of irreversible pulpitis.

Author Contributions: Conceptualization, R.Z.A. and O.A.; methodology, R.Z.A.; software, R.Z.A.; validation, R.Z.A.; formal analysis, R.Z.A. and S.A.; investigation, R.Z.A.; resources, R.Z.A.; data curation, R.Z.A.; writing—original draft preparation, R.Z.A., A.E., A.A. and O.A.; writing—review and editing, N.K., Y.H. and D.M.; visualization, R.Z.A.; supervision, O.A.; project administration, O.A.; funding acquisition, R.Z.A. All authors have read and agreed to the published version of the manuscript.

Funding: This research received no external funding.

Institutional Review Board Statement: The study was conducted according to the guidelines of the Declaration of Helsinki and approved by the Scientific Research and Postgraduate Board of Damascus University Ethics Committee, Syria (UDDS-1819-07052018/SRC-1450).

Informed Consent Statement: Informed consent was obtained from all subjects involved in the study.

Data Availability Statement: Data are available from the first author (ramizen989@gmail.com (R.Z.A.)).

Conflicts of Interest: The authors declare no conflict of interest.

References

1. Möller, Å.J.; Fabricius, L.; Dahlen, G.; Öhmang, A.E.; Heyden, G.U.Y. Influence on periapical tissues of indigenous oral bacteria and necrotic pulp tissue in monkeys. *Eur. J. Oral Sci.* **1981**, *89*, 475–484. [CrossRef] [PubMed]
2. American Association of Endodontists. Endodontic Diagnosis. [WWW Document]. Available online: https://www.aae.org/specialty/wp-content/uploads/sites/2/2017/07/endodonticdiagnosisfal2013.pdf (accessed on 5 May 2021).
3. Ricucci, D.; Loghin, S.; Siqueira, J.F., Jr. Correlation between clinical and histologic pulp diagnoses. *J. Endod.* **2014**, *40*, 1932–1939. [CrossRef] [PubMed]
4. Seltzer, S.; Bender, I.B.; Ziontz, M. The dynamics of pulp inflammation: Correlations between diagnostic data and actual histologic findings in the pulp. *Oral Surg. Oral Med. Oral Radiol.* **1963**, *16*, 846–871. [CrossRef] [PubMed]
5. Duncan, H.F.; Cooper, P.R.; Smith, A.J. Dissecting dentine–pulp injury and wound healing responses: Consequences for regenerative endodontics. *Int. Endod. J.* **2019**, *52*, 261–266. [CrossRef]
6. Hachem, C.E.; Chedid, J.C.A.; Nehme, W.; Kaloustian, M.K.; Ghosn, N.; Sahnouni, H.; Mancino, D.; Haikel, Y.; Kharouf, N. Physicochemical and antibacterial properties of conventional and two premixed root canal filling materials in primary teeth. *J. Funct. Biomater.* **2022**, *13*, 177. [CrossRef]
7. Kharouf, N.; Arntz, Y.; Eid, E.; Zghal, J.; Sauro, S.; Haike, Y.; Mancino, D. Physicochemical and antibacterial properties of novel, premixed calcium silicate-based sealer compared to powder–liquid bioceramic sealer. *J. Clin. Med.* **2020**, *9*, 3096. [CrossRef]
8. Nair, P.N.R.; Duncan, H.F.; Pitt Ford, T.R.; Luder, H.U. Histological, ultrastructural and quantitative investigations on the response of healthy human pulps to experimental capping with mineral trioxide aggregate: A randomized controlled trial. *Int. Endod. J.* **2008**, *41*, 128–150.
9. Ricucci, D.; Siqueira, J.F., Jr.; Li, Y.; Tay, F.R. Vital pulp therapy: Histopathology and histobacteriology-based guidelines to treat teeth with deep caries and pulp exposure. *J. Dent.* **2019**, *86*, 41–52. [CrossRef]
10. Wolters, W.J.; Duncan, H.F.; Tomson, P.L.; Karim, I.E.; McKenna, G.; Dorri, M.; Stangvaltaite, L.; Van Der Sluis, L.W.M. Minimally invasive endodontics: A new diagnostic system for assessing pulpitis and subsequent treatment needs. *Int. Endod. J.* **2017**, *50*, 825–829. [CrossRef]

11. Duncan, H.F. Present status and future directions—Vital pulp treatment and pulp preservation strategies. *Int. Endod. J.* **2022**, *55*, 497–511. [CrossRef]
12. Eid, A.; Mancino, D.; Rekab, M.S.; Haike, Y.; Kharouf, N. Effectiveness of three agents in pulpotomy treatment of permanent molars with incomplete root development: A randomized controlled trial. *Healthcare* **2022**, *10*, 431. [CrossRef] [PubMed]
13. European Society of Endodontology (ESE); Duncan, H.F.; Galler, K.M.; Tomson, P.L.; Simon, S.; El-Karim, I.; Kundzina, R.; Krastl, G.; Dammaschke, T.; Fransson, H.; et al. European Society of Endodontology position statement: Management of deep caries and the exposed pulp. *Int. Endod. J.* **2019**, *52*, 923–934. [PubMed]
14. Taha, N.A.; Abdelkhader, S.Z. Outcome of full pulpotomy using Biodentine in adult patients with symptoms indicative of irreversible pulpitis. *Int. Endod. J.* **2018**, *51*, 819–828. [CrossRef] [PubMed]
15. Taha, N.A.; Khazali, M.A. Partial pulpotomy in mature permanent teeth with clinical signs indicative of irreversible pulpitis: A randomized clinical trial. *J. Endod.* **2017**, *43*, 1417–1421. [CrossRef]
16. Uesrichai, N.; Nirunsittirat, A.; Chuveera, P.; Srisuwan, T.; Sastraruji, T.; Chompu-Inwai, P. Partial pulpotomy with two bioactive cements in permanent teeth of 6-to 18-year-old patients with signs and symptoms indicative of irreversible pulpitis: A noninferiority randomized controlled trial. *Int. Endod. J.* **2019**, *52*, 749–759. [CrossRef]
17. Elmsmari, F.; Ruiz, X.F.; Miró, Q.; Feijoo-Pato, N.; Durán-Sindreu, F.; Olivieri, J.G. Outcome of partial pulpotomy in cariously exposed posterior permanent teeth: A systematic review and meta-analysis. *J. Endod.* **2019**, *45*, 1296–1306. [CrossRef] [PubMed]
18. Tan, S.Y.; Yu, V.S.H.; Lim, K.C.; Tan, B.C.K.; Neo, C.L.J.; Shen, M.L.; Messer, H.H. Long-term pulpal and restorative outcomes of pulpotomy in mature permanent teeth. *J. Endod.* **2020**, *46*, 383–390. [CrossRef]
19. Mejare, I.; Axelsson, S.; Davidson, T.; Frisk, F.; Hakeberg, M.; Kvist, T.; Norlund, A.; Petersson, A.; Portenier, I.; Sandberg, H. Diagnosis of the condition of the dental pulp: A systematic review. *Int. Endod. J.* **2012**, *45*, 597–613. [CrossRef]
20. Demant, S.; Dabelsteen, S.; Bjørndal, L. A macroscopic and histological analysis of radiographically well-defined deep and extremely deep carious lesions: Carious lesion characteristics as indicators of the level of bacterial penetration and pulp response. *Int. Endod. J.* **2021**, *54*, 319–330. [CrossRef]
21. Bjørndal, L.; Demant, S.; Dabelsteen, S. Depth and activity of carious lesions as indicators for the regenerative potential of dental pulp after intervention. *J. Endod.* **2014**, *40*, S76–S81. [CrossRef]
22. Ashi, T.; Mancino, D.; Hardan, L.; Bourgi, R.; Zghal, J.; Macaluso, V.; Al-Ashkar, S.; Alkhouri, S.; Haikel, Y.; Kharouf, N. Physicochemical and antibacterial properties of bioactive retrograde filling materials. *Bioengineering* **2022**, *9*, 624. [CrossRef] [PubMed]
23. Ashi, T.; Richert, R.; Mancino, D.; Jmal, H.; Alkhouri, S.; Addiego, F.; Kharouf, N.; Haïkel, Y. Do the mechanical properties of calcium-silicate-based cements influence the stress distribution of different retrograde cavity preparations? *Materials* **2023**, *16*, 3111. [CrossRef] [PubMed]
24. Kharouf, N.; Sauro, S.; Eid, A.; Zghal, J.; Jmal, H.; Seck, A.; Maculuso, V.; Addiego, F.; Inchingolo, F.; Affolter-Zbaraszczuk, C. Physicochemical and mechanical properties of premixed calcium silicate and resin sealers. *J. Funct. Biomater.* **2022**, *14*, 9. [CrossRef]
25. Kassab, P.; El Hachem, C.; Habib, M.; Nehme, W.; Zogheib, V.; Tonini, R.; Kaloustian, M.K. The Pushout Bond Strength of Three Calcium Silicate-based Materials in Furcal Perforation Repair and the Effect of a Novel Irrigation Solution: A Comparative In Vitro Study. *J. Contemp. Dent. Pract.* **2022**, *23*, 289–294. [PubMed]
26. Careddu, R.; Duncan, H.F. A prospective clinical study investigating the effectiveness of partial pulpotomy after relating preoperative symptoms to a new and established classification of pulpitis. *Int. Endod. J.* **2021**, *54*, 2156–2172. [CrossRef]
27. Taha, N.; Ahmad, M.; Ghanim, A. Assessment of mineral trioxide aggregate pulpotomy in mature permanent teeth with carious exposures. *Int. Endod. J.* **2017**, *50*, 117–125. [CrossRef]
28. Bjørndal, L.; Simon, S.; Tomson, P.; Duncan, H.F. Management of deep caries and the exposed pulp. *Int. Endod. J.* **2019**, *52*, 949–973. [CrossRef]
29. Bjørndal, L.; Larsen, T.; Thylstrup, A. A clinical and microbiological study of deep carious lesions during stepwise excavation using long treatment intervals. *Caries Res.* **1997**, *31*, 411–417. [CrossRef]
30. Orhan, A.I.; Oz, F.T.; Ozcelik, B.; Orhan, K. A clinical and microbiological comparative study of deep carious lesion treatment in deciduous and young permanent molars. *Clin. Oral Investig.* **2008**, *12*, 369–378. [CrossRef]
31. Ballal, N.V.; Duncan, H.F.; Wiedemeier, D.; Rai, N.; Jalan, P.; Bhat, V.; Belle, V.; Zehnder, M. MMP-9 levels and NaOCl lavage in randomized trial on direct pulp capping. *J. Dent. Res.* **2022**, *101*, 414–419. [CrossRef]
32. Kazemipoor, M.; Azizi, N.; Farahat, F. Evaluation of microhardness of mineral trioxide aggregate after immediate placement of different coronal restorations: An in vitro study. *J. Dent.* **2018**, *15*, 116.
33. Cuevas-Suárez, C.E.; da Rosa, W.L.O.; Lund, R.G.; da Silva, A.F.; Piva, E. Bonding Performance of Universal Adhesives: An Updated Systematic Review and Meta-Analysis. *J. Adhe Dent.* **2019**, *21*, 7–26.
34. Linsuwanont, P.; Wimonsutthikul, K.; Pothimoke, U.; Santiwong, B. Treatment outcomes of mineral trioxide aggregate pulpotomy in vital permanent teeth with carious pulp exposure: The retrospective study. *J. Endod.* **2017**, *43*, 225–230. [CrossRef] [PubMed]
35. Murray, P.; Smith, A.; Windsor, L.; Mjör, I. Remaining dentine thickness and human pulp responses. *Int. Endod. J.* **2003**, *36*, 33–43. [CrossRef] [PubMed]
36. Matsuo, T.; Nakanishi, T.; Shimizu, H.; Ebisu, S. A clinical study of direct pulp capping applied to carious-exposed pulps. *J. Endod.* **1996**, *22*, 551–556. [CrossRef] [PubMed]

37. Cooper, P.R.; Holder, M.J.; Smith, A.J. Inflammation and regeneration in the dentin-pulp complex: A double-edged sword. *J. Endod.* **2014**, *40*, S46–S51. [CrossRef] [PubMed]
38. Schwendicke, F.; Frencken, J.E.; Bjørndal, L.; Maltz, M.; Manton, D.J.; Ricketts, D.; Van Landuyt, K.; Banerjee, V.; Campus, G.; Doméjean, S. Managing carious lesions: Consensus recommendations on carious tissue removal. *J. Adv. Dent. Res.* **2016**, *28*, 58–67. [CrossRef]
39. Bjørndal, L.; Ricucci, D. Pulp inflammation: From the reversible pulpitis to pulp necrosis during caries progression. In *The Dental Pulp: Biology, Pathology, and Regenerative Therapies*; Goldberg, M., Ed.; Springer: Berlin/Heidelberg, Germany, 2014; pp. 125–139.
40. Warfvinge, J.; Bergenholtz, G. Healing capacity of human and monkey dental pulps following experimentally-induced pulpitis. *Dent. Traumatol.* **1986**, *2*, 256–262. [CrossRef]
41. Chu, W.S.; Park, S.H.; Ahn, D.K.; Kim, S.K. Effect of local anesthesia on pulpal blood flow in mechanically stimulated teeth. *J. Korean Acad.* **2006**, *31*, 257–262. [CrossRef]
42. Oulis, C.J.; Vadiakas, G.; Vasilopoulou, A. The effectiveness of mandibular infiltration compared to mandibular block anesthesia in treating primary molars in children. *Pediatr. Dent.* **1996**, *18*, 301–305.
43. Kharouf, N.; Sauro, S.; Hardan, L.; Fawzi, A.; Suhanda, I.E.; Zghal, J.; Addiego, F.; Affolter-Zbaraszczuk, C.; Arntz, Y.; Ball, V.; et al. Impacts of Resveratrol and Pyrogallol on Physicochemical, Mechanical and Biological Properties of Epoxy-Resin Sealers. *Bioengineering* **2022**, *9*, 85. [CrossRef] [PubMed]
44. Farrayeh, A.; Akil, S.; Eid, A.; Macaluso, V.; Mancino, D.; Haïkel, Y.; Kharouf, N. Effectiveness of Two Endodontic Instruments in Calcium Silicate-Based Sealer Retreatment. *Bioengineering* **2023**, *10*, 362. [CrossRef] [PubMed]
45. Yazdi, K.A.; Ghabraei, S.; Bolhari, B.; Kafili, M.; Meraji, N.; Nekoofar, M.; Dummer, P. Microstructure and chemical analysis of four calcium silicate-based cements in different environmental conditions. *Clin. Oral Investig.* **2019**, *23*, 43–52. [CrossRef]
46. Oskoee, S.S.; Kimyai, S.; Bahari, M.; Motahari, P.; Eghbal, M.J.; Asgary, S. Comparison of shear bond strength of calcium-enriched mixture cement and mineral trioxide aggregate to composite resin. *J. Contemp. Dent. Pract.* **2011**, *12*, 457–462. [CrossRef] [PubMed]
47. American Association of Endodontists. AAE Clinical Considerations for a Regenerative Procedure. Available online: https://www.aae.org/specialty/wp-content/uploads/sites/2/2017/06/currentregenerativeendodonticconsiderations.pdf (accessed on 25 May 2018).
48. Kayahan, M.B.; Nekoofar, M.H.; Kazandağ, M.; Canpolat, C.; Malkondu, O.; Kaptan, F.; Dummer, P.M.H. Effect of acid-etching procedure on selected physical properties of mineral trioxide aggregate. *Int. Endod. J.* **2009**, *42*, 1004–1014. [CrossRef]
49. Shie, M.Y.; Huang, T.H.; Kao, C.T.; Huang, C.H.; Ding, S.J. The effect of a physiologic solution pH on properties of white mineral trioxide aggregate. *J. Endod.* **2009**, *35*, 98–101. [CrossRef]
50. Jefferson, J.C.; Manhães, F.C.; Bajo, H.; Duque, T.M. Efficiency of different concentrations of sodium hypochlorite during endodontic treatment. *Dental Press Endod. J.* **2012**, *2*, 32–37.
51. Pai, A.V. Factors influencing the occurrence and progress of sodium hypochlorite accident: A narrative and update review. *J. Conserv. Dent.* **2023**, *26*, 3.
52. Eggmann, F.; Gasser, T.J.; Hecker, H.; Amato, M.; Weiger, R.; Zaugg, L.K. Partial pulpotomy without age restriction: A retrospective assessment of permanent teeth with carious pulp exposure. *Clin. Oral Investig.* **2022**, *26*, 365–373. [CrossRef]

Disclaimer/Publisher's Note: The statements, opinions and data contained in all publications are solely those of the individual author(s) and contributor(s) and not of MDPI and/or the editor(s). MDPI and/or the editor(s) disclaim responsibility for any injury to people or property resulting from any ideas, methods, instructions or products referred to in the content.

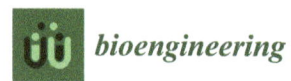

Article

Physicochemical and Antibacterial Properties of Bioactive Retrograde Filling Materials

Tarek Ashi [1,2], Davide Mancino [1,2,3], Louis Hardan [4], Rim Bourgi [4], Jihed Zghal [5,6], Valentina Macaluso [7], Sharif Al-Ashkar [8], Sleman Alkhouri [9], Youssef Haikel [1,2,3,†] and Naji Kharouf [1,2,*,†]

[1] Department of Biomaterials and Bioengineering, INSERM UMR_S 1121, Biomaterials and Bioengineering, 67000 Strasbourg, France
[2] Department of Endodontics, Faculty of Dental Medicine, Strasbourg University, 67000 Strasbourg, France
[3] Pôle de Médecine et Chirurgie Bucco-Dentaire, Hôpital Civil, Hôpitaux Universitaire de Strasbourg, 67000 Strasbourg, France
[4] Department of Restorative Dentistry, School of Dentistry, Saint-Joseph University, Beirut 1107 2180, Lebanon
[5] Laboratoire Energetique Mecanique Electromagnetisme, University of Paris Ouest, 50 Rue de Sèvres, 92410 Ville d'Avray, France
[6] ICube Laboratory, UMR 7357 CNRS, Mechanics Department, University of Strasbourg, 67000 Strasbourg, France
[7] ESTA, School of Business & Technology, 90000 Belfort, France
[8] Faculty of Dentistry, Al Sham Private University (ASPU), Damascus 0100, Syria
[9] Division Regenerative Orofacial Medicine, Department of Oral and Maxillofacial Surgery, University Medical Center Hamburg-Eppendorf, 20246 Hamburg, Germany
* Correspondence: dentistenajikharouf@gmail.com; Tel.: +33-667522841
† These authors contributed equally to this work.

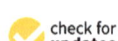

Citation: Ashi, T.; Mancino, D.; Hardan, L.; Bourgi, R.; Zghal, J.; Macaluso, V.; Al-Ashkar, S.; Alkhouri, S.; Haikel, Y.; Kharouf, N. Physicochemical and Antibacterial Properties of Bioactive Retrograde Filling Materials. *Bioengineering* 2022, 9, 624. https://doi.org/10.3390/bioengineering9110624

Academic Editor: Chengfei Zhang

Received: 8 October 2022
Accepted: 26 October 2022
Published: 28 October 2022

Publisher's Note: MDPI stays neutral with regard to jurisdictional claims in published maps and institutional affiliations.

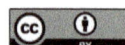

Copyright: © 2022 by the authors. Licensee MDPI, Basel, Switzerland. This article is an open access article distributed under the terms and conditions of the Creative Commons Attribution (CC BY) license (https://creativecommons.org/licenses/by/4.0/).

Abstract: The purpose of the present study was to evaluate the physicochemical properties and antibacterial activity of three calcium silicate cements. Mineral trioxide aggregate (MTA Biorep "BR"), Biodentine (BD) and Well-Root PT (WR) materials were investigated using scanning electron microscopy (SEM) at 24, 72 and 168 h of immersion in phosphate buffered saline (PBS). The antibacterial activity against *Enterococcus faecalis* (*E. faecalis*), the solubility, roughness, pH changes and water contact angle were also analyzed. All results were statistically analyzed using a one-way analysis of variance test. Statistically significant lower pH was detected for BD than WR and BR ($p < 0.05$). No statistical difference was found among the three materials for the efficacy of kill against *E. faecalis* ($p > 0.05$). Good antibacterial activity was observed (kill 50% of *bacteria*) after 24 h of contact. The wettability and the roughness of BR were higher than for the other cements ($p < 0.05$). BD was more soluble than WR and BR ($p < 0.05$). In conclusion, the use of bioceramic cements as retrograde materials may play an important role in controlling bacterial growth and in the development of calcium phosphate surface layer to support healing. Moreover, the premixed cement was easier to use than powder–liquid cement.

Keywords: calcium silicate cement; retrograde materials; premixed cement; powder–liquid cement

1. Introduction

The success of surgical endodontic treatment requires root-end filling materials that are easy to use, biocompatible, stable and economical [1–3]. The goal is to seal the apex hermetically and prevent microorganisms from entering the root canal [4,5].

Retrograde root-end filling materials have included zinc oxide eugenol cements, amalgam, glass ionomer and resins which have failed to meet the ideal requirements of root-end filling treatment [6,7].

Calcium silicate cement materials, colloquially denoted as "Bioceramic", in both forms, sealer [8] or thicker mixture [9], are considered as the ideal endodontic material for retrograde treatment due to their excellent physicochemical and biological properties [10–15], including biocompatibility and stability. These inorganic and non-corrosive ceramic cements contain tricalciums silicate and various radiopaque powders [16].

Mineral Trioxide aggregate (MTA) was the original calcium silicate cement introduced for endodontic treatment in 1993 and it is considered as the gold-standard material for various endodontic applications [10]. Other tricalcium silicate-based products have been developed, improvements on the original Portland cement invention [10]. MTA Biorep (Itena Clinical, Paris, France) is a powder–liquid product containing calcium silicate cement and calcium tungstate. Its water-based liquid, containing an organic plasticizer, improves the handling and plasticity [10].

Biodentine™ (Septodont, Saint-Maur-des-fossés, France) is a calcium silicate cement material and it has higher strength than other similar products [17]. This product consists of a powder–liquid material, where the liquid contains calcium chloride with an admixture of polycarboxylate [17]. MTA Biorep and Biodentine cements are indicated for several endodontic treatments, including pulpotomy, pulp capping, resorption, apicoectomy and open apex [9,10,18–21].

Some bioceramic cements require manual mixing and handling, powder–liquid systems, which require certain skills [16,22]. In addition, any change in the powder–liquid ratio or the mixing could affect and alter the physicochemical properties of these cements [8,23]. Premixed cements have been introduced to avoid errors during manual mixing. These premixed materials do not require any preparation before clinical application [8,16]. As mentioned in previous studies [8,16], these premixed materials are advantageous for some clinicians in the handling.

Well-Root™ PT is a novel premixed calcium aluminosilicate cement delivered in capsules for direct clinical use [24]. No information was found in the literature on the antibacterial activity and the physicochemical properties of this cement.

The purpose of the present research was to investigate the physicochemical properties and the antibacterial activity of three calcium silicate cements. The hypothesis concerned whether there would be antibacterial and physicochemical differences between the three tested materials.

2. Materials and Methods

2.1. Materials

MTA Biorep "BR" (Itena Clinical, Paris, France), Biodentine™ "BD" (Septodont, Saint-Maur-des-fossés, France) and Well-Root™ PT "WR" (Vericom, Gangwon-Do, Korea) were used in the present study, following the manufacturer's instructions (Table 1). All specimens were conserved in the dark in a container at 37 °C and 95% relative humidity for 48 h until completely set [25].

2.2. pH Measurements of the Aqueous Solution in Contact with the Cement

Five samples of each group were prepared using Teflon molds (3.8 mm in high and 3 mm in diameter). Each sample was put in contact with 10 mL distilled water at 37 °C. A pH meter, "CyberScan pH 510" (Thermo Scientific, Waltham, Massachusetts, USA), was used to measure the pH of water at 3, 24, 72 and 168 h. Before each pH test, the calibration of pH meter was performed using standard solutions at pH 10, 4 and 7 (Hanna Instruments, Lingolsheim, France). Distilled water was used to rinse and eliminate the previous solution from the pH meter electrode.

2.3. Solubility

Five samples (2 mm in height and 20 mm in diameter) of each material were analyzed following the method of a previous study [26]. The samples were weighed using a digital system, then the disks were immersed for 24 h in 50 mL of water at 37 °C. The samples were removed from distilled water and then dried at 37 °C for 24 h. Finally, the samples were weighed again to obtain the final weight. The solubility was defined from the difference in mass between the final and the initial weight.

Table 1. Manufacturer and manipulation of the tested materials.

Materials	Manufacturer	Lot	Mixing	Composition
MTA Biorep	Itena Clinical, Paris, France	53505	Powder: 1 capsule Liquid: 4 drops	Powder: Tricalcium silicate; Dicalcium silicate; Tricalcium aluminate; Calcium oxide; Calcium Tungstate Liquid: Water and Plasticizer.
Biodentine™	Septodont, Saint-Maur-des-fossés, France	B28033	Powder: 1 capsule Liquid: 5 drops	Powder: Tricalcium silicate; Dicalcium silicate; Calcium carbonate; Zirconiom dioxide; Iron oxide Liquid: Calcium chloride; Hydrosoluble polymer
Well-Root™ PT	Vericom, Gangwon-Do, Korea	WT010100	Premixed	Calcium aluminosilicate compound; Zirconium oxide; Thickening agent

2.4. Scanning Electron Microscope (SEM) of Crystallites Creation

Twelve samples for each material were created (3.8 mm in high and 3 mm in diameter). After the setting time, as described in Section 2.1, three samples from each group were stored in hermetic boxes and kept in dry condition. The remaining samples (9 samples) from each group were put in 10 mL of phosphate-buffered saline (PBS10×, Dominique Dutscher, Bernolsheim, France) at 37 °C. After 24, 72 and 168 h in PBS, 3 samples for each period were washed with distilled water for 5 min, sputter-coated with gold–palladium (20/80) [27], then, analyzed using an SEM (FEI Company, Eindhoven, The Netherlands, 10 kV) at a magnification of 5000×. Energy Dispersive X-ray (EDX) analysis was used during an acquisition time of 1 min and a working length of 10 mm to attain the spectrum of chemical elements present on the surface.

2.5. Roughness and Water Sorption Tests

Five samples from each product were created using Teflon molds (10 mm in diameter and 2 mm in height). After the setting time, as described in Section 2.1, the samples were kept in dry in the fume hood overnight. The roughness of each surface was measured using a 3D digital profilometer (Keyence, Osaka, Japan) at 2500× magnification. The average roughness (Sa) was calculated using software (Keyence 7000 VHX, Osaka, Japan).

After measuring the surface roughness, on the same samples, a contact angle device (Biolin Scientific, Espoo, Finland) was used to observe the infiltration time of a 5 µL droplet of water into the material surface. A movie was recorded to track the profile and the absorption time of the water droplet.

2.6. Antimicrobial Activity

Brain Heart Infusion medium (BHI) (Darmstadt, Germany) was used to culture *Enterococcus faecalis* (*E. faecalis*, ATCC 29212). The turbidity was adjusted to OD_{600} (nm) = 0.3. A direct contact test (DCT) was performed to investigate the antibacterial activity of the three products against *E. faecalis*. Triplicate samples were placed in 24-well culture plates. One milliliter of the bacterial medium was put to each well and incubated anaerobically for 24 h at 37 °C (constant stirring at 450 rpm). The bacterial medium without the cement materials was used as the control group. After 24 h, 10-fold serial dilutions up to 10^6 in BHI were performed on each specimen. One hundred microliters of each diluted medium was added onto a BHI agar plate, homogeneously spread and incubated at 37 °C for 24 h. Manual CFU/mL (colony forming units/mL) counting was measured the *E. faecalis* concentration.

2.7. Statistical Analysis

The results of pH, solubility, roughness and antibacterial activity were statistically analyzed using the Kruskal–Wallis test along with the Tukey Test. SigmaPlot release 11.2 (Systat Software, Inc., San Jose, CA, USA) was used with a statistical significance was set at $\alpha = 0.05$.

3. Results

3.1. pH Measurements

The pH of the solution in contact with the three cements over 7 days is shown in Figure 1. All three cements were alkaline for the solution for up to 72 h. BR and WR demonstrated statistically higher pH than BD at all time points (3, 24, 72 and 168 h) ($p < 0.05$). No significance difference was found between BR and WR ($p > 0.05$).

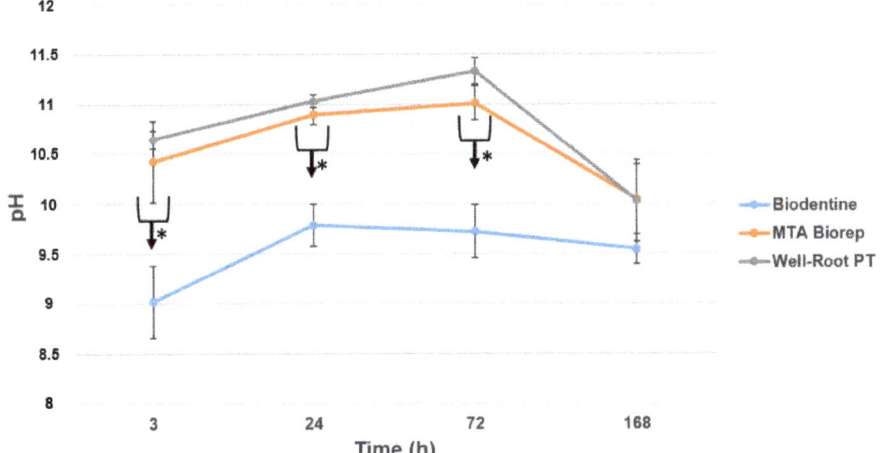

Figure 1. pH changes for the three products after 3, 24, 72 and 168 h of contact with water. * $p < 0.05$.

3.2. Solubility

The mean and standard deviation of solubility (wt.%) values are presented in Figure 2. BD was more soluble than BR and WR at 24 h ($p < 0.05$).

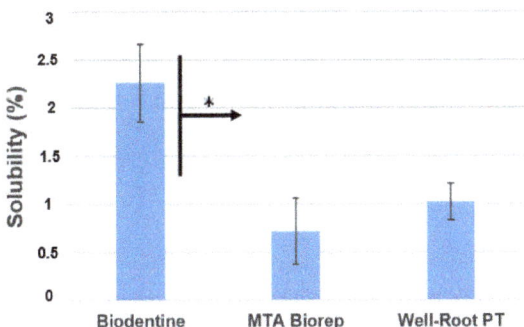

Figure 2. Solubility percentages of the different products after aging in water for 24 h at 37 °C. * $p < 0.05$.

3.3. Scanning Electron Microscope (SEM)

The crystalline structures of the three cements are shown in Figures 3 and 4. All three cements had crystalline deposits after immersion in PBS at 37 °C. At each immersion period (24, 72 and 168 h), different crystalline appearances were observed. At 24 and 72 h, WR had elongated crystals, BD and BR had globular and cubic crystals (Figure 3).

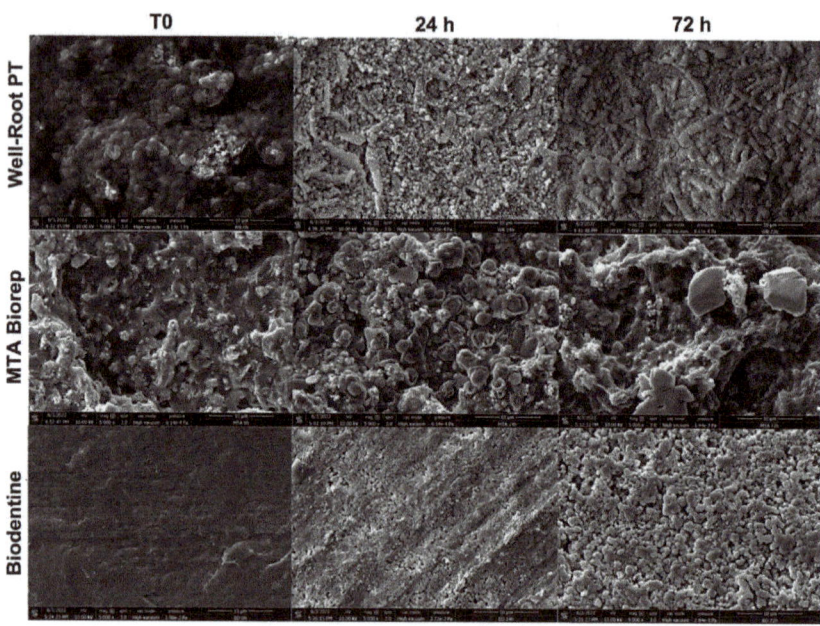

Figure 3. Scanning electron microscope images (5000× magnification) demonstrate the morphological changes of each material at 24 and 72 h of immersion in phosphate-buffered solution at 37 °C.

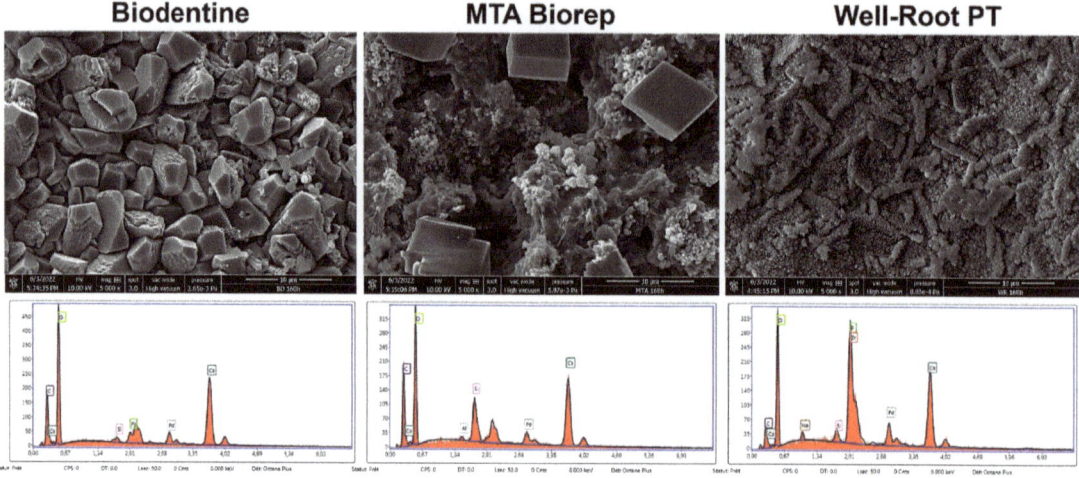

Figure 4. Scanning electron microscope images (5000× magnification) demonstrate the morphological changes and EDX spectrums of each material at 168 h of immersion in phosphate-buffered solution at 37 °C.

After 168 h, BR and BD showed cubic crystals. The cubic crystals of BR were larger (8–10 μm) than for BD (3–6 μm). WR had globular and elongated crystal features at 168 h. EDX analysis for the three cements after 168 h in PBS showed different percentages of Ca, P and Si among the three materials. Other chemical elements were detected on WR (Zr) and BR (Al) surfaces.

3.4. Roughness and Water Sorption Tests

BR demonstrated the highest hydrophilicity for a 5 μL of a drop of distilled water compared to BD and WR. Contact angles of 15° and 9° for BD and WR, respectively, were investigated after 10 s (Table 2). Whereas, the water sorption in the BR surface was faster (<10 s) than the other cement surfaces. The contact angle of the drop in contact with BR surface after 10 s was 0° (Figure 5). All tested cement surfaces were analyzed using KEYENCE 7000 VHX to measure the roughness of these surfaces. In addition, rougher surfaces were obtained for BR and BD compared with WR surfaces ($p < 0.05$) (Table 2 and Figure 5).

Table 2. Contact angles of 5 μL of distilled water on the different material surfaces after 10 s of deposition. Mean and standard deviations of the roughness (Sa) of the tested materials. Superscript letters a, b, c and x, y, z indicate statistical significance ($p < 0.05$).

Test\Materials	Biodentine	MTA Biorep	Well-Root PT	Statistical Significance
Contact angle (°)	15.2 ± 3.5^{x}	0^{y}	8.9 ± 0.4^{z}	$p < 0.05$
Roughness (Sa)	0.7 ± 0.05^{a}	0.9 ± 0.2^{b}	0.3 ± 0.02^{c}	$p < 0.05$

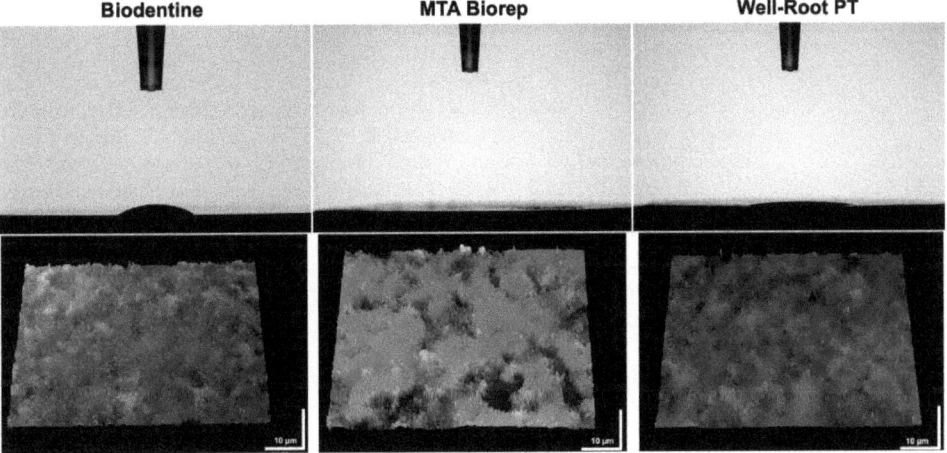

Figure 5. Contact angles of 5 μL of water drop on the different cement surfaces after 10 s. Digital micrographs of the different surfaces using KEYENCE 7000 VHX demonstrate the roughness of each material.

3.5. Antimicrobial Activity

Bacterial growth was significantly inhibited with the three cements. No significant difference was found among them for the efficiency against *E.faecalis* ($p > 0.05$). The three cements killed about 50% of the *bacteria* after 24 h, versus the control ($p < 0.05$) (Figure 6).

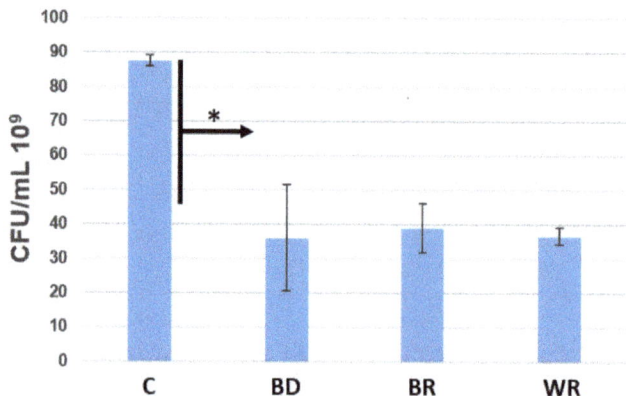

Figure 6. Number of colony-forming units/mL of *Enterococcus faecalis* in contact with Biodentine (BD), MTA Biorep (BR) and Well-Root PT (WR) after 24 h at 37 °C in anaerobic conditions. * $p < 0.05$.

4. Discussion

Since their introduction in the dental market, calcium silicate cement materials have attained popularity due to their excellent physicochemical, biological and mechanical properties and their positive outcomes in clinical applications [9,28]. Calcium silicate cement products are the ideal dentine repair materials for various endodontic applications [2,3,17,20,29]. A number of investigations have been conducted to determine the differences among the products as retrograde bioactive material.

Our present in vitro study comparing BR, BD and WR showed significant antibacterial activity and formation of crystals on their surfaces after immersion in PBS. Therefore, the null hypothesis was partially rejected.

Alkaline pH was detected with the three materials (Figure 1), but BD had a lower pH than WR and BR ($p < 0.05$). The alkalinity is key to the antibacterial activity and healing process [8,30–32]. Kharouf et al. [10] measured a high alkaline pH with MTA Biorep. Oliveira et al. [33] measured a lower pH for BD (pH = around 6–7) after 24 h than the one attained our study (pH = around 9–10), whilst Hassan et al. [34] measured higher pH values (pH = around 11–12) for BD after 24 h. The differences may be related to the methods of exposing the materials. The premixed bioceramic cement (WR) created a similar pH to the powder–liquid BR cement.

In the present study, the solubility of the three cements did not exceed the 3% mass after 24 h in distilled water; however, the ISO 6876 was not used. The results of the present study agree with those of the Al-Sherbiny study [35] for BD results and with the study of Queiroz et al. [36] for MTA Repair HP. The premixed bioceramic (WR) had a solubility similar to that of the other two cements (Figure 2). Solubility is important because if it is high, voids and gaps may be formed, which would be a pathway for the microorganisms to re-infect the root canal system [8,27]. BD demonstrated lower pH values than the other products, but the solubility of BD was higher. Weckwerth et al. [37] noted that a higher solubility does not always correlate with higher pH. The cement may release other components, which do not have any effect on pH changes and the liberation of these components increases the solubility of this material.

The direct contact test was used in this in vitro study to evaluate the antibacterial activity of the different cements. The agar contact test was not used, because in our previous study [8], we noted that these cements infiltrate the agar plates and hide the inhibition zones. *E. faecalis* was used in our experiment because this Gram-positive facultative anaerobe microorganism is the most predominant *bacterium* found in root canal infections and failure [8,38–41]. No significant differences were found among the capacity of killing bacteria of the three cements ($p > 0.05$). All the materials demonstrated high potential of killing bacteria after 24 h (kill around 50%) compared to the control group (bacterial medium). The antibacterial activity of these cements comes from the high alkaline pH [8,10,16,42,43].

All the three cements had different crystalline features (Figures 3 and 4) after immersion in PBS. Cubic crystals were observed on BR and BD samples after 7 d of immersion in PBS (Figure 4). The crystallites of BD were more numerous and smaller than BR crystallites. Elongated crystals were observed on WR surfaces. Yoo et al. [44] showed the importance of biomineralization to entomb the microorganisms in dentinal tubules, since the elimination of 100% of bacteria from the root canal system is impossible [45,46]. EDX analysis showed different chemical compositions of formed crystals onto each cement. Ca, Si and P were detected on the surfaces of the three materials, which reflects the reactions between calcium silicate and PBS. Zr presented onto WR and Al onto BR surface due to the initial composition which contain Zirconium oxide and Tricalcium aluminate, respectively. Al was not detected on WR surface which is a calcium aluminosilicate compound. Therefore, EDX could be considered as a qualitative method and the composition of these crystals could not be identified without X-ray diffraction analysis, which could be considered as limitation of this in vitro study.

A contact angle test was used to determine the capacity of absorption of 5 µL drops of distilled water. This test is an indicator of the wetting behavior of a solid material (cement) and a liquid (water). Contact angle measurement is affected by the surface roughness [47] and the chemical surface composition [48]. The roughnesss of WR surface was less than that of BR and BD ($p < 0.05$), which could be related to the particles size of each cement. After 10 s, the 5 µL drop was totally absorbed by the surface of BR which had the higher roughness values compared to BD and WR ($p < 0.05$). Whatever the considered wetting model (Wenzel or Cassie–Baxter) [48], the higher roughness and hydrophilic surface would increase the adhesion, protein adsorption and the cellular attachment, and provide a superior biocompatibility [48–50]. In contrast, a decrease in cell proliferation and growth could be related to a critical roughness ration, where the elastic energy of the cell hinders the insertion of the cells into surface trenches, where cells install over the tips of the rough surfaces leading to only point-contact, which minimizes cell–surface interaction [51].

Further studies are required to investigate the cytotoxicity, the setting time, the flowability, calcium ions releasing and the filling ability of the novel premixed cement.

5. Conclusions

Within the limitations of the present study, the three calcium silicate cement products, MTA Biorep, Biodentine and Well-Root PT, had a high antibacterial activity, formation of phosphate crystal in PBS alkaline and had comparable solubility. The premixed format was more convenient as a retrograde agent.

Author Contributions: Conceptualization, N.K.; methodology, T.A.; software, J.Z.; validation, L.H., R.B., S.A., Y.H. and S.A.-A.; formal analysis, V.M. and J.Z.; investigation, T.A.; resources, T.A.; data curation, T.A.; writing—original draft preparation, D.M., N.K. and T.A.; writing—review and editing, N.K. and T.A.; funding acquisition, N.K. All authors have read and agreed to the published version of the manuscript.

Funding: This research received no external funding.

Institutional Review Board Statement: Not applicable.

Informed Consent Statement: Not applicable.

Data Availability Statement: The data presented in this study are available on request from the corresponding author.

Acknowledgments: We acknowledge the INSERM UMR_S 1121 laboratory for providing the experimental setups.

Conflicts of Interest: The authors declare no conflict of interest.

References

1. Murata, K.; Washio, A.; Morotomi, T.; Rojasawasthien, T.; Kokabu, S.; Kitamura, C. Physicochemical Properties, Cytocompatibility, and Biocompatibility of a Bioactive Glass Based Retrograde Filling Material. *Nanomaterials* **2021**, *11*, 1828. [CrossRef]
2. Parirokh, M.; Torabinejad, M. Mineral Trioxide Aggregate: A comprehensive literature review—Part III: Clinical applications, drawbacks, and mechanism of action. *J. Endod.* **2010**, *36*, 400–413. [CrossRef]
3. Roberts, H.W.; Toth, J.M.; Berzins, D.W.; Charlton, D.G. Mineral trioxide aggregate material use in endodontic treatment: A review of the literature. *Dent. Mater.* **2008**, *24*, 149–164. [CrossRef]
4. Cohen, S.; Burns, R. *Pathways of the Pulp*, 6th ed.; Mosby-Year Book: Saint Louis, MO, USA, 1994; pp. 531–568.
5. Ingle, J.I.; Bakland, L.K.; Baumgartner, J.C. *Ingle's Endodontics 6*; BC Decker: Hamilton, CA, USA, 2008; pp. 1233–1294.
6. Viswanath, G.; Tilakchand, M.; Naik, B.D.; Kalabhavi, A.S.; Kulkarni, R.D. Comparative evaluation of antimicrobial and antifungal efficacy of bioactive root-end filling materials: An in vitro study. *J. Conserv. Dent.* **2021**, *24*, 148–152. [CrossRef]
7. Suhag, A.; Chhikara, N.; Pillania, A.; Yadav, P. Root end filling materials: A review. *Indian J. Dent. Sci.* **2018**, *4*, 320–323.
8. Kharouf, N.; Arntz, Y.; Eid, A.; Zghal, J.; Sauro, S.; Haikel, Y.; Mancino, D. Physicochemical and Antibacterial Properties of Novel Premixed Calcium Silicate-Based Sealer Compared to Powder–Liquid Bioceramic Sealer. *J. Clin. Med.* **2020**, *9*, 3096. [CrossRef]
9. Eid, A.; Mancino, D.; Rekab, M.S.; Haikel, Y.; Kharouf, N. Effectiveness of Three Agents in Pulpotomy Treatment of Permanent Molars with Incomplete Root Development: A Randomized Controlled Trial. *Healthcare* **2022**, *10*, 431. [CrossRef]
10. Kharouf, N.; Zghal, J.; Addiego, F.; Gabelout, M.; Jmal, H.; Haïkel, Y.; Bahlouli, N.; Ball, V. Tannic Acid Speeds up the Setting of Mineral Trioxide Aggregate Cements and Improves Its Surface and Bulk Properties. *J. Colloid Interface Sci.* **2021**, *589*, 318–326. [CrossRef]
11. Hardan, L.; Mancino, D.; Bourgi, R.; Alvarado-Orozco, A.; Rodríguez-Vilchis, L.E.; Flores-Ledesma, A.; Cuevas-Suárez, C.E.; Lukomska-Szymanska, M.; Eid, A.; Danhache, M.-L.; et al. Bond Strength of Adhesive Systems to Calcium Silicate-Based Materials: A Systematic Review and Meta-Analysis of In Vitro Studies. *Gels* **2022**, *8*, 311. [CrossRef]
12. Kang, T.-Y.; Choi, J.-W.; Seo, K.-J.; Kim, K.-M.; Kwon, J.-S. Physical, Chemical, Mechanical, and Biological Properties of Four Different Commercial Root-End Filling Materials: A Comparative Study. *Materials* **2021**, *14*, 1693. [CrossRef]
13. Vergaças, J.H.N.; de Lima, C.O.; Barbosa, A.F.A.; Vieira, V.T.L.; Dos Santos Antunes, H.; da Silva, E.J.N.L. Marginal gaps and voids of three root-end filling materials: A microcomputed tomographic study. *Microsc. Res. Tech.* **2022**, *85*, 617–622. [CrossRef]
14. Džanković, A.; Hadžiabdić, N.; Korać, S.; Tahmiščija, I.; Konjhodžić, A.; Hasić-Branković, L. Sealing Ability of Mineral Trioxide Aggregate, Biodentine and Glass Ionomer as Root-End Materials: A Question of Choice. *Acta Med. Acad.* **2020**, *49*, 232–239. [CrossRef]
15. Jardine, A.P.; Rosa, K.F.V.; Matoso, F.B.; Quintana, R.M.; Grazziotin-Soares, R.; Kopper, P.M.P. Marginal gaps and internal voids after root-end filling using three calcium silicate-based materials: A Micro-CT analysis. *Braz. Dent. J.* **2021**, *32*, 1–7. [CrossRef]
16. Debelian, G.; Trope, M. The use of premixed bioceramic materials in endodontics. *G. Ital. Di Endod.* **2016**, *30*, 70–80. [CrossRef]
17. Nowicka, A.; Lipski, M.; Parafiniuk, M.; Sporniak-Tutak, K.; Lichota, D.; Kosierkiewicz, A.; Kaczmarek, W.; Buczkowska-Radlińska, J. Response of human dental pulp capped with biodentine and mineral trioxide aggregate. *J. Endod.* **2013**, *39*, 743–747. [CrossRef]
18. Taha, N.A.; Al-Rawash, M.H.; Imran, Z.A. Outcome of full pulpotomy in mature permanent molars using 3 calcium silicate-based materials: A parallel, double blind, randomized controlled trial. *Int. Endod. J.* **2022**, *55*, 416–429. [CrossRef]
19. Jovanović, L.Z.; Bajkin, B.V. Scanning electron microscopy analysis of marginal adaptation of mineral trioxide aggregate, tricalcium silicate cement, and dental amalgam as a root end filling materials. *Microsc. Res. Tech.* **2021**, *84*, 2068–2074. [CrossRef]
20. Selvendran, K.E.; Ahamed, A.S.; Krishnamurthy, M.; Kumar, V.N.; Raju, V.G. Comparison of three different materials used for indirect pulp capping in permanent molars: An in vivo study. *J. Conserv. Dent.* **2022**, *25*, 68–71. [CrossRef]
21. Sanaei-Rad, P.; Bolbolian, M.; Nouri, F.; Momeni, E. Management of internal root resorption in the maxillary central incisor with fractured root using Biodentine. *Clin. Case Rep.* **2021**, *9*, e04502. [CrossRef]
22. Motwani, N.; Ikhar, A.; Nikhade, P.; Chandak, M.; Rathi, S.; Dugar, M.; Rajnekar, R. Premixed bioceramics: A novel pulp capping agent. *J. Conserv. Dent.* **2021**, *24*, 124–129. [CrossRef]
23. Cavenago, B.C.; Pereira, T.C.; Duarte, M.A.H.; Ordinola-Zapata, R.; Marciano, M.A.; Bramante, C.M.; Bernardineli, N. Influence of powder-to-water ratio on radiopacity, setting time, pH, calcium ion release and a micro-CT volumetric solubility of white mineral trioxide aggregate. *Int. Endod. J.* **2014**, *47*, 120–126. [CrossRef]
24. Jeon, J.; Choi, N.; Kim, S. Color Change in Tooth Induced by Various Calcium Silicate-Based Pulp-Capping Materials. *J. Korean Acad. Pediatr. Dent.* **2021**, *48*, 280–290. [CrossRef]
25. Kharouf, N.; Sauro, S.; Hardan, L.; Fawzi, A.; Suhanda, I.E.; Zghal, J.; Addiego, F.; Affolter-Zbaraszczuk, C.; Arntz, Y.; Ball, V.; et al. Impacts of Resveratrol and Pyrogallol on Physicochemical, Mechanical and Biological Properties of Epoxy-Resin Sealers. *Bioengineering* **2022**, *9*, 85. [CrossRef]
26. Kharouf, N.; Mancino, D.; Zghal, J.; Helle, S.; Jmal, H.; Lenertz, M.; Viart, N.; Bahlouli, N.; Meyer, F.; Haikel, Y.; et al. Dual role of Tannic acid and pyrogallol incorporated in plaster of Paris: Morphology modification and release for antimicrobial properties. *Mater. Sci. Eng. C Mater. Biol. Appl.* **2021**, *127*, 112209. [CrossRef]
27. Kharouf, N.; Sauro, S.; Jmal, H.; Eid, A.; Karrout, M.; Bahlouli, N.; Haikel, Y.; Mancino, D. Does Multi-Fiber-Reinforced Composite-Post Influence the Filling Ability and the Bond Strength in Root Canal? *Bioengineering* **2021**, *8*, 195. [CrossRef]
28. Camilleri, J. Classification of hydraulic cements used in dentistry. *Front. Dent. Med.* **2020**, *1*, 9. [CrossRef]

29. Kaur, M.; Singh, H.; Dhillon, J.S.; Batra, M.; Saini, M. MTA versus Biodentine: Review of Literature with a Comparative Analysis. *J. Clin. Diagn. Res.* **2017**, *11*, ZG01–ZG05. [CrossRef]
30. Drukteinis, S.; Peciuliene, V.; Shemesh, H.; Tusas, P.; Bendinskaite, R. Porosity Distribution in Apically Perforated Curved Root Canals Filled with Two Different Calcium Silicate Based Materials and Techniques: A Micro-Computed Tomography Study. *Materials* **2019**, *12*, 1729. [CrossRef]
31. Urban, K.; Neuhaus, J.; Donnermeyer, D.; Schäfer, E.; Dammaschke, T. Solubility and pH Value of 3 Different Root Canal Sealers: A Long-term Investigation. *J. Endod.* **2018**, *44*, 1736–1740. [CrossRef]
32. Poggio, C.; Dagna, A.; Ceci, M.; Meravini, M.-V.; Colombo, M.; Pietrocola, G. Solubility and pH of bioceramic root canal sealers: A comparative study. *J. Clin. Exp. Dent.* **2017**, *9*, e1189–e1194. [CrossRef]
33. Oliveira, L.V.; de Souza, G.L.; da Silva, G.R.; Magalhães, T.E.A.; Freitas, G.A.N.; Turrioni, A.P.; de Rezende Barbosa, G.L.; Moura, C.C.G. Biological parameters, discolouration and radiopacity of calcium silicate-based materials in a simulated model of partial pulpotomy. *Int. Endod. J.* **2021**, *54*, 2133–2144. [CrossRef]
34. Hassan, T.; Zeid, A.; Alothmani, O.S.; Yousef, M. Biodentine and Mineral Trioxide Aggregate: An Analysis of Solubility, pH Changes and Leaching Elements. *Life Sci. J.* **2015**, *12*, 1097–8135.
35. Al-Sherbiny, I.M.; Farid, M.H.; Abu-Seida, A.M.; Motawea, I.T.; Bastawy, H.A. Chemico-physical and mechanical evaluation of three calcium silicate-based pulp capping materials. *Saudi Dent. J.* **2021**, *33*, 207–214. [CrossRef]
36. Queiroz, M.B.; Torres, F.F.E.; Rodrigues, E.M.; Viola, K.S.; Bosso-Martelo, R.; Chavez-Andrade, G.M.; Guerreiro-Tanomaru, J.M.; Tanomaru-Filho, M. Physicochemical, biological, and antibacterial evaluation of tricalcium silicate-based reparative cements with different radiopacifiers. *Dent. Mater.* **2021**, *37*, 311–320. [CrossRef]
37. Weckwerth, P.H.; Machado, A.C.; Kuga, M.C.; Vivan, R.R.; Polleto Rda, S.; Duarte, M.A. Influence of radiopacifying agents on the solubility, pH and antimicrobial activity of portland cement. *Braz. Dent. J.* **2012**, *23*, 515–520. [CrossRef]
38. Alsubait, S.; Albader, S.; Alajlan, N.; Alkhunaini, N.; Niazy, A.; Almahdy, A. Comparison of the antibacterial activity of calcium silicate- and epoxy resin-based endodontic sealers against Enterococcus faecalis biofilms: A confocal laser-scanning microscopy analysis. *Odontology* **2019**, *107*, 513–520. [CrossRef]
39. Chang, S.-W.; Lee, S.-Y.; Kang, S.-K.; Kum, K.-Y.; Kim, E.-C. In vitro biocompatibility, inflammatory response, and osteogenic potential of 4 root canal sealers: Sealapex, Sankin apatite root sealer, MTA Fillapex, and iRoot SP root canal sealer. *J. Endod.* **2014**, *40*, 1642–1648. [CrossRef]
40. Portela, C.A.; Smart, K.F.; Tumanov, S.; Cook, G.M.; Villas-Bôas, S.G. Global metabolic response of Enterococcus faecalis to oxygen. *J. Bacteriol.* **2014**, *196*, 2012–2022. [CrossRef]
41. Stuart, C.H.; Schwartz, S.A.; Beeson, T.J.; Owatz, C.B. Enterococcus faecalis: Its role in root canal treatment failure and current concepts in retreatment. *J. Endod.* **2006**, *32*, 93–98. [CrossRef]
42. López-García, S.; Myong-Hyun, B.; Lozano, A.; García-Bernal, D.; Forner, L.; Llena, C.; Guerrero-Gironés, J.; Murcia, L.; Rodríguez-Lozano, F.J. Cytocompatibility, bioactivity potential, and ion release of three premixed calcium silicate-based sealers. *Clin. Oral Investig.* **2020**, *24*, 1749–1759. [CrossRef]
43. Camilleri, J. Characterization and hydration kinetics of tricalcium silicate cement for use as a dental biomaterial. *Dent. Mater.* **2011**, *27*, 836–844. [CrossRef]
44. Yoo, J.S.; Chang, S.W.; Oh, S.R.; Perinpanayagam, H.; Lim, S.M.; Yoo, Y.J.; Oh, Y.R.; Woo, S.B.; Han, S.H.; Zhu, Q.; et al. Bacterial entombment by intratubular mineralization following orthograde mineral trioxide aggregate obturation: A scanning electron microscopy study. *Int. J. Oral Sci.* **2014**, *6*, 227–232. [CrossRef]
45. Mancino, D.; Kharouf, N.; Cabiddu, M.; Bukiet, F.; Haïkel, Y. Microscopic and chemical evaluation of the filling quality of five obturation techniques in oval-shaped root canals. *Clin. Oral Investig.* **2021**, *25*, 3757–3765. [CrossRef]
46. Mancino, D.; Kharouf, N.; Hemmerlé, J.; Haïkel, Y. Microscopic and Chemical Assessments of the Filling Ability in Oval-Shaped Root Canals Using Two Different Carrier-Based Filling Techniques. *Eur. J. Dent.* **2019**, *13*, 166–171. [CrossRef]
47. Kontakiotis, E.G.; Tzanetakis, G.N.; Loizides, A.L. A comparative study of contact angles of four different root canal sealers. *J. Endod.* **2007**, *33*, 299–302. [CrossRef]
48. Ball, V. *Self-Assembly Processes at Interfaces*, 1st ed.; Akademic Press: London, UK, 2018; pp. 1–241.
49. Colombo, M.; Poggio, C.; Dagna, A.; Meravini, M.-V.; Riva, P.; Trovati, F.; Pietrocola, G. Biological and physico-chemical properties of new root canal sealers. *J. Clin. Exp. Dent.* **2018**, *10*, e120–e126. [CrossRef]
50. Hachem, C.E.; Chedid, J.C.A.; Nehme, W.; Kaloustian, M.K.; Ghosn, N.; Sahnouni, H.; Mancino, D.; Haikel, Y.; Kharouf, N. Physicochemical and Antibacterial Properties of Conventional and Two Premixed Root Canal Filling Materials in Primary Teeth. *J. Funct. Biomater.* **2022**, *13*, 177. [CrossRef]
51. Majhy, B.; Priyadarshini, P.; Sen, A.K. Effect of surface energy and roughness on cell adhesion and growth—Facile surface modification for enhanced cell culture. *RSC Adv.* **2021**, *11*, 15467–15476. [CrossRef]

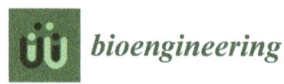

Review

Peptides in Dentistry: A Scoping Review

Louis Hardan [1,†], **Jean Claude Abou Chedid** [2,†], **Rim Bourgi** [1,3], **Carlos Enrique Cuevas-Suárez** [4,*], **Monika Lukomska-Szymanska** [5], **Vincenzo Tosco** [6], **Ana Josefina Monjarás-Ávila** [4], **Massa Jabra** [7], **Fouad Salloum-Yared** [8], **Naji Kharouf** [3,9,*], **Davide Mancino** [3,9,10] and **Youssef Haikel** [3,9,10,*]

1. Department of Restorative Dentistry, School of Dentistry, Saint Joseph University, Beirut 1107 2180, Lebanon
2. Department of Pediatric Dentistry, Faculty of Dentistry, Saint Joseph University, Beirut 1107 2180, Lebanon
3. Department of Biomaterials and Bioengineering, INSERM UMR_S 1121, University of Strasbourg, 67000 Strasbourg, France
4. Dental Materials Laboratory, Academic Area of Dentistry, Autonomous University of Hidalgo State, San Agustín Tlaxiaca 42160, Mexico
5. Department of General Dentistry, Medical University of Lodz, 251 Pomorska St., 92-213 Lodz, Poland
6. Department of Clinical Sciences and Stomatology (DISCO), Polytechnic University of Marche, 60126 Ancona, Italy
7. Faculty of Medicine, Damascus University, Damascus 0100, Syria
8. Private Practice, 54290 Trier, Germany
9. Department of Endodontics and Conservative Dentistry, Faculty of Dental Medicine, University of Strasbourg, 67000 Strasbourg, France
10. Pôle de Médecine et Chirurgie Bucco-Dentaire, Hôpital Civil, Hôpitaux Universitaire de Strasbourg, 67000 Strasbourg, France

* Correspondence: cecuevas@uaeh.edu.mx (C.E.C.-S.); dentistenajikharouf@gmail.com (N.K.); youssef.haikel@unistra.fr (Y.H.); Tel.: +52-(771)-72000 (C.E.C.-S.)
† These authors contributed equally to this work.

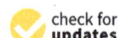

Citation: Hardan, L.; Chedid, J.C.A.; Bourgi, R.; Cuevas-Suárez, C.E.; Lukomska-Szymanska, M.; Tosco, V.; Monjarás-Ávila, A.J.; Jabra, M.; Salloum-Yared, F.; Kharouf, N.; et al. Peptides in Dentistry: A Scoping Review. *Bioengineering* **2023**, *10*, 214. https://doi.org/10.3390/bioengineering10020214

Academic Editors: Francesca Scalera and Chengfei Zhang

Received: 18 January 2023
Revised: 2 February 2023
Accepted: 3 February 2023
Published: 6 February 2023

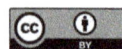

Copyright: © 2023 by the authors. Licensee MDPI, Basel, Switzerland. This article is an open access article distributed under the terms and conditions of the Creative Commons Attribution (CC BY) license (https://creativecommons.org/licenses/by/4.0/).

Abstract: Currently, it remains unclear which specific peptides could be appropriate for applications in different fields of dentistry. The aim of this scoping review was to scan the contemporary scientific papers related to the types, uses and applications of peptides in dentistry at the moment. Literature database searches were performed in the following databases: PubMed/MEDLINE, Scopus, Web of Science, Embase, and Scielo. A total of 133 articles involving the use of peptides in dentistry-related applications were included. The studies involved experimental designs in animals, microorganisms, or cells; clinical trials were also identified within this review. Most of the applications of peptides included caries management, implant osseointegration, guided tissue regeneration, vital pulp therapy, antimicrobial activity, enamel remineralization, periodontal therapy, the surface modification of tooth implants, and the modification of other restorative materials such as dental adhesives and denture base resins. The in vitro and in vivo studies included in this review suggested that peptides may have beneficial effects for treating early carious lesions, promoting cell adhesion, enhancing the adhesion strength of dental implants, and in tissue engineering as healthy promotors of the periodontium and antimicrobial agents. The lack of clinical trials should be highlighted, leaving a wide space available for the investigation of peptides in dentistry.

Keywords: antimicrobial; osseointegration; surface modification; tissue engineering

1. Introduction

Dental plaques contain over 750 different bacterial species, which are the major reason for dental caries, with streptococci being the most predominantly present. These bacteria, due to the production of acids, can demineralize and affect mineralized tooth tissues [1]. Different additives and biomaterials were used in dental treatments in order to eliminate and decrease the number of bacteria in the oral cavity and teeth tissues. Some dental materials, such as calcium silicate-based products, have been introduced in the dental market due to their antibacterial, antioxidant and remineralization properties [2]. Other solutions that have antibacterial effects are used to clean the root canal and kill resistant bacteria in the root canal system [3]. Even though they sometimes display high cytotoxicity [4,5], these materials are still currently used in dentistry.

It should be remembered that a peptide is expressed as a short polymer of amino acids (AA) [6]. According to the description of diverse authors in the literature, sizes of peptides may vary from <20, <50, to <100 [7–10]. The use of peptides has been paid attention to over the last two decades [6,11]. These peptides were used in various dental fields such as in endodontic treatment, coronal restoration, caries management, bone and dental tissue remineralization and in the modification of dental materials in order to promote the biological effects of these materials in the oral environment [6,12].

In the last periods, over 7000 native peptides (NP) have been considered by means of significant human physiological functions [13]. These peptides have functions by way of cell-penetrating, cell adhesion motifs, tumor-homing peptides, neuropeptides, structural peptides, peptide hormones, antimicrobial peptides, peptide tags, matrix metalloprotease substrates, growth factors, amyloid peptides, and erstwhile diverse NPs [10].

Nevertheless, one should state that NPs are frequently not truthfully appropriate for therapeutic usage since they have intrinsic drawbacks, including their poor physical and chemical stability, low oral bioavailability, short flowing plasma half-life, and quick removal from the circulation through the kidneys and the liver [9,13,14]. It is well described that peptides such as insulin and adrenocorticotrophic hormone were used for human therapeutic purposes in the first half of the 20th century [15]. Later on, synthetic oxytocin and vasopressin arrived in clinical use in the 1950s with the chemical elucidation of the sequences of these peptides [16].

Lately, pharmaceutical manufacturing has amplified the consideration of novel therapeutic peptides, persistently touching clinical claims [9,17]. By 2018, more than 60 peptides were approved by the Food and Drug Administration (FDA), and more than 600 were undergoing preclinical and clinical examinations [9,18]. With the current elaborations of solid-phase peptide synthesis, the production of therapeutic synthetic peptides (SP) has become achievable [9]. Accordingly, innovative synthetic approaches permit the modulation of pharmacokinetic assets and focus on specificity through AAs, the integration of non-natural AAs, backbone adjustments, and the peptide conjugates refining solubility or prolonging the half-life [8,13,14].

It is recognized that human dental masses, once fashioned, cannot be biologically replaced or repaired, and their multifaceted conformations require diverse approaches for regeneration [6]. However, it is unclear in the literature which specific peptides could be effective for applications in different fields of dentistry. Thus, the aim of this scoping review was to map the contemporary scientific papers related to the use and applications of peptides in dentistry at present.

2. Materials and Methods

The present scoping review has been described according to the PRISMA extension for scoping reviews guideline [19]. The review protocol was registered at Open Science Framework, and it is available at https://osf.io/up6ty (accessed on 18 December 2022). The systematic search was performed according to the following parameters: (i) population: peer-reviewed articles; (ii) intervention: use of natural or synthetic peptides; (iii) comparison: other substances or treatments; (iv) outcome: dental applications, (v) study design: in vitro or in vivo articles. The general question of the review was as follows: what scientific applications of products based on peptides are being used for dental applications?

2.1. Information Sources and Search

The literature database search was performed by two independent reviewers (RB and CECS) until September 2022. The search was carried out in the following databases: PubMed/MEDLINE, Scopus, Web of Science, Embase, and Scielo. The search strategy was first defined for the MEDLINE database using a controlled vocabulary and free keywords

(Table 1). The MEDLINE search strategy was then adapted to other electronic databases. The reviewers also hand-searched the reference lists of the included articles to identify additional manuscripts.

Table 1. Search strategy used in the MEDLINE database.

(Peptide) OR (Polypeptides) OR (Polypeptide) AND (Materials, Dental) OR (Dental Material) OR (Material, Dental)

2.2. Selection Process and Data Collection Process

After running the search strategy, a reference management program was used (End-Note X9, Clarivate Analytics, Philadelphia, PA, USA) to store the files of all databases. Then, duplicate articles were removed, followed by manual removal after the organization of titles in alphabetical order. All studies were initially scanned for relevance by title followed by abstract using an online software program (Rayyan, Qatar Computing Research Institute, HBKU, Doha, Qatar). The titles and abstracts of the articles were screened according to the following inclusion criterium: in vitro or in vivo studies that evaluated or reported the use of peptides for dental applications. The search was carried out on documents published in any language without restrictions on their date of publication. Reviews, case reports, case series, pilot studies, and conference abstracts were excluded. If the review authors were not sure about the eligibility of any study, it was kept for the next phase. All phases were carried out by two independent reviewers (RB and CECS) to check whether they met the inclusion criteria. The same two reviewers summarized and categorized the data using a standardized form. The information collected included the type of study, the peptide used, the application proposed and the main results.

3. Results

This scoping review is described according to the PRISMA extension for scoping reviews guideline [19]. After database screening and duplicate removal, a total of 6450 articles were recognized (Figure 1). After title and abstract screening, 156 articles remained for full-text inspection. From the 156 articles assessed for eligibility, 23 articles were excluded due to the following reasons: in 11 articles, the full text was not retrieved [20–30], 4 articles were not related to the dentistry field [31–34], 4 studies were reviews [6,12,35,36], 3 studies were not related to peptides [37–39], and 1 study was a pilot clinical trial [40]. Thus, a total of 133 articles were included in the present review.

3.1. Characteristics of Studies

The main characteristics of the studies included in the present review are presented in Table 2.

Table 2. Characteristics of the included studies.

Study and Year	Type of Study	Peptide Used	Application	Main Results
Bagno, 2007 [41]	In vitro	Two adhesive peptides: an RGD-containing peptide and a peptide recorded on human vitronectin	Implant osseointegration	It was observed that there was a capacity of the peptides to promote enhanced cell adhesion
Artzi, 2006 [42]	Experimental study	A synthetic peptide (P-15)	Guided tissue regeneration and guided bone regeneration techniques	The use of a synthetic peptide showed increased osteoconductive and biocompatible features
Bröseler, 2020 [43]	Randomized clinical trial	Self-assembling peptide (SAP) P11-4	Early buccal carious lesions	Self-assembling peptide regenerated enamel caries lesions

Table 2. Cont.

Study and Year	Type of Study	Peptide Used	Application	Main Results
Butz, 2011 [44]	Prospective in vivo study	Synthetic Peptide in a Sodium Hyaluronate Carrier (PepGen P-15 Putty)	Sinus grafting	The peptide evaluated was successful for maxillary sinus augmentation
Chung, 2013 [45]	In vitro	Asparagine–serine–serine (NSS) peptide.	Remineralization of eroded enamel.	Peptide increased the nanohardness and elastic modulus of eroded enamel
Altankhishig, 2021 [46]	In vitro and in vivo	Peptide	Vital pulp therapy	The dentin phosphophoryn-derived arginine-glycine-aspartic acid-containing peptide showed adequate properties as a bioactive material for dentin regeneration
Afami, 2021 [47]	In vitro	Ultrashort peptide hydrogel, (naphthalene-2-ly)-acetyl-diphenylalanine-dilysine-OH (NapFFεKεK-OH)	Antimicrobial activity and angiogenic growth factor release by dental pulp stem/stromal cells	Peptide-containing hydrogels have potential in tissue engineering for pulp regeneration
Babaji, 2019 [48]	In vitro	SAP P11-4 and casein phosphopeptides-amorphous calcium phosphate (CPP-ACP)	Enamel remineralization	The peptide was more effective and efficient when compared to CPP-ACP
Dettin, 2002 [49]	In vitro	Novel osteoblast-adhesive peptides	Osteoblast adhesion	The novel peptide promotes proteoglycan-mediated osteoblast adhesion efficiently
Cirera, 2019 [50]	In vivo	TGF-β1 inhibitor peptide: P144	Osseointegration of synthetic bone grafts	The healing period of osseointegrated biomaterials can be shortened when peptide biofunctionalization is used
Boda, 2020 [51]	In vitro	Mineralized nanofiber segments combined with calcium-binding bone morphogenetic protein 2 (BMP-2)-mimicking peptides	Alveolar bone regeneration	Mineralized nanofibers functionalized with peptides have the potential to regenerate craniofacial bone defects
Chen, 2017 [52]	In vivo	GL13K-peptide	Osseointegration of implants	This study showed that titanium dental implants with an antimicrobial GL13K peptide coating enables in vivo implant osseointegration
Aref, 2022 [53]	In vitro	CPP-ACP	White spot lesion	CPP-ACP could be a promising approach to manage WSLs efficiently, with subsequent universal adhesive resin infiltration
Aruna, 2015 [54]	Clinical	Gingival crevicular fluid (GCF) N-terminal telopeptides of type I collagen (NTx)	Periodontal therapy	Cross-linked NTx can be successfully estimated in the GCF of chronic periodontitis subjects
Brunton, 2013 [55]	A clinical trial	Biomimetic SAP: P11-4	Early caries lesions	Treatment of early caries lesions with P11-4 is safe, and a single application of this peptide is associated with significant enamel regeneration

Table 2. *Cont.*

Study and Year	Type of Study	Peptide Used	Application	Main Results
Fang, 2020 [56]	In vitro	Two hexapeptide coatings	Dental implants	The novel hexapeptide coating can inhibit the attachment of Porphyromonas gingivalis and prevent the formation of dental biofilm
Goldberg, 2009 [57]	In vitro	Polypeptide	Occluding dentin tubules	Peptide catalysts that mediate mineral formation can retain functionality on dentin, suggesting a wide range of preventive and treatment strategies
Amin, 2012 [58]	In vitro	Amelogenin Peptides	Osteogenic differentiation	Amelogenin-derived peptide could be a useful tool for limiting pathological bone cell growth
Godoy-Gallardo, 2015 [59]	In vitro	hLf1-11 Peptide	Antibacterial properties on titanium surfaces	A greater amount of peptide attached to the surfaces functionalized via atom transfer radical polymerization than those functionalized via silane
Dommisch, 2019 [60]	In vivo and in vitro	Antimicrobial peptides	Gingival inflammation	The study delivers evidence on the role of antimicrobial peptides as guardians of a healthy periodontium
Dommisch, 2015 [61]	Experimental study	Antimicrobial peptides	Gingivitis	Differential temporal expression for antimicrobial peptides could guarantee continuous antimicrobial activity alongside changes in the bacterial composition of the growing dental biofilm
Fernandez-Garcia, 2015 [62]	In vitro	Peptide-functionalized zirconia	Implant	Surface bioactivation of zirconia-containing constituents for dental implant applications will allow their perfected clinical implementation by incorporating signaling oligopeptides to accelerate osseointegration, improve mucosal sealing, and/or incorporate antimicrobial properties to avoid peri-implant infections
Fiorellini, 2016 [63]	In vitro	Osteopontin-derived synthetic peptide: OC-1016	Osseointegration of implants	OC-1016 was capable of meaningfully accelerating the initial stage of osseointegration and bone healing around implants
Goeke, 2018 [64]	Clinical	Antimicrobial peptides	Caries risk	The incidence of low-susceptible strains to antimicrobial peptides appears to relate to individual caries status

Table 2. Cont.

Study and Year	Type of Study	Peptide Used	Application	Main Results
Galler, 2012 [65]	In vitro	SAP hydrogel	Dental pulp tissue engineering	The use of this innovative biomaterial was considered a highly favorable candidate for upcoming treatment hypotheses in regenerative endodontics
Kirkham, 2007 [66]	In situ	SAP scaffolds	Enamel remineralization	SAP might be useful for dental tissue engineering
Kämmerer, 2011 [67]	In vitro	RGD peptides	Dental implants	Modifications of titanium surfaces with c-RGD peptides are an encouraging way to endorse endothelial cell growth
Golland, 2017 [68]	In vitro	SAP	Remineralization of white spot lesions	The application of SAP on demineralized bovine enamel indicated an irregular crystal or a lack of remineralization
Hsu, 2010 [69]	In vitro	Aspartate-serine-serine (8DSS) pep-tides	Nucleation of calcium phosphate carbonate from free ions	8DSS peptides reduced the surface roughness of demineralized enamel and promoted the uniform deposition of nano-crystalline calcium phosphate carbonate over demineralized enamel surfaces
Kwak, 2017 [70]	In vitro	Leucine-rich amelogenin peptide (LRAP)	Enamel regeneration	LRAP has the power to enhance the linear growth of mature enamel crystals
Kong, 2015 [71]	In vivo	Histatin-5 (Hst-5)	Oral Candidiasis	Hst-5 was able to clear existing lesions
Koch, 2019 [72]	In vitro	SAP: P11-4 and P11-28/29	Periodontal therapy	SAP hydrogels were effective for periodontal therapy
Hashimoto, 2011 [73]	In vitro	Peptide motif	Zirconia	A peptide motif was successful in binding zirconia
Kind, 2017 [74]	In vitro	SAP: P11-4	Remineralization of carious lesions	The application of P11-4 might facilitate the subsurface regeneration of the enamel lesion
Gonçalves, 2020 [75]	In vitro	Casein phosphopeptide-amorphous calcium phosphate (MI Paste Plus)	Enamel demineralization and dental caries	MI Paste Plus might be effective in improving oral health
Kim, 2019 [76]	In vitro and in vivo	A laminin-derived functional peptide	Implant	Peptide DN3 promotes bone healing
Kohgo, 2011 [77]	In vitro	SAP	Implant	SAP could be useful for bone regeneration around dental implants
Gungormus, 2012 [78]	Ex vivo	Amelogenin-derived peptides	Periodontal tissues	Amelogenin-derived peptide 5 promoted the regeneration of periodontal tissues

Table 2. Cont.

Study and Year	Type of Study	Peptide Used	Application	Main Results
Kakegawa, 2010 [79]	In vitro	Enamel sheath protein peptides	Construction of the enamel sheath during tooth development	A specific peptide sequence encourages the cytodifferentiation and mineralization activity of human periodontal ligaments
Kramer, 2009 [80]	In vitro	Integrin blocking peptide	Titanium surfaces	Antibody and peptide treatment reduced the number of fibroblast cells involved on the implant surfaces
Hua, 2010 [81]	In vitro	Antimicrobial peptide	Oral cavity	The antimicrobial peptide was demonstrated as an anti-Candida agent
Hua, 2010 [81]	In vitro	Antimicrobial peptide	Oral cavity	The antimicrobial peptide exhibits potent activity against both *A. actinomycetemcomitans* and *P. gingivalis* biofilms
Kohlgraf, 2010 [82]	In vitro	Human neutrophil peptide α-defensins (HNPs)	Cytokine responses	The ability of HNPs to attenuate proinflammatory cytokines was dependent upon both the defensin and antigen of *P. gingivalis*
Holmberg, 2013 [83]	In vitro	Antimicrobial peptide: GL13K	Dental and orthopedic implants	The antimicrobial activity and cytocompatibility of GL13K-biofunctionalized titanium make it a promising candidate for sustained inhibition of bacterial biofilm growth
Koidou, 2019 [84]	In vitro	Bioinspired peptide coatings	Peri-implant mucosal Seal	Peptide coatings were considered a promising candidate for inducing a peri-mucosal seal around dental implants
Knaup, 2021 [85]	In vitro	SAP: P11-4	Metal brackets	The application of the caries-protective SAP P11-4 before the bonding of brackets did not influence the shear bond strength
Kihara, 2018 [86]	In vitro	Novel synthetic peptide (A10)	Titanium surface	The novel peptide has a useful presentation that might enhance advanced clinical outcomes by means of titanium implants and abutments by preventing or reducing peri-implant disease
Jablonski-Momeni, 2020 [87]	In vitro	SAP P11-4	Early enamel lesions adjacent to orthodontic brackets	The application of p11-4 with fluoride varnish was demonstrated to be superior for the remineralization of enamel adjacent to brackets when compared to the use of fluorides alone
Kamal, 2018 [88]	In vitro	SAP P11-4	Artificially induced enamel lesions	SAP confers a higher remineralizing efficacy
Mao, 2021 [89]	In vitro	CPP-ACP	Dental caries	The use of 5% CPP-ACP reduced 39% of bacterial biofilm

Table 2. *Cont.*

Study and Year	Type of Study	Peptide Used	Application	Main Results
Makihira, 2011 [90]	In vivo	Antimicrobial peptide derived from histatin: JH8194	Dental implant	JH8194 might deliver a viable biological modification of titanium surfaces to amplify trabecular bone formation around dental implants
Li, 2014 [91]	In vitro	Synthetic and self-assembled oligopeptide amphiphile (OPA)	Mineralization of enamel	OPA was successful in the biomimetic mineralization of demineralized enamel
Liu, 2016 [92]	Experimental	Chimeric peptides comprising antimicrobial and titanium-binding motifs	Biofilm formation	Chimeric peptides provide a promising alternative to inhibit the formation of biofilms on titanium surfaces with the power to prevent peri-implantitis
Min, 2013 [93]	In vitro	Laminin-derived functional peptide, Ln2-P3	Implant	An Ln2-P3-coated implant surface enhances bone cell adhesion
Moore, 2015 [94]	Ex vivo	Multidomain peptide hydrogels	Dental pulp	Multidomain peptide hydrogels offered centrally and peripherally within whole dental pulp tissue are demonstrated to be biocompatible and preserve the architecture of the local tissue
Muruve, 2017 [95]	In vitro	PEGylated metal-binding peptide (D-K122-4-PEG)	Titanium surface	D-K122-4-PEG promotes resistance to corrosion
Nguyen, 2018 [96]	In vitro	Dentinogenic peptide	Dental pulp stem cells	The SAP promised guided dentinogenesis
Mardas, 2007 [97]	An experimental study in rats	PepGen	Bone regeneration	The anorganic bovine-derived hydroxyapatite matrix coupled with a synthetic cell-binding peptide failed to promote new bone formation
Mateescu, 2015 [98]	In vitro	Antimicrobial peptide Cateslytin	Peri-implant diseases	The new peptide could be ideal in the prevention of peri-implant diseases
Liu, 2021 [99]	In vitro	RADA16-I: (SAP)	Pulp regeneration	The novel SAP could be ideal in endodontic tissue engineering
Li, 2020 [100]	In vitro	GH12: antimicrobial peptide	Root canal irrigant	GH12 suppressed *E. faecali* in dentinal tubules
Mancino, 2022 [101]	In vitro	Catestatin-derived peptides	Oral candidiasis	The catestatin-derived peptides were considered for the treatment of oral candidiasis
Mai, 2016 [102]	In vitro	Antimicrobial peptides	Caries and pulpal infections	Antimicrobial peptide mimics offer opportunities for new therapeutics in regenerative endodontics and root canal treatments
Lv, 2015 [103]	In vitro	Amelogenin based peptide	Remineralization of initial enamel caries	The amelogenin-based peptide enhances enamel caries remineralization
Lee, 2007 [104]	In vitro and in vivo	Collagen-binding peptide	Osteogenesis	Collagen-binding peptide induced biomineralization of bone

Table 2. Cont.

Study and Year	Type of Study	Peptide Used	Application	Main Results
Liang, 2018 [105]	In vitro	8DSS peptide	Dentinal tubule occlusion	8DSS peptide induced strong dentinal tubule occlusion and can be used in dentin hypersensitivity
Lee, 2018 [106]	In vitro and in vivo	Bone formation peptide-1 (BFP1)	Bone regeneration	BFP1 was considered promising for bone repair
Na, 2005 [107]	Preformulation study	Antimicrobial decapeptide (KSL)	Antiplaque agent	KSL served as a novel antiplaque agent in the oral cavity
Magalhães, 2022 [108]	In vitro	Self-assembly peptide: P11-4	Bleached enamel	The use of P11-4 after bleaching results in the fastest recovery to baseline enamel properties
Lallier, 2003 [109]	In vitro	Collagen-binding peptide P-15	Periodontal treatment	P-15 promoted fibroblast attachment to root surfaces
Li, 2021 [110]	In vitro	Small-size peptide: RR9	Oral streptococci	RR9 might be considered a possible antimicrobial agent for periodontal disease
Matsugishi, 2021 [111]	In vitro	Rice peptide	Biofilm formation	Rice peptide hindered the biofilm formation of F. nucleatum and P. gingivalis
Li, 2022 [112]	In vitro	Amelogenin-based peptide hydrogel	Human dental pulp cells	The amelogenin peptide hydrogel enhanced mineralization and encouraged odontogenic differentiation
Mishra, 2019 [113]	A randomized clinical trial	Anorganic bone matrix/cell-binding peptide (ABM/P-15)	Human infrabony periodontal defects	The combination of ABM/P-15 was established to be a favorable material for periodontal regeneration
Padovano, 2015 [114]	In vitro	DMP1-derived peptides	Remineralization of human dentin	DMP1-derived peptides could be useful in modulating mineral deposition
Park, 2020 [115]	In vitro	BMP-mimetic peptide	Dental pulp stem cells	BMP-mimetic peptide accelerated human dental pulp stem cells
Pellissari, 2021 [116]	In vitro	Statherin-derived peptides	Biofilm development	The natural peptides from statherin are able to decrease biofilm proliferation and Candida albicans colonization
Petzold, 2012 [117]	In vivo	Proline-rich synthetic peptide	Titanium implants	Proline-rich peptides have a probable biocompatible capacity for endorsing osseointegration by lessening bone resorption
Picker, 2014 [118]	In vitro	Binding peptides	Calcium silicate hydrate	A new strong calcium silicate hydrate-binding additive influenced the physical properties of cement
Pihl, 2021 [119]	In vivo	Antimicrobial peptide: RRP9W4N	Titania implant	RRP9W4N was demonstrated to be successful in the control of infection in osseointegrating implants

Table 2. Cont.

Study and Year	Type of Study	Peptide Used	Application	Main Results
Ren, 2018 [120]	In vitro	Chitosan hydrogel containing amelogenin-derived peptide	Initial caries lesions	Chitosan hydrogel containing amelogenin-derived peptide was demonstrated to be effective in controlling caries and promoting the remineralization of the initial enamel carious lesion
Santarpia, 1991 [121]	In vivo	Histidine-rich polypeptides	Denture stomatitis	Histidine-rich polypeptides were effective in the treatment of denture stomatitis
Schmidlin, 2015 [122]	In vitro	SAP	Mineralization of artificial caries lesions	SAP improved the hardness profile of deep demineralized artificial lesions
Schmitt, 2016 [123]	In vivo	Synthetic peptide (P-15)	Osseointegration	There is no advantage in the early phase of osseointegration for dental implants with P-15-containing surfaces
Schuler, 2006 [124]	In vitro	RGDSP-peptide sequence	Titanium dental implant	There is no communication between RGD-peptide surface density and surface topography for osteoblasts
Schuster, 2020 [125]	In vitro	Hydroxyapatite/BMP-2 mimetic peptide	Bone tissue engineering	Biofunctionalization of collagen-hydroxyapatite composites with BMP-2 simulated peptides was considered cost-effective and fast for prolonged and improved jaw periosteal cell proliferation
Secchi, 2007 [126]	In vitro	Arginine-glycine-aspartic acid (RGDS) peptides	Implant	The modification of the titanium surface with RGDS peptides promoted osseointegration
Segvich, 2009 [127]	In vitro	Binding peptide sequences	Bone regeneration	The binding peptide sequences can be used in dentin and bone tissue engineering
Sfeir, 2014 [128]	In vitro	Multiphosphorylated peptides	Mineralized collagen fibrils of bone and dentin	Using phosphopeptides, there is progress in biomimetic nanostructured materials for mineralized tissue regeneration and repair
Shi, 2015 [129]	In vitro	Antimicrobial peptide-loaded coatings	Dental implant	The antimicrobial peptide-loaded coatings were demonstrated to be a potential approach for preventing peri-implantitis
Shinkai, 2010 [130]	In vitro	Synthetic peptides derived from dentin matrix protein 1 (pA and pB)	Direct pulp capping and bonding agent	The primer containing synthetic peptides derived from dentin matrix protein 1 negatively affected the bond strength to dentin

Table 2. Cont.

Study and Year	Type of Study	Peptide Used	Application	Main Results
Shinkai, 2010 [131]	In vitro	Synthetic peptides (pA and pB)	Bonding agent	A significant difference was seen in bond strength among $CaCl_2$ concentrations in Primer-I (comprising 10 wt.% $CaCl_2$) and pA/pB concentrations in Primer-II comprising 10 wt.% pA/pB, and there is a noteworthy interaction between these two factors
Shuturminska, 2017 [132]	In vitro	Statherin-derived peptide	Enamel biomineralization	The use of statherin-derived peptide was considered effective in enamel therapy
Su, 2017 [133]	In vitro	Peptide nisin	Dental adhesive	The cured nisin included in the dental adhesive showed a noteworthy inhibitory effect on the growth of S. mutans
Suaid, 2010 [134]	Histologic and histomorphometric study	Anorganic bone matrix–synthetic cell-binding peptide 15	Periodontal class III furcation defects	The use of anorganic bone matrix–synthetic cell-binding peptide 15 was effective in bone formation
Sugawara, 2016 [135]	In vitro	Platelet-activating peptide	Titanium surface	An epithelial basement membrane was formed on the titanium surface when platelet activating peptide was used
Sun, 2016 [136]	Clinical	Peptidome	Early childhood caries	The magnetic bead-founded matrix-assisted laser desorption/ionization time-of-flight mass spectrometry was considered an effective technique for screening distinctive peptides from the saliva of junior patients with early childhood caries
Takahashi, 2002 [137]	In vitro	Dipeptide: aspartylaspartate and glutamylglutamate	Periodontal pathogens	Dipeptides can be employed as growth substrates for P. intermedia, P. gingivalis, F. nucleatum, and P. nigrescens
Tanhaieian, 2020 [138]	In vitro	Recombinant peptide	Dental diseases	The recombinant peptide was demonstrated effective as an antimicrobial agent against E. faecalis and oral streptococci
Üstuün, 2019 [139]	In vitro	SAP: P11-4	Artificial enamel lesions	P11-4 was demonstrated to have the best remineralization efficacy
Wag, 2020 [140]	In vivo	Neural peptide	Angiogenesis and osteogenesis around oral implants	Alpha-calcitonin gene-related peptide up-regulated the expression of Hippo-YAP and downstream genes in order to encourage osteogenesis and angiogenesis around the implants

Table 2. Cont.

Study and Year	Type of Study	Peptide Used	Application	Main Results
Wang, 2015 [141]	In vitro	Peptide DJK-5	Dentin canals	The peptide DJK-5 showed an imperative antibacterial property against mono- and multispecies biofilms in dentin canals
Warnke, 2013 [142]	In vitro	Human beta-defensins (HBDs), small cationic antimicrobial peptides	Dental implants	HBD-2 is not only biocompatible with but further encourages the proliferation of human mesenchymal stem cells
Wener, 2009 [143]	In vitro	Laminin-derived peptide	Dental implants	Laminin-derived peptide improved and enhanced the integration of soft tissue on titanium implants used in dentistry
Winfred, 2014 [144]	In vitro	Cationic peptides	Endodontic procedures	Cationic peptides prevented the spread of endodontic infections
Wu, 2022 [145]	In vitro	TGF-β1 binding peptide–modified bioglass	Endodontic therapy	TGF-β1 binding peptide–modified bioglass was effective for regeneration in endodontic therapy
Xue Xie, 2019 [146]	In vitro	Antimicrobial peptide	Dental adhesive system	Antimicrobial peptide-hydrophilic adhesive delivers an advanced adhesive/dentin interface
Xue Xie, 2020 [147]	In vitro	Antimicrobial peptide	Dental adhesive system	Peptide-conjugated dentin adhesives were effective in secondary caries treatment and improved the durability of dental composites
Yakufu, 2020 [147]	In vitro	Osteogenic growth peptide (OGP)	Osteogenesis activity	OGP was promising in dental and orthopedic applications
Yamamoto, 2012 [148]	In vivo	Peptide including Arg-Gly-Asp (RGD) sequence	Periodontal ligament cells	Glial cell line-derived neurotrophic factor, which was hindered by pre-treatment with the peptide-embracing Arg-Gly-Asp (RGD) sequence, enhanced the appearance of bone sialoprotein and fibronectin on human periodontal ligament cells
Yamashita, 2010 [149]	In vitro	Anabolic peptide	Periodontal regeneration	Anabolic peptide has a positive influence on bone cells
Yang, 2017 [150]	In vitro	Peptide-modified tannic acid	Hydroxyapatite surface	Peptide-modified tannic acid inhibited the adhesion of bacteria
Yang, 2018 [151]	In vitro	Salivary acquired pellicle (SAPe)-inspired peptide DDDEEK	Biofilms	SAPe-inspired peptide DDDEEK has a great advantage in the field of implant materials

Table 2. *Cont.*

Study and Year	Type of Study	Peptide Used	Application	Main Results
Yang, 2017 [152]	In vitro and in vivo	Bioinspired peptide-decorated tannic acid	Remineralization of tooth enamel	Bioinspired peptide-decorated tannic acid has a good influence on the remineralization of tooth enamel
Yang, 2019 [153]	In vitro	Dual-functional polypeptide	Implant materials	Dual-functional polypeptide has a potential application in the treatment of hard tissue-related diseases
Yang, 2019 (b) [154]	In vitro and in vivo	Immunomodulatory peptide 1018	Plaque biofilms	Immunomodulatory peptide 1018 was effective as an anti-biofilm agent
Yang, 2017 (b) [155]	In vitro	DpSpSEEKC peptide	Demineralized tooth enamel	DpSpSEEKC restored demineralized tooth enamel
Yang, 2020 [156]	In vitro	Cell-adhesion peptides via polydopamine crosslinking	Zirconia abutment surfaces	Cell-adhesion peptides improved soft tissue integration around zirconia abutments via polydopamine crosslinking
Yazici, 2013 [157]	In vitro	Modular peptides	Titanium implant	Modular peptides on titanium surfaces improved the bioactivity of fibroblast and osteoblast cells on implant-grade materials
Ye, 2017 [158]	In vitro	Peptide-based approach	Adhesive-dentin interface	The peptide-based remineralization approach was effective in designing integrated tissue-biomaterial interfaces
Ye, 2019 [159]	In vitro	*D-enantiomeric* and *L-enantiomeric* antimicrobial peptides	Root canal wall biofilms	*D-enantiomeric* peptides exhibited more antimicrobial potent activity than *L-enantiomeric* peptides against *E. faecalis* biofilms on the canal space
Yonehara, 1986 [160]	In vivo	Opioids and opioid peptides	Tooth pulp stimulation	There is an interaction between substance P and enkephalin systems in the superficial layer of the brain-stem trigeminal sensory nuclear complex for the regulation of dental pain transmission. In addition, the native application of naloxone (5×10^{-7} M) partly antagonized the inhibitory effects of locally applied morphine and the opioid peptide
Yoshinari, 2005 [161]	In vitro	Antimicrobial peptide histatin 5	Poly (methyl methacrylate) denture base	*C. albicans* colonization on histatin-adsorbed PMMA was knowingly less than the control

Table 2. Cont.

Study and Year	Type of Study	Peptide Used	Application	Main Results
Yoshinari, 2010 [162]	In vitro	Antimicrobial and titanium-binding peptides	Titanium surfaces	Antimicrobial and titanium-binding peptides were encouraging for the reduction of biofilm formation on titanium surfaces
Yuca, 2021 [163]	In vitro	Dual-peptide tethered polymer system	Dental adhesives	The adhesive system formed of co-tethered peptides revealed both localized calcium phosphate remineralization and strong metabolic inhibition of S. mutans
Zhang, 2022 [164]	In-vitro	Dual-sensitive antibacterial peptide	Dental caries	This peptide prevented damage from bacteria and, thus, from dental caries
Zhang, 2016 [165]	In vitro	D-Enantiomeric peptide	Oral biofilms	D-enantiomeric peptide was effective against oral biofilms
Zhao, 2020 [166]	In vitro	Antimicrobial peptide nisin	Dental adhesive	3% (w/v) nisin-incorporated Single Bond Universal substantially inhibited the development of both saliva-derived multispecies biofilms and monospecific S. mutans biofilms without hindering the bonding performance
Zhou, 2008 [167]	In vitro	Genetically engineered peptides for inorganics	Tooth repair	Genetically engineered peptides for inorganics were effective in tooth repair
Zhou, 2015 [168]	In vitro	Antimicrobial peptide	Titanium surfaces	Antimicrobial peptide provided a promising bifunctional surface
Gungormus, 2021 [169]	In vitro	Peptide-assisted pre-bonding	Remineralization of dentin	Pre-bonding remineralization of dentin using peptide during 10 min notably enhanced the stiffness of dentin and the resistance to hydrolysis. In addition, it can reduce shrinkage due to drying
Koidou, 2018 [84]	In vitro	Laminin 332- and ameloblastin-derived peptides (Lam, Ambn)	Peri-implant mucosal seal	Laminin 332- and ameloblastin-derived peptides were demonstrated to be effective in producing a peri-mucosal seal around dental implants
Gug, 2022 [170]	In vivo	CPNE7-derived functional peptide	Dentin regeneration of dental caries	CPNE7-derived functional peptide repaired caries by dentin regeneration

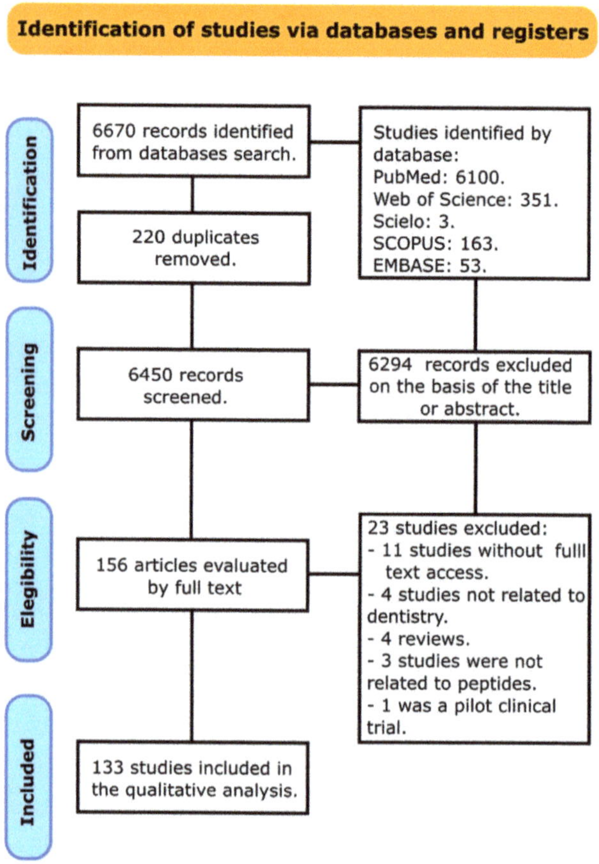

Figure 1. Flowchart summarizing the selection process of articles.

The studies included experiments in animals and/or using bacteria or cells; also, several clinical trials were found. Most of the applications of the peptides included caries management, implant osseointegration, guided tissue regeneration, vital pulp therapy, antimicrobial activity, enamel remineralization, occlusion of dentin tubules, periodontal therapy, the surface modification of dental implants, and the modification of dental materials such as dental adhesives and denture base resins.

3.2. Synthesis of Results and Summary of Evidence

The in vitro and in vivo studies included in the present review stated that peptides may have beneficial effects for treating early carious lesions. Additionally, the use of peptides seems to be beneficial for promoting cell adhesion and enhancing the adhesion strength of dental implants. In addition, peptides were useful for tissue engineering for cell-based pulp regeneration. Peptides were also successfully used as healthy promotors of the periodontium, acting as inflammatory mediators. Finally, most peptides were used as effective antimicrobial agents.

4. Discussion

A scoping review was performed regarding the use and applications of peptides in the dental field at present. Appropriately, most of the applications of the peptides included caries management, implant osseointegration, guided tissue regeneration, vital pulp therapy, antimicrobial activity, enamel remineralization, occlusion of dentin tubules, periodontal therapy, the surface modification of dental implants, and the modification of dental materials such as dental adhesives and denture base resins.

One should keep in mind that dental caries is considered the most common disease worldwide [171], and it can lead to the destruction of dental surfaces by means of acidogenic bacteria changing sugars to acids [43]. Dissolution of the mineral tooth structure begins with caries formation, therefore generating a demineralized subsurface lesion body, similar to white spots [172], followed by the development of irreversible cavitation of the mineralized surface layer [173,174]. Treatment of manifested caries involves an oral hygiene regulation and a follow-up visit to identify whether the caries has been prevented or has advanced into a cavity, which is subsequently treated by means of restoration [173]. The use of fluoride varnish can prevent caries formation by reinforcing the inorganic surface layer, consequently inhibiting the progression of caries [175–177]. Fluoride ions are preserved within the inorganic surface layer covering the demineralized carious lesion due to the high correspondence to hydroxyapatite [178]. Subsequently, the demineralized subsurface zone is not penetrated by fluoride; yet this is where remineralization would be essential in an attempt to regenerate decayed enamel tissue [43]. For this reason, novel methods for the treatment of caries have been introduced to mimic the structure of the enamel matrix, such as guided enamel regeneration (GER) [179].

It should be noted that self-assembling peptide (SAP) technology was designated on the reasonable design of a short hydrophilic peptide in combination with GER that builds into fibers, establishing a three-dimensional (3D) scaffold [180–182]. The surface features of the fibers might fluctuate, concurring with the physiological desires of the treated tissue [66,183]. This could be explained by the rational design criteria [183]. When treating early caries lesions, SAP P11-4 fibers have been adjusted to suitably bind ionic calcium and template hydroxyapatite formation, thus, accompanying remineralization in a comparable approach of amelogenin that supports the construction of the enamel. From this analysis, the SAP P11-4 fibers might be known as a biomimetic agent [66,74]. This could be in agreement with the finding of this review that demonstrated the potential effect of peptide P11-4 in caries management.

With regards to implant osseointegration, pure titanium is commercially used for implants in the dental field due to its possible resistance to corrosion, biocompatibility, and suitable mechanical properties [184–186]. Researchers have detected peri-implant bone resorption produced by peri-implantitis, which is considered the key reason for the failure of osseointegrated dental implants [187,188]. In this manner, surface modification of dental implants has been a topic of interest for researchers since titanium is an inert material that decreases the aptitude for remedial tissue therapy to succeed and resists bacterial settlement [189–191]. To counteract peri-implantitis and advance osseointegration, different type of coatings have been investigated [192]. Surfaces incorporating chlorhexidine, antimicrobial agents and antibiotics such as gentamicin, and surfaces incorporating chlorhexidine, poly-lysine, sliver, and chitosan have all been established for coating the titanium surface of implants [52]. However, some drawbacks could be noted with antibiotic-coated titanium, such as the controversial opinion about their bacterial resistance and host cytotoxicity [193]. In 2015, Zhou et al. demonstrated that antimicrobial peptides provided a promising bifunctional titanium surface and enhanced its bactericidal activity and cytocompatibility [168]. Likewise, a previous report suggested that after 6 weeks of implantation in rabbit femurs, titanium dental implants with an antimicrobial peptide GL13K coating allowed in vivo dental implant osseointegration at similar bone growth rates to gold-standard non-coated dental implants [52]. This could be explained by the fact that GL13K is bactericidal in solution against *Escherichia coli*, *Pseudomonas aeruginosa*, *Porphyromonas gingivalis* and *Streptococcus gordonii* [83,194,195]. Similarly, Yoshinari et al. proved that the antimicrobial and titanium-binding peptides were favorable for the diminution of biofilm formation on titanium surfaces [162]. In addition, a laminin-derived peptide was demonstrated to improve and enhance the integration of soft tissue on dental titanium implants [143].

Furthermore, an epithelial basement membrane was formed on a titanium surface when platelet-activating peptide was used [135]. All in all, this could clearly support the result of this review that the use of peptides seems to be beneficial for promoting cell adhesion and enhancing the adhesion strength of dental implants.

In addition, this analysis determined that peptides were useful for guided tissue regeneration [42]. This could be achieved when a combination of a synthetic peptide named P-15 (analog of collagen) and an anorganic bovine bone mineral (ABM) was used. ABM enhanced cell attachment by differentiation and cell binding, thus enhancing osseous formation and ensuing an accelerated periodontal ligament fibroblast attachment [109,196]. Adding to P-15, biocompatible and osteoconductive filler material was thus detected [42].

A major task in the use of tissue engineering for therapy in dentistry involves the initiation of tooth and bone regeneration. The dentin phosphophoryn-derived arginine-glycine-aspartic acid-containing peptide was demonstrated as a biodegradable, biocompatible, and bioactive material for dentin regeneration. These results could be clarified by the short AA sequences of the peptide used and by its 3D conformation essential for acquiring this function [46]. Accordingly, the peptide can be used in vital pulp therapy when a specific sequence is used.

Further, most peptides were used as effective antimicrobial agents. Peptide hydrogels have shown that ultrashort peptides (<8 amino acids) might self-assemble into hydrogels. These ultrashort peptides might be intended to integrate antimicrobial motifs, such as positively charged lysine residues; thus, the peptides have integral antimicrobial features [47]. The scheme and synthesis of biocompatible hydrogels with antimicrobial activity are of numerous interests for tissue engineering drives comprising the replacement of tissue in infected root canals [65,197,198]. Moreover, antimicrobial peptides were used in coated titanium surfaces [168], dental adhesives [147], caries infection [102], and plaque biofilm inhibition [36].

Peptides were also successful for enamel remineralization. It is imperative to note that the acidic nature of dental cavities created by a massive amount of sugar intake leads to bacterial colonization and a reduction in the pH. Accordingly, the demineralization of the enamel surface begins [48]. In order to prevent this issue, numerous remineralizing agents were presented [48]. A perfect agent should be free of toxicity and qualified to initiate remineralization without any harm to the dental surface. Matrix-facilitated mineralization equal to a natural process should be carried out, though this ability is absent in almost all these agents [199]. The arrival of SAP P11-4 has overwhelmed this restriction. It has the ability to regenerate enamel. In addition, these agents initiate remineralization by making 3D constructions mimic the extracellular matrix of the dental surface [200]. Therefore, when talking about enamel remineralization, clinicians should focus on SAP due to its efficient and effective outcomes obtained in this review.

The occlusion of dentin tubules is considered possible with the help of peptides. This theory became conceivable when mineral particles were observed on dentinal tubules, thus reducing dentinal permeability and enhancing the seal of the material-tooth interfaces [57]. Bonding agents and desensitizers have been demonstrated to be effective for occluding tubules by mineral precipitation; however, these techniques are sensitive, and the long-term performance of the resin is doubtful [201,202]. As a balancing method for the protein mediation of hydroxyapatite mineralization, streamlined synthetic cationic macromolecules comprising poly(L-lysine) (PLL) that cover primary and secondary amine groups are organizationally comparable to the functional areas of the natural proteins and have further been presented to encourage silicification [203]. This review implies that this peptide-catalyst-mediated method of mineral formation for occluding tubules and/or reinforcing dentin-bonding resins might retain function on the dentin surface, advising a wide range of protective and treatment plans.

Peptides have also been successfully used as healthy promotors of the periodontium, acting as inflammatory mediators. Periodontitis is a chronic inflammatory and tissue-destructive illness. Meanwhile, the oral cavity with its polymicrobial effect makes it problematic to treat; thus, new healing approaches are mandatory. In a minimally invasive way, SAP delivers the benefit of being functional at a defect site without creating a toxic area [204]. Furthermore, their tunable mechanical characteristics and reasonably designed physicochemical features permit a high variety of encapsulated drugs [205]. Some peptides called P11-4 and P11-28/29 were considered SAP-applicable for periodontal therapy, due to their biocompatibility, injectability, tunable mechanical and physicochemical properties, and cargo-loading capacity [72].

Finally, peptides were used in the modification of dental materials such as dental adhesives and denture base resins. Recurrent decay that grows at the composite-tooth interface was demonstrated to be a disadvantage when using resin-based composite [163]. Primarily, the composite-tooth interface becomes coated by a low-viscosity adhesive system; however, when a fragile seal to the dentin is obtained, damage from enzymes, acids, and oral fluids will be achieved. This impairment is chief in crevices that are occupied by cariogenic bacteria such as *Streptococcus mutans* [206–209]. Various bacterial-inhibition strategies have been incorporated into adhesive systems, but none of these strategies address the multifaceted interplay of the mechanical and physicochemical influences of the durability of the adhesive seal at the composite-tooth interface. Antimicrobial peptides have been coupled into the adhesive system using non-bonded interactions [146], and subsequently, antimicrobial peptides were conjugated into the network of the adhesive system in order to improve the antimicrobials' effectiveness [147]. An antimicrobial peptide AMP2-derivative (AMPM7) sequence using a functional spacer was used for integration into a monomer site. This adhesive system formed of co-tethered peptides demonstrated both localized calcium phosphate remineralization and strong metabolic inhibition of *S. mutans* [163]. An adhesive system incorporated with an antimicrobial peptide inhibited bacterial attack, and a hydroxyapatite-binding peptide promoted the remineralization of damaged tooth structures [146,163]. In 2017, Su et al. demonstrated that a cured antimicrobial peptide with nisin-incorporated dental adhesive showed a significant inhibitory effect on the growth of *S. mutans* [133], and recently, a paper showed that 3% (w/v) of nisin-incorporated universal adhesive system substantially inhibited the growth of both saliva-derived multispecies biofilms and *S. mutans* monospecific biofilms without hindering the bonding performance [166].

Moreover, it was demonstrated that *C. albicans* colonization on the denture's base was significantly less than the control when histatin-adsorbed PMMA (poly methyl methacrylate), an antimicrobial peptide, was used [161]. Another report suggested that histidine-rich polypeptides were effective in the treatment of denture stomatitis [121], thus evidencing the important use of peptides in removable prostheses.

Some limitations relative to the applications of peptides in the dental field can be cited. One restriction is the absence of homogeneity of the type and obtention of the peptides used in the different applications described in the present review. Another limitation that can be highlighted is that due to the heterogeneity of the analytical techniques used for distinguishing the peptides, analyzing data using any statistical analysis was avoided.

5. Conclusions

The use of peptides has been gaining increasing attention in contemporary dentistry. Dental research evidence suggests that peptides have several applications, including osseointegration, guided tissue regeneration, vital pulp therapy, antimicrobial activity, enamel remineralization, and the surface modification of dental implants. The lack of clinical trials should be highlighted, leaving a wide space available for the investigation of peptides in dentistry.

Author Contributions: Conceptualization, L.H., R.B., Y.H. and C.E.C.-S.; methodology, L.H., R.B., N.K. and C.E.C.-S.; software, L.H., R.B. and C.E.C.-S.; validation, D.M., J.C.A.C., M.J., N.K., V.T. and Y.H.; formal analysis, L.H., R.B. and C.E.C.-S.; investigation, L.H., R.B., N.K., M.L.-S., F.S.-Y. and D.M.; resources, A.J.M.-Á., Y.H., M.J., N.K., F.S.-Y., M.L.-S. and D.M.; data curation, L.H., R.B.,Y.H. and C.E.C.-S.; writing—original draft preparation, L.H., R.B., Y.H. and C.E.C.-S.; writing—review and editing, M.L.-S., L.H., N.K. and Y.H.; visualization, N.K., A.J.M.-Á., M.J., J.C.A.C., V.T., L.H., R.B. and M.J.; supervision, L.H.; project administration, L.H. All authors have read and agreed to the published version of the manuscript.

Funding: This research received no external funding.

Institutional Review Board Statement: Not applicable.

Informed Consent Statement: Not applicable.

Data Availability Statement: The data presented in this study are available on reasonable request from the first author (L.H.).

Acknowledgments: Authors L.H. and R.B. would like to acknowledge the Saint Joseph University of Beirut, Lebanon. Furthermore, the referees would also recognize the University of Hidalgo State, Mexico, the Polytechnic University of Marche, the Medical University of Lodz, and the University of Strasbourg for accompanying this research.

Conflicts of Interest: The authors declare no conflict of interest.

References

1. Kharouf, N.; Haikel, Y.; Ball, V. Polyphenols in Dental Applications. *Bioengineering* **2020**, *7*, 72. [CrossRef]
2. Hachem, C.E.; Chedid, J.C.A.; Nehme, W.; Kaloustian, M.K.; Ghosn, N.; Sahnouni, H.; Mancino, D.; Haikel, Y.; Kharouf, N. Physicochemical and Antibacterial Properties of Conventional and Two Premixed Root Canal Filling Materials in Primary Teeth. *J. Funct. Biomater.* **2022**, *13*, 177. [CrossRef] [PubMed]
3. Kharouf, N.; Pedullà, E.; La Rosa, G.R.M.; Bukiet, F.; Sauro, S.; Haikel, Y.; Mancino, D. In Vitro Evaluation of Different Irrigation Protocols on Intracanal Smear Layer Removal in Teeth with or without Pre-Endodontic Proximal Wall Restoration. *J. Clin. Med.* **2020**, *9*, 3325. [CrossRef] [PubMed]
4. Malta, C.P.; Barcelos, R.C.S.; Segat, H.J.; Burger, M.E.; Bier, C.A.S.; Morgental, R.D. Toxicity of Bioceramic and Resinous Endodontic Sealers Using an Alternative Animal Model: Artemia Salina. *J. Conserv. Dent.* **2022**, *25*, 185. [CrossRef]
5. Sismanoglu, S.; Ercal, P. The Cytotoxic Effects of Various Endodontic Irrigants on the Viability of Dental Mesenchymal Stem Cells. *Aust. Endod. J.* **2022**, *48*, 305–312. [CrossRef]
6. Bermúdez, M.; Hoz, L.; Montoya, G.; Nidome, M.; Pérez-Soria, A.; Romo, E.; Soto-Barreras, U.; Garnica-Palazuelos, J.; Aguilar-Medina, M.; Ramos-Payán, R. Bioactive Synthetic Peptides for Oral Tissues Regeneration. *Front. Mater.* **2021**, *8*, 655495. [CrossRef]
7. Lien, S.; Lowman, H.B. Therapeutic Peptides. *Trends Biotechnol.* **2003**, *21*, 556–562. [CrossRef]
8. Sato, A.K.; Viswanathan, M.; Kent, R.B.; Wood, C.R. Therapeutic Peptides: Technological Advances Driving Peptides into Development. *Curr. Opin. Biotechnol.* **2006**, *17*, 638–642. [CrossRef] [PubMed]
9. Vlieghe, P.; Lisowski, V.; Martinez, J.; Khrestchatisky, M. Synthetic Therapeutic Peptides: Science and Market. *Drug Discov. Today* **2010**, *15*, 40–56. [CrossRef]
10. Hamley, I.W. Small Bioactive Peptides for Biomaterials Design and Therapeutics. *Chem. Rev.* **2017**, *117*, 14015–14041. [CrossRef]
11. Scavello, F.; Kharouf, N.; Lavalle, P.; Haikel, Y.; Schneider, F.; Metz-Boutigue, M.-H. The Antimicrobial Peptides Secreted by the Chromaffin Cells of the Adrenal Medulla Link the Neuroendocrine and Immune Systems: From Basic to Clinical Studies. *Front. Immunol.* **2022**, *in press*. [CrossRef]
12. Alkilzy, M.; Santamaria, R.; Schmoeckel, J.; Splieth, C. Treatment of Carious Lesions Using Self-Assembling Peptides. *Adv. Dent. Res.* **2018**, *29*, 42–47. [CrossRef]
13. Fosgerau, K.; Hoffmann, T. Peptide Therapeutics: Current Status and Future Directions. *Drug Discov. Today* **2015**, *20*, 122–128. [CrossRef] [PubMed]
14. Lau, J.L.; Dunn, M.K. Therapeutic Peptides: Historical Perspectives, Current Development Trends, and Future Directions. *Bioorg. Med. Chem.* **2018**, *26*, 2700–2707. [CrossRef]
15. Banting, F.G.; Best, C.H.; Collip, J.B.; Campbell, W.R.; Fletcher, A.A. Pancreatic Extracts in the Treatment of Diabetes Mellitus. *Can. Med. Assoc. J.* **1922**, *12*, 141.
16. Stürmer, E. Vasopressin, Oxytocin and Synthetic Analogues: The Use of Bioassays. *J. Pharm. Biomed. Anal.* **1989**, *7*, 199–210. [CrossRef]
17. Dang, T.; Süssmuth, R.D. Bioactive Peptide Natural Products as Lead Structures for Medicinal Use. *Acc. Chem. Res.* **2017**, *50*, 1566–1576. [CrossRef] [PubMed]
18. Erak, M.; Bellmann-Sickert, K.; Els-Heindl, S.; Beck-Sickinger, A.G. Peptide Chemistry Toolbox–Transforming Natural Peptides into Peptide Therapeutics. *Bioorg. Med. Chem.* **2018**, *26*, 2759–2765. [CrossRef]
19. Tricco, A.C.; Lillie, E.; Zarin, W.; O'Brien, K.K.; Colquhoun, H.; Levac, D.; Moher, D.; Peters, M.D.; Horsley, T.; Weeks, L. PRISMA Extension for Scoping Reviews (PRISMA-ScR): Checklist and Explanation. *Ann. Intern. Med.* **2018**, *169*, 467–473. [CrossRef] [PubMed]

20. Bertoldi, C.; Labriola, A.; Generali, L. Dental Root Surface Treatment with Ethylenediaminetetraacetic Acid Does Not Improve Enamel Matrix Derivative Peptide Treatment within Intrabony Defects: A Retrospective Study. *J. Biol. Regul. Homeost. Agents* **2019**, *33*, 1945–1947.
21. Hossein, B.G.; Sadr, A.; Espigares, J.; Hariri, I.; Nakashima, S.; Hamba, H.; Shafiei, F.; Moztarzadeh, F.; Tagami, J. Study on the Influence of Leucine-Rich Amelogenin Peptide (LRAP) on the Remineralization of Enamel Defects via Micro-Focus X-ray Computed Tomography and Nanoindentation. *Biomed. Mater.* **2015**, *10*, 035007. [CrossRef]
22. Gonçalves, F.M.C.; Delbem, A.C.B.; Gomes, L.F.; Emerenciano, N.G.; Pessan, J.P.; Romero, G.D.A.; Cannon, M.L.; Danelon, M. Effect of Fluoride, Casein Phosphopeptide-Amorphous Calcium Phosphate and Sodium Trimetaphosphate Combination Treatment on the Remineralization of Caries Lesions: An in Vitro Study. *Arch. Oral Biol.* **2021**, *122*, 105001. [CrossRef]
23. Kim, H.; Lee, W.S.; Jeong, J.; Kim, D.S.; Lee, S.; Kim, S. Effect of Elastin-like Polypeptide Incorporation on the Adhesion Maturation of Mineral Trioxide Aggregates. *J. Biomed. Mater. Res. B Appl. Biomater.* **2020**, *108*, 2847–2856. [CrossRef]
24. Li, C.; Yang, P.; Kou, Y.; Zhang, D.; Li, M. The Polypeptide OP3-4 Induced Osteogenic Differentiation of Bone Marrow Mesenchymal Stem Cells via Protein Kinase B/Glycogen Synthase Kinase 3β/β-Catenin Pathway and Promoted Mandibular Defect Bone Regeneration. *Arch. Oral Biol.* **2021**, *130*, 105243. [CrossRef]
25. Minguela, J.; Müller, D.; Mücklich, F.; Llanes, L.; Ginebra, M.; Roa, J.; Mas-Moruno, C. Peptidic Biofunctionalization of Laser Patterned Dental Zirconia: A Biochemical-Topographical Approach. *Mater. Sci. Eng. C* **2021**, *125*, 112096. [CrossRef]
26. Niu, J.Y.; Yin, I.X.; Wu, W.K.K.; Li, Q.-L.; Mei, M.L.; Chu, C.H. Efficacy of the Dual-Action GA-KR12 Peptide for Remineralising Initial Enamel Caries: An in Vitro Study. *Clin. Oral Investig.* **2022**, *26*, 2441–2451. [CrossRef]
27. Pietruski, J.; Pietruska, M.; Stokowska, W.; Pattarelli, G. Evaluation of Polypeptide Growth Factors in the Process of Dental Implant Osseointegration. *Rocz. Akad. Med. Bialymstoku 1995* **2001**, *46*, 19–27.
28. Wang, R.; Nisar, S.; Vogel, Z.; Liu, H.; Wang, Y. Dentin Collagen Denaturation Status Assessed by Collagen Hybridizing Peptide and Its Effect on Bio-Stabilization of Proanthocyanidins. *Dent. Mater.* **2022**, *38*, 748–758. [CrossRef]
29. Yamaguchi, M.; Kojima, T.; Kanekawa, M.; Aihara, N.; Nogimura, A.; Kasai, K. Neuropeptides Stimulate Production of Interleukin-1β, Interleukin-6, and Tumor Necrosis Factor-α in Human Dental Pulp Cells. *Inflamm. Res.* **2004**, *53*, 199–204. [CrossRef]
30. Park, C.; Song, M.; Kim, S.; Min, B. Vitronectin-Derived Peptide Promotes Reparative Dentin Formation. *J. Dent. Res.* **2022**, *101*, 1481–1489. [CrossRef]
31. Yaguchi, A.; Hiramatsu, H.; Ishida, A.; Oshikawa, M.; Ajioka, I.; Muraoka, T. Hydrogel-Stiffening and Non-Cell Adhesive Properties of Amphiphilic Peptides with Central Alkylene Chains. *Chem. Eur. J.* **2021**, *27*, 9295–9301. [CrossRef]
32. Xie, S.; Allington, R.W.; Svec, F.; Fréchet, J.M. Rapid Reversed-Phase Separation of Proteins and Peptides Using Optimized 'Moulded'Monolithic Poly (Styrene–Co-Divinylbenzene) Columns. *J. Chromatogr. A* **1999**, *865*, 169–174. [CrossRef]
33. Pastor, J.J.; Fernández, I.; Rabanal, F.; Giralt, E. A New Method for the Preparation of Unprotected Peptides on Biocompatible Resins with Application in Combinatorial Chemistry. *Org. Lett.* **2002**, *4*, 3831–3833. [CrossRef]
34. Mizuno, M.; Goto, K.; Miura, T.; Hosaka, D.; Inazu, T. A Novel Peptide Synthesis Using Fluorous Chemistry. *Chem. Commun.* **2003**, *8*, 972–973. [CrossRef]
35. Khurshid, Z.; Naseem, M.; Sheikh, Z.; Najeeb, S.; Shahab, S.; Zafar, M.S. Oral Antimicrobial Peptides: Types and Role in the Oral Cavity. *Saudi Pharm. J.* **2016**, *24*, 515–524. [CrossRef]
36. Park, S.-C.; Park, Y.; Hahm, K.-S. The Role of Antimicrobial Peptides in Preventing Multidrug-Resistant Bacterial Infections and Biofilm Formation. *Int. J. Mol. Sci.* **2011**, *12*, 5971–5992. [CrossRef]
37. Li, C.; Bhatt, P.; Johnston, T. Evaluation of a Mucoadhesive Buccal Patch for Delivery of Peptides: In Vitro Screening of Bioadhesion. *Drug Dev. Ind. Pharm.* **1998**, *24*, 919–926. [CrossRef]
38. Kokkonen, H.; Cassinelli, C.; Verhoef, R.; Morra, M.; Schols, H.; Tuukkanen, J. Differentiation of Osteoblasts on Pectin-Coated Titanium. *Biomacromolecules* **2008**, *9*, 2369–2376. [CrossRef]
39. Glimcher, M.; Levine, P. Studies of the Proteins, Peptides and Free Amino Acids of Mature Bovine Enamel. *Biochem. J.* **1966**, *98*, 742. [CrossRef]
40. Takayama, S.; Kato, T.; Imamura, K.; Kita, D.; Ota, K.; Suzuki, E.; Sugito, H.; Saitoh, E.; Taniguchi, M.; Saito, A. Effect of a Mouthrinse Containing Rice Peptide CL (14-25) on Early Dental Plaque Regrowth: A Randomized Crossover Pilot Study. *BMC Res. Notes* **2015**, *8*, 531. [CrossRef]
41. Bagno, A.; Piovan, A.; Dettin, M.; Chiarion, A.; Brun, P.; Gambaretto, R.; Fontana, G.; Di Bello, C.; Palù, G.; Castagliuolo, I. Human Osteoblast-like Cell Adhesion on Titanium Substrates Covalently Functionalized with Synthetic Peptides. *Bone* **2007**, *40*, 693–699. [CrossRef]
42. Artzi, Z.; Weinreb, M.; Tal, H.; Nemcovsky, C.E.; Rohrer, M.D.; Prasad, H.S.; Kozlovsky, A. Experimental Intrabony and Periodontal Defects Treated with Natural Mineral Combined With a Synthetic Cell-Binding Peptide in the Canine: Morphometric Evaluations. *J. Periodontol.* **2006**, *77*, 1658–1664. [CrossRef]
43. Bröseler, F.; Tietmann, C.; Bommer, C.; Drechsel, T.; Heinzel-Gutenbrunner, M.; Jepsen, S. Randomised Clinical Trial Investigating Self-Assembling Peptide P11-4 in the Treatment of Early Caries. *Clin. Oral Investig.* **2020**, *24*, 123–132. [CrossRef]
44. Butz, F.; Bächle, M.; Ofer, M.; Marquardt, K.; Kohal, R.J. Sinus Augmentation with Bovine Hydroxyapatite/Synthetic Peptide in a Sodium Hyaluronate Carrier (PepGen P-15 Putty): A Clinical Investigation of Different Healing Times. *Int. J. Oral Maxillofac. Implant.* **2011**, *26*, 1317–1323.

45. Chung, H.-Y.; Huang, K.-C. Effects of Peptide Concentration on Remineralization of Eroded Enamel. *J. Mech. Behav. Biomed. Mater.* **2013**, *28*, 213–221. [CrossRef]
46. Altankhishig, B.; Polan, M.A.A.; Qiu, Y.; Hasan, M.R.; Saito, T. Dentin Phosphophoryn-Derived Peptide Promotes Odontoblast Differentiation In Vitro and Dentin Regeneration In Vivo. *Materials* **2021**, *14*, 874. [CrossRef] [PubMed]
47. Afami, M.E.; El Karim, I.; About, I.; Coulter, S.M.; Laverty, G.; Lundy, F.T. Ultrashort Peptide Hydrogels Display Antimicrobial Activity and Enhance Angiogenic Growth Factor Release by Dental Pulp Stem/Stromal Cells. *Materials* **2021**, *14*, 2237. [CrossRef]
48. Babaji, P.; Melkundi, M.; Bhagwat, P.; Mehta, V. An in Vitro Evaluation of Remineralizing Capacity of Self-Assembling Peptide (SAP) P11-4 and Casein Phosphopeptides-Amorphous Calcium Phosphate (CPP-ACP) on Artificial Enamel. *Pesqui. Bras. Odontopediatr. Clín. Integr.* **2019**, *19*, e4504. [CrossRef]
49. Dettin, M.; Conconi, M.T.; Gambaretto, R.; Pasquato, A.; Folin, M.; Di Bello, C.; Parnigotto, P.P. Novel Osteoblast-adhesive Peptides for Dental/Orthopedic Biomaterials. *J. Biomed. Mater. Res.* **2002**, *60*, 466–471. [CrossRef] [PubMed]
50. Cirera, A.; Manzanares, M.C.; Sevilla, P.; Ortiz-Hernandez, M.; Galindo-Moreno, P.; Gil, J. Biofunctionalization with a TGFβ-1 Inhibitor Peptide in the Osseointegration of Synthetic Bone Grafts: An in Vivo Study in Beagle Dogs. *Materials* **2019**, *12*, 3168. [CrossRef]
51. Boda, S.K.; Almoshari, Y.; Wang, H.; Wang, X.; Reinhardt, R.A.; Duan, B.; Wang, D.; Xie, J. Mineralized Nanofiber Segments Coupled with Calcium-Binding BMP-2 Peptides for Alveolar Bone Regeneration. *Acta Biomater.* **2019**, *85*, 282–293. [CrossRef]
52. Chen, X.; Zhou, X.; Liu, S.; Wu, R.; Aparicio, C.; Wu, J. In Vivo Osseointegration of Dental Implants with an Antimicrobial Peptide Coating. *J. Mater. Sci. Mater. Med.* **2017**, *28*, 76. [CrossRef] [PubMed]
53. Aref, N.S.; Alrasheed, M.K. Casein Phosphopeptide Amorphous Calcium Phosphate and Universal Adhesive Resin as a Complementary Approach for Management of White Spot Lesions: An In-Vitro Study. *Prog. Orthod.* **2022**, *23*, 10. [CrossRef]
54. Aruna, G. Estimation of N-Terminal Telopeptides of Type I Collagen in Periodontal Health, Disease and after Nonsurgical Periodontal Therapy in Gingival Crevicular Fluid: A Clinico-Biochemical Study. *Indian J. Dent. Res.* **2015**, *26*, 152. [CrossRef]
55. Brunton, P.; Davies, R.; Burke, J.; Smith, A.; Aggeli, A.; Brookes, S.; Kirkham, J. Treatment of Early Caries Lesions Using Biomimetic Self-Assembling Peptides—A Clinical Safety Trial. *Br. Dent. J.* **2013**, *215*, E6. [CrossRef]
56. Fang, D.; Yuran, S.; Reches, M.; Catunda, R.; Levin, L.; Febbraio, M. A Peptide Coating Preventing the Attachment of Porphyromonas Gingivalis on the Surfaces of Dental Implants. *J. Periodontal Res.* **2020**, *55*, 503–510. [CrossRef]
57. Goldberg, A.; Advincula, M.; Komabayashi, T.; Patel, P.; Mather, P.; Goberman, D.; Kazemi, R. Polypeptide-Catalyzed Biosilicification of Dentin Surfaces. *J. Dent. Res.* **2009**, *88*, 377–381. [CrossRef] [PubMed]
58. Amin, H.D.; Olsen, I.; Knowles, J.C.; Donos, N. Differential Effect of Amelogenin Peptides on Osteogenic Differentiation in Vitro: Identification of Possible New Drugs for Bone Repair and Regeneration. *Tissue Eng. Part A* **2012**, *18*, 1193–1202. [CrossRef] [PubMed]
59. Godoy-Gallardo, M.; Mas-Moruno, C.; Yu, K.; Manero, J.M.; Gil, F.J.; Kizhakkedathu, J.N.; Rodriguez, D. Antibacterial Properties of HLf1–11 Peptide onto Titanium Surfaces: A Comparison Study between Silanization and Surface Initiated Polymerization. *Biomacromolecules* **2015**, *16*, 483–496. [CrossRef] [PubMed]
60. Dommisch, H.; Skora, P.; Hirschfeld, J.; Olk, G.; Hildebrandt, L.; Jepsen, S. The Guardians of the Periodontium—Sequential and Differential Expression of Antimicrobial Peptides during Gingival Inflammation. Results from In Vivo and In Vitro Studies. *J. Clin. Periodontol.* **2019**, *46*, 276–285. [CrossRef]
61. Dommisch, H.; Staufenbiel, I.; Schulze, K.; Stiesch, M.; Winkel, A.; Fimmers, R.; Dommisch, J.; Jepsen, S.; Miosge, N.; Adam, K. Expression of Antimicrobial Peptides and Interleukin-8 during Early Stages of Inflammation: An Experimental Gingivitis Study. *J. Periodontal Res.* **2015**, *50*, 836–845. [CrossRef]
62. Fernandez-Garcia, E.; Chen, X.; Gutierrez-Gonzalez, C.F.; Fernandez, A.; Lopez-Esteban, S.; Aparicio, C. Peptide-Functionalized Zirconia and New Zirconia/Titanium Biocermets for Dental Applications. *J. Dent.* **2015**, *43*, 1162–1174. [CrossRef] [PubMed]
63. Fiorellini, J.P.; Glindmann, S.; Salcedo, J.; Weber, H.-P.; Park, C.-J.; Sarmiento, H.L. The Effect of Osteopontin and an Osteopontin-Derived Synthetic Peptide Coating on Osseointegration of Implants in a Canine Model. *Int. J. Periodontics Restor. Dent.* **2016**, *36*, e88–e94. [CrossRef]
64. Goeke, J.E.; Kist, S.; Schubert, S.; Hickel, R.; Huth, K.C.; Kollmuss, M. Sensitivity of Caries Pathogens to Antimicrobial Peptides Related to Caries Risk. *Clin. Oral Investig.* **2018**, *22*, 2519–2525. [CrossRef] [PubMed]
65. Galler, K.M.; Hartgerink, J.D.; Cavender, A.C.; Schmalz, G.; D'Souza, R.N. A Customized Self-Assembling Peptide Hydrogel for Dental Pulp Tissue Engineering. *Tissue Eng. Part A* **2012**, *18*, 176–184. [CrossRef]
66. Kirkham, J.; Firth, A.; Vernals, D.; Boden, N.; Robinson, C.; Shore, R.; Brookes, S.; Aggeli, A. Self-Assembling Peptide Scaffolds Promote Enamel Remineralization. *J. Dent. Res.* **2007**, *86*, 426–430. [CrossRef]
67. Kämmerer, P.; Heller, M.; Brieger, J.; Klein, M.; Al-Nawas, B.; Gabriel, M. Immobilisation of Linear and Cyclic RGD-Peptides on Titanium Surfaces and Their Impact on Endothelial Cell Adhesion and Proliferation. *Eur. Cell Mater.* **2011**, *21*, 364–372. [CrossRef]
68. Golland, L.; Schmidlin, P.R.; Schätzle, M. The Potential of Self-Assembling Peptides for Enhancement of in Vitro Remineralisation of White Spot Lesions as Measured by Quantitative Laser Fluorescence. *Oral Health Prev. Dent.* **2017**, *15*, 147–152. [PubMed]
69. Hsu, C.; Chung, H.; Yang, J.-M.; Shi, W.; Wu, B. Influence of 8DSS Peptide on Nano-Mechanical Behavior of Human Enamel. *J. Dent. Res.* **2011**, *90*, 88–92. [CrossRef]
70. Kwak, S.; Litman, A.; Margolis, H.; Yamakoshi, Y.; Simmer, J. Biomimetic Enamel Regeneration Mediated by Leucine-Rich Amelogenin Peptide. *J. Dent. Res.* **2017**, *96*, 524–530. [CrossRef]

71. Kong, E.F.; Tsui, C.; Boyce, H.; Ibrahim, A.; Hoag, S.W.; Karlsson, A.J.; Meiller, T.F.; Jabra-Rizk, M.A. Development and in Vivo Evaluation of a Novel Histatin-5 Bioadhesive Hydrogel Formulation against Oral Candidiasis. *Antimicrob. Agents Chemother.* **2016**, *60*, 881–889. [CrossRef] [PubMed]
72. Koch, F.; Ekat, K.; Kilian, D.; Hettich, T.; Germershaus, O.; Lang, H.; Peters, K.; Kreikemeyer, B. A Versatile Biocompatible Antibiotic Delivery System Based on Self-Assembling Peptides with Antimicrobial and Regenerative Potential. *Adv. Healthc. Mater.* **2019**, *8*, 1900167. [CrossRef] [PubMed]
73. Hashimoto, K.; Yoshinari, M.; Matsuzaka, K.; Shiba, K.; Inoue, T. Identification of Peptide Motif That Binds to the Surface of Zirconia. *Dent. Mater. J.* **2011**, *30*, 935–940. [CrossRef] [PubMed]
74. Kind, L.; Stevanovic, S.; Wuttig, S.; Wimberger, S.; Hofer, J.; Müller, B.; Pieles, U. Biomimetic Remineralization of Carious Lesions by Self-Assembling Peptide. *J. Dent. Res.* **2017**, *96*, 790–797. [CrossRef]
75. Gonçalves, F.M.C.; Delbem, A.C.B.; Gomes, L.F.; Emerenciano, N.G.; dos Passos Silva, M.; Cannon, M.L.; Danelon, M. Combined Effect of Casein Phosphopeptide-Amorphous Calcium Phosphate and Sodium Trimetaphosphate on the Prevention of Enamel Demineralization and Dental Caries: An in Vitro Study. *Clin. Oral Investig.* **2021**, *25*, 2811–2820. [CrossRef]
76. Kim, S.; Choi, J.-Y.; Jung, S.Y.; Kang, H.K.; Min, B.-M.; Yeo, I.-S.L. A Laminin-Derived Functional Peptide, PPFEGCIWN, Promotes Bone Formation on Sandblasted, Large-Grit, Acid-Etched Titanium Implant Surfaces. *Int. J. Oral Maxillofac. Implant.* **2019**, *34*, 836–844. [CrossRef] [PubMed]
77. Kohgo, T.; Yamada, Y.; Ito, K.; Yajima, A.; Yoshimi, R.; Okabe, K.; Baba, S.; Ueda, M. Bone Regeneration with Self-Assembling Peptide Nanofiber Scaffolds in Tissue Engineering for Osseointegration of Dental Implants. *Int. J. Periodontics Restor. Dent.* **2011**, *31*, e9–e16.
78. Gungormus, M.; Oren, E.E.; Horst, J.A.; Fong, H.; Hnilova, M.; Somerman, M.J.; Snead, M.L.; Samudrala, R.; Tamerler, C.; Sarikaya, M. Cementomimetics—Constructing a Cementum-like Biomineralized Microlayer via Amelogenin-Derived Peptides. *Int. J. Oral Sci.* **2012**, *4*, 69–77. [CrossRef] [PubMed]
79. Kakegawa, A.; Oida, S.; Gomi, K.; Nagano, T.; Yamakoshi, Y.; Fukui, T.; Kanazashi, M.; Arai, T.; Fukae, M. Cytodifferentiation Activity of Synthetic Human Enamel Sheath Protein Peptides. *J. Periodontal Res.* **2010**, *45*, 643–649. [CrossRef]
80. Kramer, P.R.; JanikKeith, A.; Cai, Z.; Ma, S.; Watanabe, I. Integrin Mediated Attachment of Periodontal Ligament to Titanium Surfaces. *Dent. Mater.* **2009**, *25*, 877–883. [CrossRef]
81. Hua, J.; Yamarthy, R.; Felsenstein, S.; Scott, R.W.; Markowitz, K.; Diamond, G. Activity of Antimicrobial Peptide Mimetics in the Oral Cavity: I. Activity against Biofilms of Candida Albicans. *Mol. Oral Microbiol.* **2010**, *25*, 418–425. [CrossRef]
82. Kohlgraf, K.G.; Ackermann, A.; Lu, X.; Burnell, K.; Bélanger, M.; Cavanaugh, J.E.; Xie, H.; Progulske-Fox, A.; Brogden, K.A. Defensins Attenuate Cytokine Responses yet Enhance Antibody Responses to Porphyromonas Gingivalis Adhesins in Mice. *Future Microbiol.* **2010**, *5*, 115–125. [CrossRef]
83. Holmberg, K.V.; Abdolhosseini, M.; Li, Y.; Chen, X.; Gorr, S.-U.; Aparicio, C. Bio-Inspired Stable Antimicrobial Peptide Coatings for Dental Applications. *Acta Biomater.* **2013**, *9*, 8224–8231. [CrossRef] [PubMed]
84. Koidou, V.P.; Argyris, P.P.; Skoe, E.P.; Siqueira, J.M.; Chen, X.; Zhang, L.; Hinrichs, J.E.; Costalonga, M.; Aparicio, C. Peptide Coatings Enhance Keratinocyte Attachment towards Improving the Peri-Implant Mucosal Seal. *Biomater. Sci.* **2018**, *6*, 1936–1945. [CrossRef] [PubMed]
85. Knaup, T.; Korbmacher-Steiner, H.; Jablonski-Momeni, A. Effect of the Caries-Protective Self-Assembling Peptide P11-4 on Shear Bond Strength of Metal Brackets. *J. Orofac. Orthop. Kieferorthopädie* **2021**, *82*, 329–336. [CrossRef]
86. Kihara, H.; Kim, D.M.; Nagai, M.; Nojiri, T.; Nagai, S.; Chen, C.-Y.; Lee, C.; Hatakeyama, W.; Kondo, H.; Da Silva, J. Epithelial Cell Adhesion Efficacy of a Novel Peptide Identified by Panning on a Smooth Titanium Surface. *Int. J. Oral Sci.* **2018**, *10*, 21. [CrossRef]
87. Jablonski-Momeni, A.; Nothelfer, R.; Morawietz, M.; Kiesow, A.; Korbmacher-Steiner, H. Impact of Self-Assembling Peptides in Remineralisation of Artificial Early Enamel Lesions Adjacent to Orthodontic Brackets. *Sci. Rep.* **2020**, *10*, 15132. [CrossRef] [PubMed]
88. Kamal, D.; Hassanein, H.; Elkassas, D.; Hamza, H. Comparative Evaluation of Remineralizing Efficacy of Biomimetic Self-Assembling Peptide on Artificially Induced Enamel Lesions: An in Vitro Study. *J. Conserv. Dent.* **2018**, *21*, 536. [CrossRef]
89. Mao, B.; Xie, Y.; Yang, H.; Yu, C.; Ma, P.; You, Z.; Tsuo, C.; Chen, Y.; Cheng, L.; Han, Q. Casein Phosphopeptide-Amorphous Calcium Phosphate Modified Glass Ionomer Cement Attenuates Demineralization and Modulates Biofilm Composition in Dental Caries. *Dent. Mater. J.* **2021**, *40*, 84–93. [CrossRef]
90. Makihira, S.; Nikawa, H.; Shuto, T.; Nishimura, M.; Mine, Y.; Tsuji, K.; Okamoto, K.; Sakai, Y.; Sakai, M.; Imari, N. Evaluation of Trabecular Bone Formation in a Canine Model Surrounding a Dental Implant Fixture Immobilized with an Antimicrobial Peptide Derived from Histatin. *J. Mater. Sci. Mater. Med.* **2011**, *22*, 2765–2772. [CrossRef]
91. Li, Q.-L.; Ning, T.-Y.; Cao, Y.; Zhang, W.; Mei, M.L.; Chu, C.H. A Novel Self-Assembled Oligopeptide Amphiphile for Biomimetic Mineralization of Enamel. *BMC Biotechnol.* **2014**, *14*, 32. [CrossRef] [PubMed]
92. Liu, Z.; Ma, S.; Duan, S.; Xuliang, D.; Sun, Y.; Zhang, X.; Xu, X.; Guan, B.; Wang, C.; Hu, M. Modification of Titanium Substrates with Chimeric Peptides Comprising Antimicrobial and Titanium-Binding Motifs Connected by Linkers to Inhibit Biofilm Formation. *ACS Appl. Mater. Interfaces* **2016**, *8*, 5124–5136. [CrossRef]
93. Min, S.-K.; Kang, H.K.; Jang, D.H.; Jung, S.Y.; Kim, O.B.; Min, B.-M.; Yeo, I.-S. Titanium Surface Coating with a Laminin-Derived Functional Peptide Promotes Bone Cell Adhesion. *BioMed Res. Int.* **2013**, *2013*, 638348. [CrossRef]

94. Moore, A.; Perez, S.; Hartgerink, J.; D'Souza, R.; Colombo, J. Ex Vivo Modeling of Multidomain Peptide Hydrogels with Intact Dental Pulp. *J. Dent. Res.* **2015**, *94*, 1773–1781. [CrossRef] [PubMed]
95. Muruve, N.; Feng, Y.; Platnich, J.; Hassett, D.; Irvin, R.; Muruve, D.; Cheng, F. A Peptide-Based Biological Coating for Enhanced Corrosion Resistance of Titanium Alloy Biomaterials in Chloride-Containing Fluids. *J. Biomater. Appl.* **2017**, *31*, 1225–1234. [CrossRef]
96. Nguyen, P.K.; Gao, W.; Patel, S.D.; Siddiqui, Z.; Weiner, S.; Shimizu, E.; Sarkar, B.; Kumar, V.A. Self-Assembly of a Dentinogenic Peptide Hydrogel. *ACS Omega* **2018**, *3*, 5980–5987. [CrossRef] [PubMed]
97. Mardas, N.; Stavropoulos, A.; Karring, T. Calvarial Bone Regeneration by a Combination of Natural Anorganic Bovine-derived Hydroxyapatite Matrix Coupled with a Synthetic Cell-binding Peptide (PepGen^{TM}): An Experimental Study in Rats. *Clin. Oral Implant. Res.* **2008**, *19*, 1010–1015. [CrossRef]
98. Mateescu, M.; Baixe, S.; Garnier, T.; Jierry, L.; Ball, V.; Haikel, Y.; Metz-Boutigue, M.H.; Nardin, M.; Schaaf, P.; Etienne, O. Antibacterial Peptide-Based Gel for Prevention of Medical Implanted-Device Infection. *PLoS ONE* **2015**, *10*, e0145143. [CrossRef] [PubMed]
99. Liu, Y.; Fan, L.; Lin, X.; Zou, L.; Li, Y.; Ge, X.; Fu, W.; Zhang, Z.; Xiao, K.; Lv, H. Functionalized Self-Assembled Peptide RAD/Dentonin Hydrogel Scaffold Promotes Dental Pulp Regeneration. *Biomed. Mater.* **2021**, *17*, 015009. [CrossRef] [PubMed]
100. Li, Y.; Wang, Y.; Chen, X.; Jiang, W.; Jiang, X.; Zeng, Y.; Li, X.; Feng, Z.; Luo, J.; Zhang, L. Antimicrobial Peptide GH12 as Root Canal Irrigant Inhibits Biofilm and Virulence of Enterococcus Faecalis. *Int. Endod. J.* **2020**, *53*, 948–961. [CrossRef]
101. Mancino, D.; Kharouf, N.; Scavello, F.; Hellé, S.; Salloum-Yared, F.; Mutschler, A.; Mathieu, E.; Lavalle, P.; Metz-Boutigue, M.-H.; Haïkel, Y. The Catestatin-Derived Peptides Are New Actors to Fight the Development of Oral Candidosis. *Int. J. Mol. Sci.* **2022**, *23*, 2066. [CrossRef] [PubMed]
102. Mai, S.; Mauger, M.T.; Niu, L.; Barnes, J.B.; Kao, S.; Bergeron, B.E.; Ling, J.; Tay, F.R. Potential Applications of Antimicrobial Peptides and Their Mimics in Combating Caries and Pulpal Infections. *Acta Biomater.* **2017**, *49*, 16–35. [CrossRef]
103. Lv, X.; Yang, Y.; Han, S.; Li, D.; Tu, H.; Li, W.; Zhou, X.; Zhang, L. Potential of an Amelogenin Based Peptide in Promoting Reminerlization of Initial Enamel Caries. *Arch. Oral Biol.* **2015**, *60*, 1482–1487. [CrossRef]
104. Lee, J.-Y.; Choo, J.-E.; Choi, Y.-S.; Park, J.-B.; Min, D.-S.; Lee, S.-J.; Rhyu, H.K.; Jo, I.-H.; Chung, C.-P.; Park, Y.-J. Assembly of Collagen-Binding Peptide with Collagen as a Bioactive Scaffold for Osteogenesis in Vitro and in Vivo. *Biomaterials* **2007**, *28*, 4257–4267. [CrossRef]
105. Liang, K.; Xiao, S.; Liu, H.; Shi, W.; Li, J.; Gao, Y.; He, L.; Zhou, X.; Li, J. 8DSS Peptide Induced Effective Dentinal Tubule Occlusion in Vitro. *Dent. Mater.* **2018**, *34*, 629–640. [CrossRef]
106. Lee, S.J.; Won, J.-E.; Han, C.; Yin, X.Y.; Kim, H.K.; Nah, H.; Kwon, I.K.; Min, B.-H.; Kim, C.-H.; Shin, Y.S. Development of a Three-Dimensionally Printed Scaffold Grafted with Bone Forming Peptide-1 for Enhanced Bone Regeneration with in Vitro and in Vivo Evaluations. *J. Colloid Interface Sci.* **2019**, *539*, 468–480. [CrossRef] [PubMed]
107. Na, D.H.; Faraj, J.; Capan, Y.; Leung, K.P.; DeLuca, P.P. Chewing Gum of Antimicrobial Decapeptide (KSL) as a Sustained Antiplaque Agent: Preformulation Study. *J. Control. Release* **2005**, *107*, 122–130. [CrossRef] [PubMed]
108. Magalhães, G.d.A.P.; Fraga, M.A.A.; de Souza Araújo, I.J.; Pacheco, R.R.; Correr, A.B.; Puppin-Rontani, R.M. Effect of a Self-Assembly Peptide on Surface Roughness and Hardness of Bleached Enamel. *J. Funct. Biomater.* **2022**, *13*, 79. [CrossRef] [PubMed]
109. Lallier, T.E.; Palaiologou, A.A.; Yukna, R.A.; Layman, D.L. The Putative Collagen-binding Peptide P-15 Promotes Fibroblast Attachment to Root Shavings but Not Hydroxyapatite. *J. Periodontol.* **2003**, *74*, 458–467. [CrossRef] [PubMed]
110. Li, M.; Yang, Y.; Lin, C.; Zhang, Q.; Gong, L.; Wang, Y.; Zhang, X. Antibacterial Properties of Small-Size Peptide Derived from Penetratin against Oral Streptococci. *Materials* **2021**, *14*, 2730. [CrossRef]
111. Matsugishi, A.; Aoki-Nonaka, Y.; Yokoji-Takeuchi, M.; Yamada-Hara, M.; Mikami, Y.; Hayatsu, M.; Terao, Y.; Domon, H.; Taniguchi, M.; Takahashi, N. Rice Peptide with Amino Acid Substitution Inhibits Biofilm Formation by Porphyromonas Gingivalis and Fusobacterium Nucleatum. *Arch. Oral Biol.* **2021**, *121*, 104956. [CrossRef]
112. Li, X.; Yu, Z.; Jiang, S.; Dai, X.; Wang, G.; Wang, Y.; Yang, Z.; Gao, J.; Zou, H. An Amelogenin-Based Peptide Hydrogel Promoted the Odontogenic Differentiation of Human Dental Pulp Cells. *Regen. Biomater.* **2022**, *9*, rbac039.
113. Mishra, P.R.N.; Kolte, A.P.; Kolte, R.A.; Pajnigara, N.G.; Shah, K.K. Comparative Evaluation of Open Flap Debridement Alone and in Combination with Anorganic Bone Matrix/Cell-Binding Peptide in the Treatment of Human Infrabony Defects: A Randomized Clinical Trial. *J. Indian Soc. Periodontol.* **2019**, *23*, 42.
114. Padovano, J.; Ravindran, S.; Snee, P.; Ramachandran, A.; Bedran-Russo, A.; George, A. DMP1-Derived Peptides Promote Remineralization of Human Dentin. *J. Dent. Res.* **2015**, *94*, 608–614. [PubMed]
115. Park, J.H.; Gillispie, G.J.; Copus, J.S.; Zhang, W.; Atala, A.; Yoo, J.J.; Yelick, P.C.; Lee, S.J. The Effect of BMP-Mimetic Peptide Tethering Bioinks on the Differentiation of Dental Pulp Stem Cells (DPSCs) in 3D Bioprinted Dental Constructs. *Biofabrication* **2020**, *12*, 035029.
116. Pellissari, C.V.G.; Jorge, J.H.; Marin, L.M.; Sabino-Silva, R.; Siqueira, W.L. Statherin-Derived Peptides as Antifungal Strategy against Candida Albicans. *Arch. Oral Biol.* **2021**, *125*, 105106. [CrossRef]
117. Petzold, C.; Monjo, M.; Rubert, M.; Reinholt, F.P.; Gomez-Florit, M.; Ramis, J.M.; Ellingsen, J.E.; Lyngstadaas, S.P. Effect of Proline-Rich Synthetic Peptide–Coated Titanium Implants on Bone Healing in a Rabbit Model. *Oral Craniofac. Tissue Eng.* **2012**, *2*, 35–43. [CrossRef]

118. Picker, A.; Nicoleau, L.; Nonat, A.; Labbez, C.; Cölfen, H. Identification of Binding Peptides on Calcium Silicate Hydrate: A Novel View on Cement Additives. *Adv. Mater.* **2014**, *26*, 1135–1140. [CrossRef] [PubMed]
119. Pihl, M.; Galli, S.; Jimbo, R.; Andersson, M. Osseointegration and Antibacterial Effect of an Antimicrobial Peptide Releasing Mesoporous Titania Implant. *J. Biomed. Mater. Res. B Appl. Biomater.* **2021**, *109*, 1787–1795. [PubMed]
120. Ren, Q.; Li, Z.; Ding, L.; Wang, X.; Niu, Y.; Qin, X.; Zhou, X.; Zhang, L. Anti-Biofilm and Remineralization Effects of Chitosan Hydrogel Containing Amelogenin-Derived Peptide on Initial Caries Lesions. *Regen. Biomater.* **2018**, *5*, 69–76.
121. Santarpia, R.P., III; Pollock, J.J.; Renner, R.P.; Gwinnett, A.J. In Vivo Antifungal Efficacy of Salivary Histidine-Rich Polypeptides: Preliminary Findings in a Denture Stomatitis Model System. *J. Prosthet. Dent.* **1991**, *66*, 693–699. [CrossRef] [PubMed]
122. Schmidlin, P.; Zobrist, K.; Attin, T.; Wegehaupt, F. In Vitro Re-Hardening of Artificial Enamel Caries Lesions Using Enamel Matrix Proteins or Self-Assembling Peptides. *J. Appl. Oral Sci.* **2016**, *24*, 31–36. [CrossRef]
123. Schmitt, C.M.; Koepple, M.; Moest, T.; Neumann, K.; Weisel, T.; Schlegel, K.A. In Vivo Evaluation of Biofunctionalized Implant Surfaces with a Synthetic Peptide (P-15) and Its Impact on Osseointegration. A Preclinical Animal Study. *Clin. Oral Implant. Res.* **2016**, *27*, 1339–1348. [CrossRef] [PubMed]
124. Schuler, M.; Owen, G.R.; Hamilton, D.W.; de Wild, M.; Textor, M.; Brunette, D.M.; Tosatti, S.G. Biomimetic Modification of Titanium Dental Implant Model Surfaces Using the RGDSP-Peptide Sequence: A Cell Morphology Study. *Biomaterials* **2006**, *27*, 4003–4015. [CrossRef] [PubMed]
125. Schuster, L.; Ardjomandi, N.; Munz, M.; Umrath, F.; Klein, C.; Rupp, F.; Reinert, S.; Alexander, D. Establishment of Collagen: Hydroxyapatite/BMP-2 Mimetic Peptide Composites. *Materials* **2020**, *13*, 1203. [CrossRef] [PubMed]
126. Secchi, A.G.; Grigoriou, V.; Shapiro, I.M.; Cavalcanti-Adam, E.A.; Composto, R.J.; Ducheyne, P.; Adams, C.S. RGDS Peptides Immobilized on Titanium Alloy Stimulate Bone Cell Attachment, Differentiation and Confer Resistance to Apoptosis. *J. Biomed. Mater. Res. Part Off. J. Soc. Biomater. Jpn. Soc. Biomater. Aust. Soc. Biomater. Korean Soc. Biomater.* **2007**, *83*, 577–584. [CrossRef] [PubMed]
127. Segvich, S.J.; Smith, H.C.; Kohn, D.H. The Adsorption of Preferential Binding Peptides to Apatite-Based Materials. *Biomaterials* **2009**, *30*, 1287–1298. [CrossRef]
128. Sfeir, C.; Fang, P.-A.; Jayaraman, T.; Raman, A.; Xiaoyuan, Z.; Beniash, E. Synthesis of Bone-like Nanocomposites Using Multiphosphorylated Peptides. *Acta Biomater.* **2014**, *10*, 2241–2249. [CrossRef]
129. Shi, J.; Liu, Y.; Wang, Y.; Zhang, J.; Zhao, S.; Yang, G. Biological and Immunotoxicity Evaluation of Antimicrobial Peptide-Loaded Coatings Using a Layer-by-Layer Process on Titanium. *Sci. Rep.* **2015**, *5*, 16336. [CrossRef]
130. Shinkai, K.; Taira, Y.; Suzuki, M.; Kato, C.; Yamauchi, J.; Suzuki, S.; Katoh, Y. Dentin Bond Strength of an Experimental Adhesive System Containing Calcium Chloride, Synthetic Peptides Derived from Dentin Matrix Protein 1 (PA and PB), and Hydroxyapatite for Direct Pulp Capping and as a Bonding Agent. *Odontology* **2010**, *98*, 110–116. [CrossRef]
131. Shinkai, K.; Taira, Y.; Suzuki, M.; Kato, C.; Yamauchi, J.; Suzuki, S.; Katoh, Y. Effect of the Concentrations of Calcium Chloride and Synthetic Peptides in Primers on Dentin Bond Strength of an Experimental Adhesive System. *Dent. Mater. J.* **2010**, *29*, 738–746. [CrossRef] [PubMed]
132. Shuturminska, K.; Tarakina, N.V.; Azevedo, H.S.; Bushby, A.J.; Mata, A.; Anderson, P.; Al-Jawad, M. Elastin-like Protein, with Statherin Derived Peptide, Controls Fluorapatite Formation and Morphology. *Front. Physiol.* **2017**, *8*, 368. [CrossRef] [PubMed]
133. Su, M.; Yao, S.; Gu, L.; Huang, Z.; Mai, S. Antibacterial Effect and Bond Strength of a Modified Dental Adhesive Containing the Peptide Nisin. *Peptides* **2018**, *99*, 189–194. [CrossRef]
134. Suaid, F.A.; Macedo, G.O.; Novaes, A.B., Jr.; Borges, G.J.; Souza, S.L.; Taba, M., Jr.; Palioto, D.B.; Grisi, M.F. The Bone Formation Capabilities of the Anorganic Bone Matrix–Synthetic Cell-Binding Peptide 15 Grafts in an Animal Periodontal Model: A Histologic and Histomorphometric Study in Dogs. *J. Periodontol.* **2010**, *81*, 594–603. [CrossRef] [PubMed]
135. Sugawara, S.; Maeno, M.; Lee, C.; Nagai, S.; Kim, D.M.; Da Silva, J.; Nagai, M.; Kondo, H. Establishment of Epithelial Attachment on Titanium Surface Coated with Platelet Activating Peptide. *PLoS ONE* **2016**, *11*, e0164693. [CrossRef] [PubMed]
136. Sun, X.; Huang, X.; Tan, X.; Si, Y.; Wang, X.; Chen, F.; Zheng, S. Salivary Peptidome Profiling for Diagnosis of Severe Early Childhood Caries. *J. Transl. Med.* **2016**, *14*, 240. [CrossRef]
137. Takahashi, N.; Sato, T. Dipeptide Utilization by the Periodontal Pathogens Porphyromonas Gingivalis, Prevotella Intermedia, Prevotella Nigrescens and Fusobacterium Nucleatum. *Oral Microbiol. Immunol.* **2002**, *17*, 50–54. [CrossRef]
138. Tanhaieian, A.; Pourgonabadi, S.; Akbari, M.; Mohammadipour, H.-S. The Effective and Safe Method for Preventing and Treating Bacteria-Induced Dental Diseases by Herbal Plants and a Recombinant Peptide. *J. Clin. Exp. Dent.* **2020**, *12*, e523. [CrossRef]
139. Üstün, N.; Aktören, O. Analysis of Efficacy of the Self-assembling Peptide-based Remineralization Agent on Artificial Enamel Lesions. *Microsc. Res. Tech.* **2019**, *82*, 1065–1072. [CrossRef]
140. Wang, B.; Wu, B.; Jia, Y.; Jiang, Y.; Yuan, Y.; Man, Y.; Xiang, L. Neural Peptide Promotes the Angiogenesis and Osteogenesis around Oral Implants. *Cell. Signal.* **2021**, *79*, 109873. [CrossRef]
141. Wang, D.; Shen, Y.; Hancock, R.E.; Ma, J.; Haapasalo, M. Antimicrobial Effect of Peptide DJK-5 Used Alone or Mixed with EDTA on Mono-and Multispecies Biofilms in Dentin Canals. *J. Endod.* **2018**, *44*, 1709–1713. [CrossRef]
142. Warnke, P.H.; Voss, E.; Russo, P.A.; Stephens, S.; Kleine, M.; Terheyden, H.; Liu, Q. Antimicrobial Peptide Coating of Dental Implants: Biocompatibility Assessment of Recombinant Human Beta Defensin-2 for Human Cells. *Int. J. Oral Maxillofac. Implant.* **2013**, *28*, 982–988. [CrossRef] [PubMed]

143. Werner, S.; Huck, O.; Frisch, B.; Vautier, D.; Elkaim, R.; Voegel, J.-C.; Brunel, G.; Tenenbaum, H. The Effect of Microstructured Surfaces and Laminin-Derived Peptide Coatings on Soft Tissue Interactions with Titanium Dental Implants. *Biomaterials* **2009**, *30*, 2291–2301. [CrossRef]
144. Winfred, S.B.; Meiyazagan, G.; Panda, J.J.; Nagendrababu, V.; Deivanayagam, K.; Chauhan, V.S.; Venkatraman, G. Antimicrobial Activity of Cationic Peptides in Endodontic Procedures. *Eur. J. Dent.* **2014**, *8*, 254–260. [CrossRef]
145. Wu, J.; Mao, S.; Xu, L.; Qiu, D.; Wang, S.; Dong, Y. Odontogenic Differentiation Induced by TGF-B1 Binding Peptide–Modified Bioglass. *J. Dent. Res.* **2022**, *101*, 1190–1197. [CrossRef]
146. Xie, S.-X.; Boone, K.; VanOosten, S.K.; Yuca, E.; Song, L.; Ge, X.; Ye, Q.; Spencer, P.; Tamerler, C. Peptide Mediated Antimicrobial Dental Adhesive System. *Appl. Sci.* **2019**, *9*, 557. [CrossRef]
147. Xie, S.-X.; Song, L.; Yuca, E.; Boone, K.; Sarikaya, R.; VanOosten, S.K.; Misra, A.; Ye, Q.; Spencer, P.; Tamerler, C. Antimicrobial Peptide–Polymer Conjugates for Dentistry. *ACS Appl. Polym. Mater.* **2020**, *2*, 1134–1144. [CrossRef]
148. Yamamoto, N.; Maeda, H.; Tomokiyo, A.; Fujii, S.; Wada, N.; Monnouchi, S.; Kono, K.; Koori, K.; Teramatsu, Y.; Akamine, A. Expression and Effects of Glial Cell Line-derived Neurotrophic Factor on Periodontal Ligament Cells. *J. Clin. Periodontol.* **2012**, *39*, 556–564. [CrossRef]
149. Yamashita, M.; Lazarov, M.; Jones, A.A.; Mealey, B.L.; Mellonig, J.T.; Cochran, D.L. Periodontal Regeneration Using an Anabolic Peptide with Two Carriers in Baboons. *J. Periodontol.* **2010**, *81*, 727–736. [CrossRef] [PubMed]
150. Yang, X.; Huang, P.; Wang, H.; Cai, S.; Liao, Y.; Mo, Z.; Xu, X.; Ding, C.; Zhao, C.; Li, J. Antibacterial and Anti-Biofouling Coating on Hydroxyapatite Surface Based on Peptide-Modified Tannic Acid. *Colloids Surf. B Biointerfaces* **2017**, *160*, 136–143. [CrossRef] [PubMed]
151. Yang, X.; Li, Z.; Xiao, H.; Wang, N.; Li, Y.; Xu, X.; Chen, Z.; Tan, H.; Li, J. A Universal and Ultrastable Mineralization Coating Bioinspired from Biofilms. *Adv. Funct. Mater.* **2018**, *28*, 1802730. [CrossRef]
152. Yang, X.; Yang, B.; He, L.; Li, R.; Liao, Y.; Zhang, S.; Yang, Y.; Xu, X.; Zhang, D.; Tan, H. Bioinspired Peptide-Decorated Tannic Acid for in Situ Remineralization of Tooth Enamel: In Vitro and in Vivo Evaluation. *ACS Biomater. Sci. Eng.* **2017**, *3*, 3553–3562. [CrossRef] [PubMed]
153. Yang, X.; Zhang, D.; Liu, G.; Wang, J.; Luo, Z.; Peng, X.; Zeng, X.; Wang, X.; Tan, H.; Li, J. Bioinspired from Mussel and Salivary Acquired Pellicle: A Universal Dual-Functional Polypeptide Coating for Implant Materials. *Mater. Today Chem.* **2019**, *14*, 100205. [CrossRef]
154. Yang, Y.; Xia, L.; Haapasalo, M.; Wei, W.; Zhang, D.; Ma, J.; Shen, Y. A Novel Hydroxyapatite-Binding Antimicrobial Peptide against Oral Biofilms. *Clin. Oral Investig.* **2019**, *23*, 2705–2712. [CrossRef] [PubMed]
155. Yang, Y.; Yang, B.; Li, M.; Wang, Y.; Yang, X.; Li, J. Salivary Acquired Pellicle-Inspired DpSpSEEKC Peptide for the Restoration of Demineralized Tooth Enamel. *Biomed. Mater.* **2017**, *12*, 025007. [CrossRef]
156. Yang, Z.; Liu, M.; Yang, Y.; Zheng, M.; Liu, X.; Tan, J. Biofunctionalization of Zirconia with Cell-Adhesion Peptides via Polydopamine Crosslinking for Soft Tissue Engineering: Effects on the Biological Behaviors of Human Gingival Fibroblasts and Oral Bacteria. *RSC Adv.* **2020**, *10*, 6200–6212. [CrossRef]
157. Yazici, H.; Fong, H.; Wilson, B.; Oren, E.; Amos, F.; Zhang, H.; Evans, J.; Snead, M.; Sarikaya, M.; Tamerler, C. Biological Response on a Titanium Implant-Grade Surface Functionalized with Modular Peptides. *Acta Biomater.* **2013**, *9*, 5341–5352. [CrossRef]
158. Ye, Q.; Spencer, P.; Yuca, E.; Tamerler, C. Engineered Peptide Repairs Defective Adhesive–Dentin Interface. *Macromol. Mater. Eng.* **2017**, *302*, 1600487. [CrossRef]
159. Ye, W.; Yeghiasarian, L.; Cutler, C.W.; Bergeron, B.E.; Sidow, S.; Xu, H.H.; Niu, L.; Ma, J.; Tay, F.R. Comparison of the Use of D-Enantiomeric and l-Enantiomeric Antimicrobial Peptides Incorporated in a Calcium-Chelating Irrigant against Enterococcus Faecalis Root Canal Wall Biofilms. *J. Dent.* **2019**, *91*, 103231. [CrossRef]
160. Yonehara, N.; Shibutani, T.; Tsai, H.-Y.; Inoki, R. Effects of Opioids and Opioid Peptide on the Release of Substance P-like Material Induced by Tooth Pulp Stimulation in the Trigeminal Nucleus Caudalis of the Rabbit. *Eur. J. Pharmacol.* **1986**, *129*, 209–216. [CrossRef]
161. Yoshinari, M.; Kato, T.; Matsuzaka, K.; Hayakawa, T.; Inoue, T.; Oda, Y.; Okuda, K.; Shimono, M. Adsorption Behavior of Antimicrobial Peptide Histatin 5 on PMMA. *J. Biomed. Mater. Res. Part B Appl. Biomater. Off. J. Soc. Biomater. Jpn. Soc. Biomater. Aust. Soc. Biomater. Korean Soc. Biomater.* **2006**, *77*, 47–54. [CrossRef]
162. Yoshinari, M.; Kato, T.; Matsuzaka, K.; Hayakawa, T.; Shiba, K. Prevention of Biofilm Formation on Titanium Surfaces Modified with Conjugated Molecules Comprised of Antimicrobial and Titanium-Binding Peptides. *Biofouling* **2010**, *26*, 103–110. [CrossRef]
163. Yuca, E.; Xie, S.-X.; Song, L.; Boone, K.; Kamathewatta, N.; Woolfolk, S.K.; Elrod, P.; Spencer, P.; Tamerler, C. Reconfigurable Dual Peptide Tethered Polymer System Offers a Synergistic Solution for Next Generation Dental Adhesives. *Int. J. Mol. Sci.* **2021**, *22*, 6552. [CrossRef] [PubMed]
164. Zhang, P.; Wu, S.; Li, J.; Bu, X.; Dong, X.; Chen, N.; Li, F.; Zhu, J.; Sang, L.; Zeng, Y. Dual-Sensitive Antibacterial Peptide Nanoparticles Prevent Dental Caries. *Theranostics* **2022**, *12*, 4818. [CrossRef]
165. Zhang, T.; Wang, Z.; Hancock, R.E.; De La Fuente-Núñez, C.; Haapasalo, M. Treatment of Oral Biofilms by a D-Enantiomeric Peptide. *PLoS ONE* **2016**, *11*, e0166397. [CrossRef]
166. Zhao, M.; Qu, Y.; Liu, J.; Mai, S.; Gu, L. A Universal Adhesive Incorporating Antimicrobial Peptide Nisin: Effects on Streptococcus Mutans and Saliva-Derived Multispecies Biofilms. *Odontology* **2020**, *108*, 376–385. [CrossRef] [PubMed]

167. Zhou, B.; Liu, Y.; Wei, W.; Mao, J. GEPIs-HA Hybrid: A Novel Biomaterial for Tooth Repair. *Med. Hypotheses* **2008**, *71*, 591–593. [CrossRef] [PubMed]
168. Zhou, L.; Lai, Y.; Huang, W.; Huang, S.; Xu, Z.; Chen, J.; Wu, D. Biofunctionalization of Microgroove Titanium Surfaces with an Antimicrobial Peptide to Enhance Their Bactericidal Activity and Cytocompatibility. *Colloids Surf. B Biointerfaces* **2015**, *128*, 552–560. [CrossRef]
169. Gungormus, M.; Tulumbaci, F. Peptide-Assisted Pre-Bonding Remineralization of Dentin to Improve Bonding. *J. Mech. Behav. Biomed. Mater.* **2021**, *113*, 104119. [CrossRef]
170. Gug, H.R.; Park, Y.-H.; Park, S.-J.; Jang, J.Y.; Lee, J.-H.; Lee, D.-S.; Shon, W.-J.; Park, J.-C. Novel Strategy for Dental Caries by Physiologic Dentin Regeneration with CPNE7 Peptide. *Arch. Oral Biol.* **2022**, *143*, 105531. [CrossRef] [PubMed]
171. Murray, C.J.; Vos, T.; Lozano, R.; Naghavi, M.; Flaxman, A.D.; Michaud, C.; Ezzati, M.; Shibuya, K.; Salomon, J.A.; Abdalla, S. Disability-Adjusted Life Years (DALYs) for 291 Diseases and Injuries in 21 Regions, 1990–2010: A Systematic Analysis for the Global Burden of Disease Study 2010. *Lancet* **2012**, *380*, 2197–2223. [CrossRef]
172. González-Cabezas, C. The Chemistry of Caries: Remineralization and Demineralization Events with Direct Clinical Relevance. *Dent. Clin.* **2010**, *54*, 469–478. [CrossRef] [PubMed]
173. Innes, N.; Schwendicke, F. Restorative Thresholds for Carious Lesions: Systematic Review and Meta-Analysis. *J. Dent. Res.* **2017**, *96*, 501–508. [CrossRef] [PubMed]
174. Dirks, O.B. Posteruptive Changes in Dental Enamel. *J. Dent. Res.* **1966**, *45*, 503–511. [CrossRef]
175. Da Pontte, A.C.A.; Damião, A.O.M.C.; Rosa, A.M.; Da Silva, A.N.; Fachin, A.V.; Cortecazzi, A., Jr.; Marinho, A.L.D.; Prudente, A.C.L.; Pulgas, A.T.; Machado, A.D.; et al. Consensus Guidelines for the Management of Inflammatory Bowel Disease. *Arq. Gastroenterol.* **2010**, *47*, 313–325. [CrossRef]
176. Gao, S.S.; Zhang, S.; Mei, M.L.; Lo, E.C.-M.; Chu, C.-H. Caries Remineralisation and Arresting Effect in Children by Professionally Applied Fluoride Treatment–a Systematic Review. *BMC Oral Health* **2016**, *16*, 12. [CrossRef]
177. Lenzi, T.L.; Montagner, A.F.; Soares, F.Z.M.; de Oliveira Rocha, R. Are Topical Fluorides Effective for Treating Incipient Carious Lesions? A Systematic Review and Meta-Analysis. *J. Am. Dent. Assoc.* **2016**, *147*, 84–91. [CrossRef]
178. Lussi, A.; Hellwig, E.; Klimek, J. Fluorides—Mode of Action and Recommendations for Use. *Schweiz. Monatsschr. Zahnmed.* **2012**, *122*, 1030.
179. Alkilzy, M.; Tarabaih, A.; Santamaria, R.; Splieth, C. Self-Assembling Peptide P11-4 and Fluoride for Regenerating Enamel. *J. Dent. Res.* **2018**, *97*, 148–154. [CrossRef] [PubMed]
180. Aggeli, A.; Bell, M.; Boden, N.; Carrick, L.M.; Strong, A.E. Self-Assembling Peptide Polyelectrolyte Β-Sheet Complexes Form Nematic Hydrogels. *Angew. Chem.* **2003**, *115*, 5761–5764. [CrossRef]
181. Aggeli, A.; Bell, M.; Boden, N.; Keen, J.; Knowles, P.; McLeish, T.; Pitkeathly, M.; Radford, S. Responsive Gels Formed by the Spontaneous Self-Assembly of Peptides into Polymeric β-Sheet Tapes. *Nature* **1997**, *386*, 259–262. [CrossRef] [PubMed]
182. Davies, R.; Aggeli, A.; Beevers, A.; Boden, N.; Carrick, L.; Fishwick, C.; McLeish, T.; Nyrkova, I.; Semenov, A. Self-Assembling β-Sheet Tape Forming Peptides. *Supramol. Chem.* **2006**, *18*, 435–443. [CrossRef]
183. Kyle, S.; Aggeli, A.; Ingham, E.; McPherson, M.J. Recombinant Self-Assembling Peptides as Biomaterials for Tissue Engineering. *Biomaterials* **2010**, *31*, 9395–9405. [CrossRef]
184. Dabdoub, S.; Tsigarida, A.; Kumar, P. Patient-Specific Analysis of Periodontal and Peri-Implant Microbiomes. *J. Dent. Res.* **2013**, *92*, 168S–175S. [CrossRef] [PubMed]
185. Arciniegas, M.; Aparicio, C.; Manero, J.; Gil, F. Low Elastic Modulus Metals for Joint Prosthesis: Tantalum and Nickel–Titanium Foams. *J. Eur. Ceram. Soc.* **2007**, *27*, 3391–3398. [CrossRef]
186. Branemark, P.-I. Osseointegrated Implants in the Treatment of the Edentulous Jaw. Experience from a 10-Year Period. *Scand. J. Plast. Reconstr. Surg. Suppl.* **1977**, *16*, 1–132.
187. Schwartz-Arad, D.; Kidron, N.; Dolev, E. A Long-term Study of Implants Supporting Overdentures as a Model for Implant Success. *J. Periodontol.* **2005**, *76*, 1431–1435. [CrossRef]
188. Lindquist, L.; Carlsson, G.; Jemt, T. A Prospective 15-year Follow-up Study of Mandibular Fixed Prostheses Supported by Osseointegrated Implants. Clinical Results and Marginal Bone Loss. *Clin. Oral Implant. Res.* **1996**, *7*, 329–336. [CrossRef]
189. Bumgardner, J.D.; Adatrow, P.; Haggard, W.O.; Norowski, P.A. Emerging Antibacterial Biomaterial Strategies for the Prevention of Peri-Implant Inflammatory Diseases. *Int. J. Oral Maxillofac. Implant.* **2011**, *26*, 553–560.
190. Le Guéhennec, L.; Soueidan, A.; Layrolle, P.; Amouriq, Y. Surface Treatments of Titanium Dental Implants for Rapid Osseointegration. *Dent. Mater.* **2007**, *23*, 844–854. [CrossRef]
191. Schliephake, H.; Scharnweber, D. Chemical and Biological Functionalization of Titanium for Dental Implants. *J. Mater. Chem.* **2008**, *18*, 2404–2414. [CrossRef]
192. Chen, X.; Li, Y.; Aparicio, C.; Nazarpour, S.; Chaker, M. *Thin Films and Coatings in Biology*; Biological and Medical Physics–Biomedical Engineering Series; Springer: Berlin/Heidelberg, Germany, 2013.
193. Neu, H.C. The Crisis in Antibiotic Resistance. *Science* **1992**, *257*, 1064–1073. [CrossRef] [PubMed]
194. Abdolhosseini, M.; Nandula, S.R.; Song, J.; Hirt, H.; Gorr, S.-U. Lysine Substitutions Convert a Bacterial-Agglutinating Peptide into a Bactericidal Peptide That Retains Anti-Lipopolysaccharide Activity and Low Hemolytic Activity. *Peptides* **2012**, *35*, 231–238. [CrossRef]

195. Hirt, H.; Gorr, S.-U. Antimicrobial Peptide GL13K Is Effective in Reducing Biofilms of Pseudomonas Aeruginosa. *Antimicrob. Agents Chemother.* **2013**, *57*, 4903–4910. [CrossRef]
196. Bhatnagar, R.S.; Qian, J.J.; Wedrychowska, A.; Sadeghi, M.; Wu, Y.M.; Smith, N. Design of Biomimetic Habitats for Tissue Engineering with P-15, a Synthetic Peptide Analogue of Collagen. *Tissue Eng.* **1999**, *5*, 53–65. [CrossRef] [PubMed]
197. Steindorff, M.M.; Lehl, H.; Winkel, A.; Stiesch, M. Innovative Approaches to Regenerate Teeth by Tissue Engineering. *Arch. Oral Biol.* **2014**, *59*, 158–166. [CrossRef] [PubMed]
198. Wang, H.; Wang, S.; Cheng, L.; Jiang, Y.; Melo, M.A.S.; Weir, M.D.; Oates, T.W.; Zhou, X.; Xu, H.H. Novel Dental Composite with Capability to Suppress Cariogenic Species and Promote Non-Cariogenic Species in Oral Biofilms. *Mater. Sci. Eng. C* **2019**, *94*, 587–596. [CrossRef] [PubMed]
199. Pinheiro, S.L.; Azenha, G.R.; Araujo, G.; Puppin Rontani, R. Effectiveness of Casein Phosphopeptide-Amorphous Calcium Phosphate and Lysozyme, Lactoferrin, and Lactoperoxidase in Reducing Streptococcus Mutans. *Gen. Dent.* **2017**, *65*, 47–50.
200. Divyapriya, G.; Yavagal, P.C.; Veeresh, D. Casein Phosphopeptide-Amorphous Calcium Phosphate in Dentistry: An Update. *Int. J. Oral Health Sci.* **2016**, *6*, 18. [CrossRef]
201. Hardan, L.; Bourgi, R.; Kharouf, N.; Mancino, D.; Zarow, M.; Jakubowicz, N.; Haikel, Y.; Cuevas-Suárez, C.E. Bond Strength of Universal Adhesives to Dentin: A Systematic Review and Meta-Analysis. *Polymers* **2021**, *13*, 814. [CrossRef]
202. Elizalde-Hernández, A.; Hardan, L.; Bourgi, R.; Isolan, C.P.; Moreira, A.G.; Zamarripa-Calderón, J.E.; Piva, E.; Cuevas-Suárez, C.E.; Devoto, W.; Saad, A.; et al. Effect of Different Desensitizers on Shear Bond Strength of Self-Adhesive Resin Cements to Dentin. *Bioengineering* **2022**, *9*, 372. [CrossRef]
203. Rodríguez, F.; Glawe, D.D.; Naik, R.R.; Hallinan, K.P.; Stone, M.O. Study of the Chemical and Physical Influences upon in Vitro Peptide-Mediated Silica Formation. *Biomacromolecules* **2004**, *5*, 261–265. [CrossRef] [PubMed]
204. Branco, M.C.; Schneider, J.P. Self-Assembling Materials for Therapeutic Delivery. *Acta Biomater.* **2009**, *5*, 817–831. [CrossRef] [PubMed]
205. Gao, J.; Tang, C.; Elsawy, M.A.; Smith, A.M.; Miller, A.F.; Saiani, A. Controlling Self-Assembling Peptide Hydrogel Properties through Network Topology. *Biomacromolecules* **2017**, *18*, 826–834. [CrossRef] [PubMed]
206. Spencer, P.; Ye, Q.; Song, L.; Parthasarathy, R.; Boone, K.; Misra, A.; Tamerler, C. Threats to Adhesive/Dentin Interfacial Integrity and next Generation Bio-enabled Multifunctional Adhesives. *J. Biomed. Mater. Res. B Appl. Biomater.* **2019**, *107*, 2673–2683. [CrossRef]
207. Hardan, L.; Lukomska-Szymanska, M.; Zarow, M.; Cuevas-Suárez, C.E.; Bourgi, R.; Jakubowicz, N.; Sokolowski, K.; D'Arcangelo, C. One-Year Clinical Aging of Low Stress Bulk-Fill Flowable Composite in Class II Restorations: A Case Report and Literature Review. *Coatings.* **2021**, *11*, 504. [CrossRef]
208. Hardan, L.; Bourgi, R.; Cuevas-Suárez, C.E.; Zarow, M.; Kharouf, N.; Mancino, D.; Villares, C.F.; Skaba, D.; Lukomska-Szymanska, M. The Bond Strength and Anti-bacterial Activity of the Universal Dentin Bonding System: A Systematic Review and Meta-Analysis. *Microorganisms* **2021**, *9*, 1230. [CrossRef]
209. Bourgi, R.; Daood, U.; Bijle, M.N.; Fawzy, A.; Ghaleb, M.; Hardan, L. Reinforced Universal Adhesive by Ribose Crosslinker: A Novel Strategy in Adhesive Dentistry. *Polymers* **2021**, *13*, 704. [CrossRef]

Disclaimer/Publisher's Note: The statements, opinions and data contained in all publications are solely those of the individual author(s) and contributor(s) and not of MDPI and/or the editor(s). MDPI and/or the editor(s) disclaim responsibility for any injury to people or property resulting from any ideas, methods, instructions or products referred to in the content.

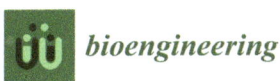

Article

The Contribution of Various In Vitro Methodologies to Comprehending the Filling Ability of Root Canal Pastes in Primary Teeth

Claire El Hachem [1], Jean Claude Abou Chedid [1], Walid Nehme [2], Marc Krikor Kaloustian [3], Nabil Ghosn [4], Morgane Rabineau [5,6], Naji Kharouf [6,7,*], Youssef Haikel [6,7,8] and Davide Mancino [6,7,8]

1. Department of Pediatric Dentistry, Faculty of Dentistry, Saint Joseph University, Beirut 1107 2180, Lebanon; claire.elhachem@gmail.com (C.E.H.); jcabouchedid@gmail.com (J.C.A.C.)
2. Department of Endodontics, Arthur A. Dugoni School of Dentistry, University of the Pacific, 155 5th Street, San Francisco, CA 94103, USA; wnehme@pacific.edu
3. Department of Endodontics, Faculty of Dentistry, Saint Joseph University, Beirut 1107 2180, Lebanon; mkaloustian75@gmail.com
4. Craniofacial Research Laboratory, Faculty of Dental Medicine, Saint Joseph University, Beirut 1107 2180, Lebanon; nabil.ghosn@usj.edu.lb
5. Faculté de Chirurgie Dentaire, Fédération de Médecine Translationnelle de Strasbourg and Fédération des Matériaux et Nanoscience d'Alsace, Université de Strasbourg, 67000 Strasbourg, France; morgane.rabineau@inserm.fr
6. Department of Biomaterials and Bioengineering, INSERM UMR_S 1121, Strasbourg University, 67000 Strasbourg, France; youssef.haikel@unistra.fr (Y.H.); mancino@unistra.fr (D.M.)
7. Department of Endodontics, Faculty of Dental Medicine, Strasbourg University, 67000 Strasbourg, France
8. Pôle de Médecine et Chirurgie Bucco-Dentaire, Hôpital Civil, Hôpitaux Universitaire de Strasbourg, 67000 Strasbourg, France
* Correspondence: dentistenajikharouf@gmail.com; Tel.: +33-667-522-841

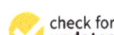

Citation: El Hachem, C.; Chedid, J.C.A.; Nehme, W.; Kaloustian, M.K.; Ghosn, N.; Rabineau, M.; Kharouf, N.; Haikel, Y.; Mancino, D. The Contribution of Various In Vitro Methodologies to Comprehending the Filling Ability of Root Canal Pastes in Primary Teeth. *Bioengineering* 2023, 10, 818. https://doi.org/10.3390/bioengineering10070818

Academic Editor: Chengfei Zhang

Received: 3 June 2023
Revised: 6 July 2023
Accepted: 7 July 2023
Published: 9 July 2023

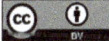

Copyright: © 2023 by the authors. Licensee MDPI, Basel, Switzerland. This article is an open access article distributed under the terms and conditions of the Creative Commons Attribution (CC BY) license (https://creativecommons.org/licenses/by/4.0/).

Abstract: A void-free obturation during root canal treatment on primary teeth is currently very difficult to attain. In this study, the pulpectomy filling abilities of Bio-C Pulpecto (Angelus, Basil, Londrina, Paraná, Brazil) and of zinc oxide eugenol, or "ZOE" (DenPro, Prevest, New York, NY, USA), were compared using several in vitro techniques. Therefore, 30 primary anterior teeth were used in the present in vitro study. Analysis of variance (ANOVA), including a multiple comparison procedure (Holm-Sidak method, Dunn's Method, or Tukey test), was used. On micro-CT, Bio-C Pulpecto exhibited higher void percentages than did ZOE (10.3 ± 3.8%, and 3.5 ± 1.3%, respectively) ($p < 0.05$). With digital microscopy, higher total void percentages were found in the BC (13.2 ± 26.7%) group compared to the ZOE (2.7 ± 2.8%) group ($p < 0.05$). With the CLSM, mean tubular penetration depths were higher for Bio-C Pulpecto than for ZOE in all canal thirds ($p < 0.05$). SEM images demonstrated no tags into dentinal tubules in either group throughout the three thirds. Moreover, higher statistically significant flowability was found for Bio-C (2.657 ± 0.06 mm) compared to ZOE (1.8 ± 0.13 mm) ($p < 0.05$). The findings of this study indicate that neither ZOE nor Bio-C Pulpecto appears to meet the criteria for an ideal root canal filling paste for primary teeth. This study laid the groundwork for future research by determining how micro-CT, digital microscopy, SEM, and CLSM contribute to our understanding of the filling process of primary teeth. More thorough research on the mechanism of root canal obturation on primary teeth is required to achieve a long-term successful root canal therapy in young children.

Keywords: calcium silicate material; confocal laser scanning microscopy; deciduous tooth; digital microscopy; flowability; micro-CT; pulpectomy primary teeth; root canal filling; SEM; zinc oxide eugenol

1. Introduction

With the introduction of mechanical shaping [1], new irrigation protocols [2], and new filling materials and techniques [3], root canal therapy for primary teeth is rapidly developing. Success is still not always assured, and in the present clinical pulpectomy practice, attaining a void-free root canal obturation is difficult [4]. It is crucial to choose the filling paste with the best biological, mechanical, and physicochemical properties to obtain dense 3D obturation, avoid shrinking or irritating the periapical tissues, and ensure that the filling paste resorbs concurrently with the roots without damaging the underlying tooth successor [5].

Zinc oxide eugenol (ZOE powder and liquid), calcium hydroxide paste alone or mixed with iodoform combined with rotary Lentulo spirals, premixed syringes, and endodontic pluggers/reamers were suggested to enhance the quality of obturation on primary teeth [6,7]. However, there is currently still no agreement on the best root canal filling material for primary teeth, and each substance has disadvantages. ZOE sets into a thick mass that resists resorption, may irritate periapical tissues, and can cause deviation of the permanent tooth bud [8]. Calcium hydroxide-based materials may result in intracanal and external resorption, resulting in long-term failure of the treatment [9].

New endodontic forms of cement, called bioceramics, have been gaining popularity due to their physicochemical and biological characteristics, such as their alkaline pH, shrink-free property, chemical stability in the biological environment, and biocompatibility [10,11]. In permanent teeth, these bioactive materials, which exhibit biological activity [12], have many clinical indications such as pulpotomies, pulp capping, resorption, perforation repair, and root canal fillings [13–16]. Pediatric dentists have recently endorsed them as well. The first resorbable bioceramic root canal filling for primary teeth is called Bio-C Pulpecto (Angelus, Basil, Londrina, Paraná, Brazil). It is made up of silicon dioxide, calcium tungstate, titanium oxide, ester glycol salicylate, toluene sulphonamide, and calcium silicate [5].

To assess the quality of a root canal filling, there are various in vitro methods, and each method enables an understanding of a certain aspect of the obturation. The most precise non-invasive imaging method that has received widespread support from studies and enables a quantitative assessment of internal structural changes in root canal morphology is micro-Computed Tomography (μCt) [17,18]. Microscopes, despite being destructive, are essential for understanding the mechanism of endodontic materials' penetration into dentinal tubules; options include using a confocal laser scanning microscope (CLSM) [19] and/or scanning electron microscope (SEM) [20]. CLSM reveals information about the sealer penetration and distribution inside the dentinal tubules of root canal walls by including a fluorescent dye marker with the pastes, while SEM allows evaluation of sealer adaptation with root canal walls and marginal gaps. In primary dentition, there are very few publications that integrate several in vitro evaluation techniques to assess the ability of root canal filling pastes used [21,22].

In the pediatric endodontic literature, there is an agreement about the difficulty of obtaining a void-free obturation with long-term success. In a meta-analysis totalizing 263 teeth, the authors stated that there is currently no scientific evidence of the superiority of any one root canal filling material for endodontic treatment of necrotic primary teeth [23]. Studies confirmed that a good hermetic seal with minimum voids is directly related to the material's capacity to adhere to the walls of the root canal and the method used to deliver this material into the root canal [6,24]. It was also reported that primary teeth filling pastes lead to overfilled canals and resorption within the root [25].

This study's main objective was to evaluate the pulpectomy filling abilities of zinc oxide eugenol and Bio-C Pulpecto. For each material, the percentage of voids/total filling, the flowability, the penetration depths, and the dentinal tags were assessed utilizing micro-CT, CLSM, digital microscopy, and SEM. The goal was to evaluate the data from each procedure and classify them so that clinicians could fully understand all facets of root canal filling on primary teeth. The null hypothesis is that there is no difference in the filling ability of zinc oxide eugenol and Bio-C Pulpecto when assessed with micro-CT, CLSM, digital microscopy, and SEM.

2. Materials and Methods

2.1. Teeth Selection

The ethics committee of the Saint Joseph University of Beirut, Lebanon (USJ-2019-237) approved this study. One hundred primary anterior teeth with minimal root resorption, belonging to children aged 3 to 6 and extracted for reasons unrelated to this study as part of treatment plans at the University of X's Department of Pediatric Dentistry, were collected and kept in formocresol 0.1%. Teeth with previous pulpotomy or pulpectomy, internal resorption, and advanced root resorption were excluded after inspection under an operating microscope. Therefore, 30 primary anterior teeth were included in this study. Using the IBM SPSS statistics software (version 27.0), the sample size was calculated. To ensure more than 80% power and an alpha error probability of 0.05, two groups of 15 canals each were formed.

2.2. Teeth Preparation

Patency was verified with a size 10 K-file (Dentsply Sirona, Ballaigues, Switzerland) following access cavity preparation. A diamond disc (Kerr Dental, Bioggio, Switzerland) was used to section the crowns to standardize the root length at 12 mm, and the working length (WL) was determined, 1 mm short of the apical foramen, with a size 15 K-file (Dentsply Sirona, Ballaigues, Switzerland). For the shaping, R-motion® 21 mm file (30/0.04) (FKG Dentaire SA, La Chaux-de-Fonds, Switzerland) was used to prepare all the canals. Using a 30G side-vented needle (NaviTip, Ultradent), 12 mL of 1% NaOCl was flushed inside the canals. Mechanical activation of the irrigant with XP-endo Finisher (FKG) operated at 1000 rpm, as suggested by the manufacturer, was carried out for 30 s in all canals; the tip was placed 1 mm short of the WL without binding. After drying the canals with sterile paper points, 1 mL of 17% EDTA was injected and left for 1 min inside the canals. Following the same protocol, EDTA was activated. For the final irrigation, 3 mL of saline was used. Canals were dried with paper points.

2.3. Root Canal Obturation

According to the filling materials, the teeth were divided into 2 groups. Furthermore, to perform analysis under CLSM, each filling paste was manually labeled with rhodamine B powder (Sigma-Aldrich, St. Louis, MO, USA) to an approximate concentration of 0.1% to provide fluorescence and allow confocal laser microscopy assessment [26].

Group 1: Zinc oxide eugenol was used in the form of powder liquid and was mixed in a ration 2:1 to obtain a creamy consistency. The labeled cement was inserted into the canal 1 mm short of the WL, with a size 30 Lentulo spiral (Dentsply Maillefer, Ballaigues, Switzerland) used for at least five seconds inside the canal in little pecking motions.

Group 2. Bio-C Pulpecto (BC), a premixed bioceramic material, was emptied on a plexiglass, marked with the fluorescent dye, refilled into the syringe, and injected directly into the canals.

To validate the quality of the filling in terms of length and density, a buccolingual and a distomesial digital radiograph were taken. None of the teeth exhibited a poor quality of obturation; therefore, none were discarded.

Afterward, the access cavity was sealed with Teflon tape and reinforced zinc oxide eugenol (Intermediate Restorative Material, IRM; Dentsply Sirona, Charlotte, NC, USA). The teeth were then incubated in the dark in a container (Memmert GmbH, Büchenbach, Germany) at 37 °C for 14 days with full saturated humidity to ensure the final setting.

2.4. Micro CT Scanning

For tooth imaging, a micro-CT Platform (EA2496, Montrouge, France) was used to investigate the 30 teeth. Each tooth was individually scanned with a micro-CT scanner

(Quantum FX; PerkinElmer Health Sciences; Hopkinton) to measure the void volume (μm^3) in each third in order to assess the filling percentage and voids in the coronal, middle, and apical thirds. The field of view was set at 10 mm to acquire 3D images with an isotropic resolution of 20 μm. Acquisition settings were 160 kV, 90 mA, and 360° scanning rotation.

DICOM data were imported into 3D Slicer 5.1 software. The following semi-automated threshold-based segmentations were realized:

- Complete root with filling
- Complete filling with voids
- Filling without voids

Boolean operations were performed to get the following 3D segmentation:

- C: Canal (filling + voids)
- F: Filling without voids
- V: Voids

The software's Models module transformed the aforementioned 3D segmentations into 3D models and automatically measured each model's volume.

The following calculation was used to determine the percentage of voids in the obturation:

$$V/C \times 100$$

To calculate the percentage of filling and voids in the coronal, middle, and apical sections, the total length of the canal was measured, divided by 3, and then 2 custom plane sections perpendicular to the long axis of the canal were realized to separate the coronal, middle, and apical models at equidistant lengths. C, F, and V were calculated for each part as follows [27]:

- Cc, Fc, and Vc for the coronal part
- Cm, Fm, and Vm for the middle part
- Ca, Fa, and Va for the apical part

The same formula was used to calculate the percentage of voids in canal thirds [27].

The percentage of filling and voids was evaluated using a threshold method and 3D models in the coronal, middle, and apical sections (Figure 1).

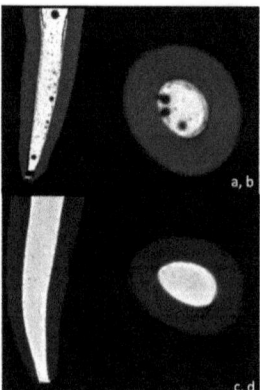

Figure 1. Micro-CT cross sections and reconstructed 3D image showing Bio-C Pulpecto (**a,b**) and ZOE (**c,d**).

2.5. Sectioning

The root canals of the 30 teeth were cross-sectioned at 1 mm and 5 mm from the root apex using a diamond disk (Buehler, Lake Bluff, IL, USA) and a slow speed (25,000 rpm) handpiece. After mounting the specimens onto glass slides, the coronal surface was polished with sandpapers of 600, 1200, 2400, and 4000-grit silicon carbide paper (Escil, Chassieu, France) under running water. The sample examined by confocal laser microscopy has a thickness of 2 mm [19].

2.6. Digital Microscopy Observations

Specimen polished surfaces (n = 90, three surfaces for each tooth) were first examined under a digital microscope VHX-5000 (KEYENCE, Osaka, Japan), and one image was captured for each specimen at 100× magnification. The micrographs were coded by an expert examiner who was not involved in the experiment, displaying the canal wall surface of both groups at the coronal, middle, and apical thirds, for blinded analysis using the VHX-5000 software (KEYENCE, Osaka, Japan) to measure the total area of the filling materials and of the internal and external voids in μm^3 following a previous study [28] (Figure 2). After that, the percentages of voids were calculated and statistically analyzed.

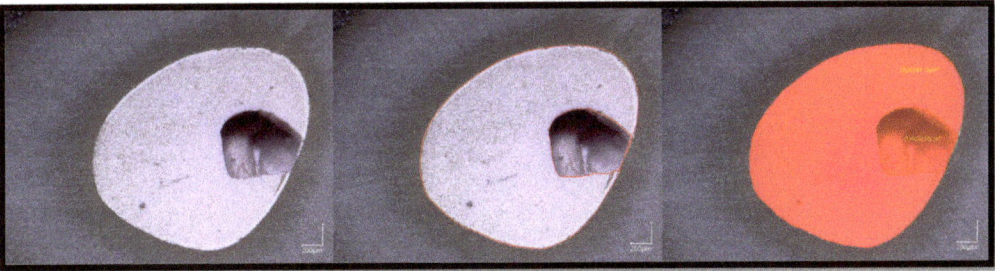

Figure 2. Methodology for measuring the area of filling materials and voids with the VHX-5000 program.

2.7. Confocal Laser Scanning Microscopy Analysis

Confocal laser scanning microscope (Zeiss, LSM 710, Göttingen, Germany) with an objective 10× Plan NeoFluor and a 514 nm excitation wavelength compatible with rhodamine dye was used to examine all the canals (n = 90, three surfaces for each tooth). The entire dentinal tubule penetration area was determined using ImageJ software (NIH). The deepest penetration from the canal wall to the point of maximum sealer penetration was calculated using ImageJ software. Each measurement was performed twice to assure accuracy and reproducibility. The penetration depths at 8 circumferential sites were averaged to obtain the mean sealer penetration depths in μm with the highest degree of accuracy at the coronal, middle, and apical sections for Bio-C Pulpecto and ZOE.

2.8. Scanning Electron Microscope Observations

From each group, six samples, including the three thirds, were chosen to closely inspect the areas where filling paste and dentin met. To observe the materials' tags into the dentinal tubules, the polished surfaces were etched with 37% phosphoric acid for 10 s and immersed in 2.5% NaOCl for 3 min [29]. After that, the specimens were dehydrated in a graded series of ethanol solutions (50, 70, 95, and 100%) for 10 min each before being coated with a gold-palladium alloy (20/80 weight percent) using Hummer JR sputtering equipment (Technics, Rocklin, CA, USA). The produced samples were examined using a Quanta 250 FEG scanning electron microscope (FEI Company, Eindhoven, The Netherlands) with an electron acceleration voltage of 10 kV and a magnification of 100–4000 [30]. These samples were examined under SEM to verify the findings obtained using CLSM and digital microscopy.

2.9. Flow Test

Additionally, a flow test was conducted using the method outlined in ISO 6876/2012: 50 µL of each mixed sealer (in triplicate) was dispensed on a separate glass plate (40 × 40 × 5 mm). A second glass plate was carefully placed on top of the sealer after 3 min of mixing. Then, a weight of 100 g was applied centrally on top of the second glass plate. After 10 min, using a digital caliper (Dexter, Elkhart, IN, USA), the compressed sealer's maximum and lowest diameters were measured. The test was repeated to determine the mean diameter if there was a discrepancy of greater than 1 mm between the two measurements [31].

2.10. Statistical Analysis

SigmaPlot (release 11.2, Systat Software, Inc., San Jose, CA, USA) was used for statistical analysis. The Shapiro–Wilk test was used to verify the normality of the data in all groups. Analysis of variance (ANOVA), including a multiple comparison procedure (Holm-Sidak method, Dunn's Method, or Tukey test), was used to determine whether significant differences existed in the void evaluations between the different techniques and materials. A statistical significance level of $p = 0.05$ was adopted in all tests.

3. Results

3.1. Micro-CT

When comparing overall void percentages, Bio-C Pulpecto exhibited higher void percentages compared to ZOE (10.3 ± 3.8%, and 3.5 ± 1.3%), respectively ($p < 0.001$). Additionally, the apical third of the ZOE group had higher void percentages than the coronal and middle thirds ($p = 0.006$), but there was no statistically significant difference between the middle and coronal thirds ($p > 0.05$). There were no statistically significant differences between the three thirds of the Bio-C Pulpecto group ($p = 0.192$) (Table 1).

Table 1. Mean and standard deviations of void percentages in ZOE and BC groups after micro-CT analysis. Zinc oxide eugenol (ZOE), Bio-C Pulpecto (BC), coronal (C), middle (M), and apical (A).

	Coronal (%)	Middle (%)	Apical (%)	Statistical Analysis
ZOE	2.7 ± 1.3	2.3 ± 1.8	6.7 ± 4.9	A > C, A > M
BC	7.5 ± 4	8.9 ± 7.7	17.2 ± 14.8	No
Statistical analysis	$p < 0.001$	$r = 0.002$	$p = 0.049$	

3.2. Digital Microscopy

The same tendency was found for the results of Keyence compared to micro-CT outcomes. Higher total void percentages were found in the BC group compared to the ZOE group in the coronal, middle, and apical thirds (Table 2). BC demonstrated higher void percentages compared to ZOE at the apical ($p < 0.001$), middle ($p = 0.002$), and coronal ($p = 0.019$) thirds (Table 2 and Figure 3).

Table 2. Mean and standard deviations of void percentages in ZOE and BC groups after digital microscope analysis. Zinc oxide eugenol (ZOE), Bio-C Pulpecto (BC), coronal (C), middle (M), and apical (A).

	Coronal (%)		Middle (%)		Apical (%)	
	Close	Open	Close	Open	Close	Open
ZOE	2.6 ± 2.1	0.2 ± 0.4	1.6 ± 1.8	0.3 ± 0.8	1.48 ± 1.77	1.7 ± 3.7
BC	4.4 ± 7.4	5 ± 7.7	2.2 ± 1.6	4.8 ± 5	13.7 ± 32.7	9.4 ± 13.6
Statistical analysis	$p = 0.019$		$p = 0.002$		$p < 0.001$	

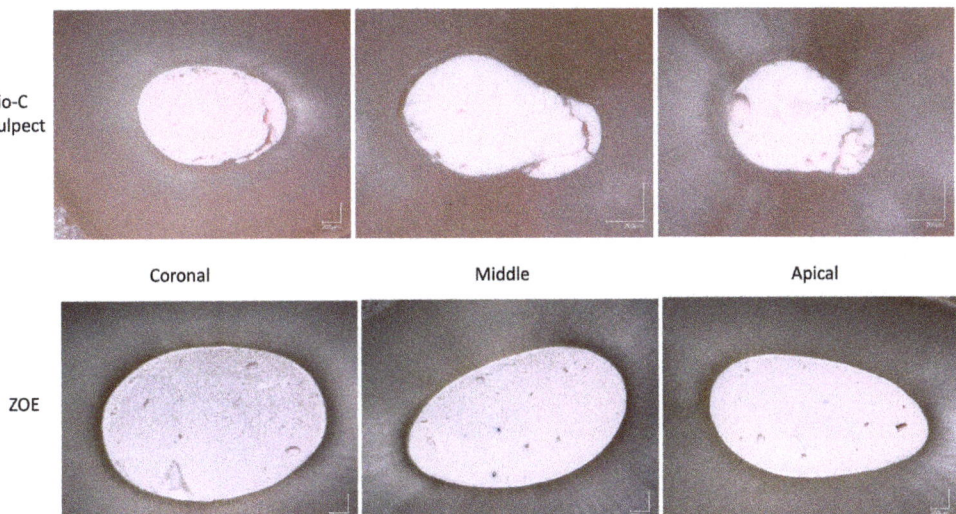

Figure 3. Digital microscopy images for Bio-C Pulpecto and ZOE in the coronal, middle, and apical thirds.

3.3. Confocal Laser Scanning Microscope

Mean tubular penetration depths were higher for Bio-C Pulpecto than for ZOE in the coronal (277 ± 124 µm and 122 ± 62 µm), middle (247 ± 118 µm and 112 ± 55 µm), and apical thirds (218 ± 114 µm and 102 ± 52 µm), respectively (Table 3).

Table 3. Mean and standard deviations of void percentages in ZOE and BC groups after confocal microscope analysis. Zinc oxide eugenol (ZOE); Bio-C Pulpecto (BC), Coronal (C); Middle (M) and Apical (A).

	Coronal (%)	Middle (%)	Apical (%)	Statistical Analysis
ZOE	122 ± 62	112 ± 55	102 ± 52	C > A
BC	277 ± 124	247 ± 118	218 ± 114	C > A
Statistical analysis	$p < 0.001$	$p < 0.001$	$p < 0.001$	

In addition, in the ZOE and BC groups, statistically higher material infiltrations values were observed in the coronal third compared to the apical third (($p = 0.012$) and ($p < 0.001$), respectively), while no statistically significant differences were found between the apical/middle and coronal/middle ($p > 0.05$) (Figure 4).

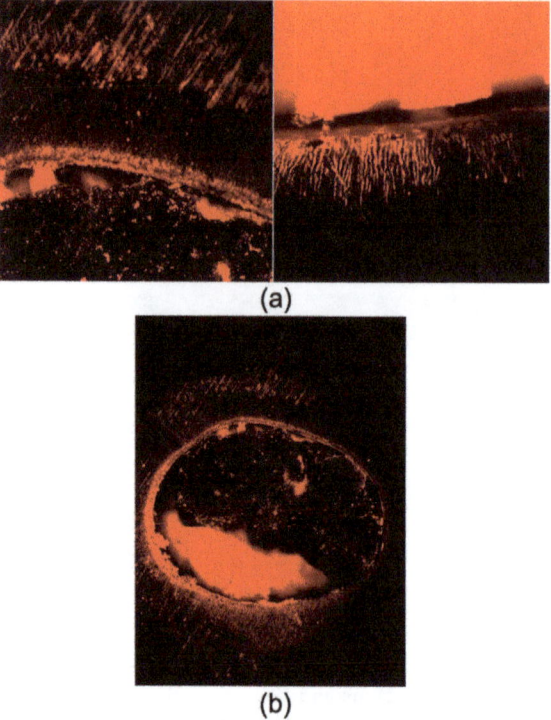

Figure 4. (**a**) ZOE and Bio-C Pulpecto penetration into dentinal tubules; (**b**) methodology for calculating mean penetration depth into dentinal tubules.

3.4. Scanning Electron Microscope (SEM vs. CLSM)

In contrast with the confocal results, SEM images demonstrated no tags into dentinal tubules in either group throughout the three thirds (Figure 5).

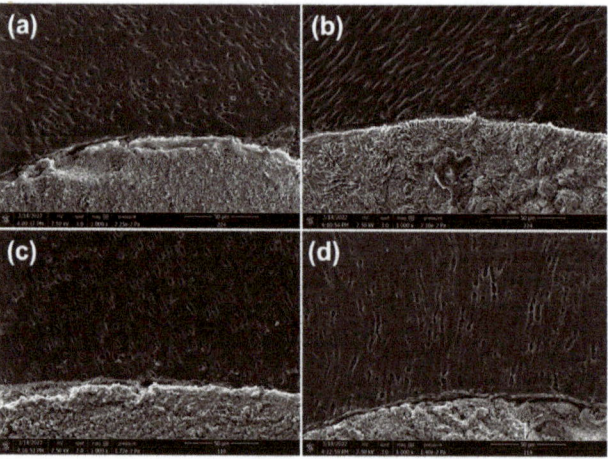

Figure 5. Representative SEM images showing no tags into dentinal tubules for ZOE in the middle (**a**) and apical thirds (**b**) or for Bio-C Pulpecto in the middle (**c**) and apical thirds (**d**).

3.5. Flow Test

Higher statistically significant flowability was found for Bio-C (2.657 ± 0.06 mm) compared to ZOE (1.8 ± 0.13 mm) ($p < 0.001$).

4. Discussion

Root canal treatment for primary teeth has seen significant development recently [32]. The best root canal filling material and procedure are still up for debate, though. Despite its disadvantages and potential toxicity, zinc oxide eugenol is nonetheless utilized routinely and with great success [8]. Nonetheless, the hunt for biocompatible and bioactive materials has led to the recent development of bioceramics, such as the non-setting Bio-C Pulpecto for primary teeth [5]. In this study, we used a variety of in vitro evaluation techniques to examine the filling ability of zinc oxide eugenol (ZOE) and Bio-C Pulpecto. Since there was a significant difference between ZOE and Bio-C Pulpecto according to all in vitro evaluation techniques, the null hypothesis was partially rejected ($p < 0.05$).

The goal of this study was to assess and categorize the data obtained from micro-CT, digital microscopy, CLSM, and SEM so that clinicians could comprehend every aspect of root canal filling on primary teeth. The novelty of this study consists of its combination of numerous in vitro methodologies to evaluate the filling capabilities of root canal pastes used on primary teeth and its choice of the filling material, namely a bioceramic created exclusively for primary teeth. Therefore, each technique would enable comprehension of a certain component of the obturation and provide never-before-published data.

The first methodology adopted in this study to compare the filling ability of ZOE and Bio-C Pulpecto was micro-CT imaging. Micro-CT is used to analyze tooth structure objectively, allowing for quantitative and qualitative image analysis [33,34]. Additionally, it enables the accurate reconstruction of 3D models and can distinguish between tooth structures, voids, and obturation materials [35]. Both materials produced voids in all canal thirds, with Bio-C Pulpecto revealing higher void percentages than ZOE ($10.3 \pm 3.8\%$, and $3.5 \pm 1.3\%$). This was per the results of numerous studies, regardless of the filling material, that agree on the difficulty of achieving a void-free obturation due to the complex root canal anatomy of human teeth [36,37].

In addition, in primary dentition, the obturation relies exclusively on a resorbable filling paste, without the support of a gutta-percha cone, which renders the 3D obturation even more difficult, especially with the abundance of lateral canals, isthmus, and canal curvatures [32,38]. In one of the few previous micro-CT studies on primary teeth filling, the authors suggested that using a syringe to inject the paste produced fewer voids than using a lentulo spiral [7]. This could explain why, in this study, there was an increase in apical voids for the ZOE group ($p < 0.05$), whereas there was no discernible difference between coronal, middle, and apical thirds for the Bio-C Pulpecto group ($p > 0.05$). In fact, in an attempt to enhance the quality of root canal obturation on primary teeth and decrease the void volume, some authors proposed ultrasonic activation of the filling paste for a better infiltration in the intricate primary teeth anatomy [39]. More micro-CT studies should be conducted to find the most efficient filling technique for primary teeth.

The samples were then sectioned and further analyzed with different microscopes.

Using the digital microscope, the filling volume and voids were quantified and measured in the coronal, middle, and apical sections for both groups. The results corroborate the micro-CT findings showing higher total void percentages in Bio-C Pulpecto ($13.2 \pm 26.7\%$) compared to ZOE ($2.7 \pm 2.8\%$) ($p < 0.05$). However, in contrast to micro-CT, no statistically significant differences were found between the three thirds for both materials ($p > 0.05$), while micro-CT demonstrated a significant difference between the three thirds of the ZOE group. This could be related to the high resolution and precision provided by micro-CT, which can detect more details, as well as to the ability of micro-CT to investigate the void in volume (3D) while the digital microscope could be used to investigate only in the slices (one section for each third), which is a limitation of the digital microscope in void investigation [31]. The two methodologies allow for quantitative evaluation of total filling percentage, voids, and detection of flaws in the bulk filling of root canal pastes for primary teeth. Therefore, both techniques showed the same tendency for both materials with higher detection for the micro-CT method.

A fluorescent rhodamine marker mixed with pastes was used to visualize the penetration and distribution of the sealers within the dentinal tubules of root canal walls using a CLSM [19]. Mean tubular penetration depths were higher for Bio-C Pulpecto than for ZOE in all canal thirds. This could be attributed to the physicochemical properties of Bio-C Pulpecto, its high contact angle, and its solubility, presumably allowing it to easily diffuse into the dentinal tubules [5]. This finding was also verified by conducting a flowability test that showed higher mean values for Bio-C Pulpecto than for ZOE. Studies agree that the penetration depth inside dentinal tubules is directly related to the properties of the materials such as setting time and flowability [40]. Moreover, under CLSM, for both materials, the depth of sealer penetration into dentinal tubules decreased from the coronal to the apical part ($p < 0.05$). This could be attributed to the obturation technique since both the lentulo spiral and the pressure syringe techniques lead to voids in the apical part [39]. This may also be accounted for by the apical region's lower density and diameter of dentinal tubules [41]. Future studies should focus on developing filling pastes with enhanced abilities to penetrate the dentinal tubule, encapsulate the bacteria inside, and favor interaction between the material and the dentinal fluid.

To visualize the adaptation of filling pastes to canal walls and marginal gaps and to detect the material tags in dentinal tubules, some samples were further observed under SEM. The intermolecular surface energy and cleanliness of the dentin, as well as the surface tension and wetting capacity of the sealer, all interact to determine the degree of adhesion [30]. The retention of filling material by root canal walls is improved by sealer plugs placed into the dentinal tubules because they mechanically interlock [42]. In the current study, in contrast to CLSM infiltration images, SEM images demonstrated no tags into dentinal tubules in either group throughout the three thirds. This could be due to the irrigation protocol being insufficient in eliminating the debris and smear layer and also to the consistency of the paste and the filling technique [30]. This could also be related to the detachment of the fluorescent dye from the filling paste, which gives the fake impression of an infiltrated dentinal tubule. Some authors even concluded that bioceramic sealers should not be utilized in conjunction with Rhodamine for CLSM assessment after it was reported that the kind of fluorophore changes the calcium silicate sealers' performance when using CLSM [43]. In addition, we can hypothesize that the several in vitro steps that were performed to prepare the samples for SEM observations, including sectioning, polishing, and chemical preparations to eliminate the smear layer and to dry the samples, could alter this observation and could dissolve the material tags.

Overall, the findings of this study indicate that neither ZOE nor Bio-C Pulpecto appears to meet the criteria for an ideal root canal filling paste for primary teeth. The purpose of this study was to create the groundwork for future research by determining how micro-CT, digital microscopy, SEM, and CLSM contribute to our understanding of the filling process. In this study, ZOE was superior to Bio-C Pulpecto according to micro-CT and digital microscopy, whereas CLSM and SEM produced contradictory findings, with CLSM indicating tubular infiltration for both pastes and SEM disproving this claim by demonstrating no dentinal tags for either group. It should be nonetheless noted that microscopes are invasive and allow only partial evaluation of root fillings and that some may create irreversible damage to the specimens [44,45]. These factors might lead to inaccuracies because some filling material might be lost during sample preparation [46].

To create better materials for pediatric endodontics, additional evidence-based research is urgently required to completely understand whether the issue is with the filling pastes, the filling technique, or most likely both, and how to fix it. More thorough research on the mechanism of root canal obturation on primary teeth is required. Numerous studies indicate that for the time being, it is impossible to obturate primary teeth in a confined, dense 3D space, putting the effectiveness of root canal therapy on primary teeth in jeopardy [47–49].

5. Conclusions

Current primary tooth filling pastes, including ZOE or Bio-C Pulpecto, do not meet the criteria for the ideal root canal filling material. Micro-CT and digital microscopy revealed that ZOE was superior to Bio-C Pulpecto; however, CLSM and SEM provided inconsistent results, with CLSM showing tubular infiltration for both pastes and SEM refuting this assertion by showing no dentinal tags for either group. The qualities and methods of filling materials should be the focus of future research. Most significantly, the studies need to find a way to improve the effectiveness of root canal filling pastes for primary teeth using all current in vitro imaging or microscopic techniques.

Author Contributions: Conceptualization, C.E.H., M.K.K. and W.N.; methodology, M.K.K., N.K. and C.E.H.; software, N.K.; validation, N.K., D.M., J.C.A.C., M.R. and Y.H.; data curation, N.G.; writing—original draft preparation, C.E.H.; writing—review and editing, N.K., W.N. and D.M.; supervision, J.C.A.C., W.N., Y.H., D.M. and N.K.; project administration, C.E.H. and N.K. All authors have read and agreed to the published version of the manuscript.

Funding: This research received no external funding.

Institutional Review Board Statement: This in vitro study was approved by the institutional ethics committee of Saint Joseph University, Beirut, Lebanon (USJ-2019-237).

Informed Consent Statement: Not applicable.

Data Availability Statement: Not applicable.

Conflicts of Interest: The authors declare no conflict of interest.

References

1. Esentürk, G.; Akkas, E.; Cubukcu, E.; Nagas, E.; Uyanik, O.; Cehreli, Z.C. A Micro-Computed Tomographic Assessment of Root Canal Preparation with Conventional and Different Rotary Files in Primary Teeth and Young Permanent Teeth. *Int. J. Paediatr. Dent.* **2020**, *30*, 202–208. [CrossRef] [PubMed]
2. Hachem, C.E.; Nehme, W.; Kaloustian, M.K.; Ghosn, N.; Daou, M.; Zogheib, C.; Karam, M.; Mhanna, R.; Macaluso, V.; Kharouf, N.; et al. The Effectiveness of Different Irrigation Techniques on Debris and Smear Layer Removal in Primary Mandibular Second Molars: An In Vitro Study. *J. Contemp. Dent. Pract.* **2022**, *23*, 1173–1179. [CrossRef]
3. Walia, T.; Ghanbari, A.H.; Mathew, S.; Ziadlou, A.H. An in Vitro Comparison of Three Delivery Techniques for Obturation of Root Canals in Primary Molars. *Eur. Arch. Paediatr. Dent.* **2017**, *18*, 17–23. [CrossRef]
4. Silva Junior, M.F.; Wambier, L.M.; Gevert, M.V.; Chibinski, A.C.R. Effectiveness of Iodoform-Based Filling Materials in Root Canal Treatment of Deciduous Teeth: A Systematic Review and Meta-Analysis. *Biomater. Investig. Dent.* **2022**, *9*, 52–74. [CrossRef]
5. Hachem, C.E.; Chedid, J.C.A.; Nehme, W.; Kaloustian, M.K.; Ghosn, N.; Sahnouni, H.; Mancino, D.; Haikel, Y.; Kharouf, N. Physicochemical and Antibacterial Properties of Conventional and Two Premixed Root Canal Filling Materials in Primary Teeth. *J. Funct. Biomater.* **2022**, *13*, 177. [CrossRef] [PubMed]
6. Najjar, R.S.; Alamoudi, N.M.; El-Housseiny, A.A.; Al Tuwirqi, A.A.; Sabbagh, H.J. A Comparison of Calcium Hydroxide/Iodoform Paste and Zinc Oxide Eugenol as Root Filling Materials for Pulpectomy in Primary Teeth: A Systematic Review and Meta-Analysis. *Clin. Exp. Dent. Res.* **2019**, *5*, 294–310. [CrossRef]
7. Aragão, A.C.; Pintor, A.V.B.; Marceliano-Alves, M.; Primo, L.G.; Silva, A.S.D.S.; Lopes, R.T.; Neves, A.D.A. Root Canal Obturation Materials and Filling Techniques for Primary Teeth: In Vitro Evaluation in Polymer-Based Prototyped Incisors. *Int. J. Paediatr. Dent.* **2020**, *30*, 381–389. [CrossRef]
8. Barja-Fidalgo, F.; Moutinho-Ribeiro, M.; Oliveira, M.A.A.; de Oliveira, B.H. A Systematic Review of Root Canal Filling Materials for Deciduous Teeth: Is There an Alternative for Zinc Oxide-Eugenol? *ISRN Dentistry* **2011**, *2011*, 367318. [CrossRef] [PubMed]
9. Lima, C.C.B.; Conde Júnior, A.M.; Rizzo, M.S.; Moura, R.D.; Moura, M.S.; Lima, M.D.M.; Moura, L.F.A.D. Biocompatibility of Root Filling Pastes Used in Primary Teeth. *Int. Endod. J.* **2015**, *48*, 405–416. [CrossRef]
10. Haapasalo, M.; Parhar, M.; Huang, X.; Wei, X.; Lin, J.; Shen, Y. Clinical Use of Bioceramic Materials. *Endod. Top.* **2015**, *32*, 97–117. [CrossRef]
11. López-García, S.; Rodríguez-Lozano, F.J.; Sanz, J.L.; Forner, L.; Pecci-Lloret, M.P.; Lozano, A.; Murcia, L.; Sánchez-Bautista, S.; Oñate-Sánchez, R.E. Biological Properties of Ceraputty as a Retrograde Filling Material: An in Vitro Study on HPDLSCs. *Clin. Oral. Investig.* **2023**, 1–11. [CrossRef]

12. Kharouf, N.; Sauro, S.; Eid, A.; Zghal, J.; Jmal, H.; Seck, A.; Macaluso, V.; Addiego, F.; Inchingolo, F.; Affolter-Zbaraszczuk, C.; et al. Physicochemical and Mechanical Properties of Premixed Calcium Silicate and Resin Sealers. *J. Funct. Biomater.* **2022**, *14*, 9. [CrossRef]
13. Çelik, B.N.; Mutluay, M.S.; Arıkan, V.; Sarı, Ş. The Evaluation of MTA and Biodentine as a Pulpotomy Materials for Carious Exposures in Primary Teeth. *Clin. Oral. Investig.* **2019**, *23*, 661–666. [CrossRef]
14. Makhlouf, M.; Kaloustian, M.; Claire, E.H.; Habib, M.; Zogheib, C. Sealing Ability of Two Calcium Silicate-Based Materials in the Repair of Furcal Perforations: A Laboratory Comparative Study. *J. Contemp. Dent. Pract.* **2020**, *21*, 1091–1097. [CrossRef] [PubMed]
15. Kassab, P.; El Hachem, C.; Habib, M.; Nehme, W.; Zogheib, C.; Tonini, R.; Kaloustian, M.K. The Pushout Bond Strength of Three Calcium Silicate-Based Materials in Furcal Perforation Repair and the Effect of a Novel Irrigation Solution: A Comparative In Vitro Study. *J. Contemp. Dent. Pract.* **2022**, *23*, 289–294. [PubMed]
16. Taha, N.A.; Abdulkhader, S.Z. Full Pulpotomy with Biodentine in Symptomatic Young Permanent Teeth with Carious Exposure. *J. Endod.* **2018**, *44*, 932–937. [CrossRef] [PubMed]
17. Almeida, A.; Romeiro, K.; Cassimiro, M.; Gominho, L.; Dantas, E.; Silva, S.; Albuquerque, D. Micro-CT Analysis of Dentinal Microcracks on Root Canals Filled with a Bioceramic Sealer and Retreated with Reciprocating Instruments. *Sci. Rep.* **2020**, *10*, 15264. [CrossRef]
18. Barasuol, J.C.; Alcalde, M.P.; Bortoluzzi, E.A.; Duarte, M.a.H.; Cardoso, M.; Bolan, M. Shaping Ability of Hand, Rotary and Reciprocating Files in Primary Teeth: A Micro-CT Study in Vitro. *Eur. Arch. Paediatr. Dent.* **2021**, *22*, 195–201. [CrossRef]
19. Hwang, J.H.; Chung, J.; Na, H.-S.; Park, E.; Kwak, S.; Kim, H.-C. Comparison of Bacterial Leakage Resistance of Various Root Canal Filling Materials and Methods: Confocal Laser-Scanning Microscope Study. *Scanning* **2015**, *37*, 422–428. [CrossRef]
20. Mancino, D.; Kharouf, N.; Cabiddu, M.; Bukiet, F.; Haïkel, Y. Microscopic and Chemical Evaluation of the Filling Quality of Five Obturation Techniques in Oval-Shaped Root Canals. *Clin. Oral. Investig.* **2021**, *25*, 3757–3765. [CrossRef]
21. Drukteinis, S.; Drukteiniene, A.; Drukteinis, L.; Martens, L.C.; Rajasekharan, S. Flowable Urethane Dimethacrylate-Based Filler for Root Canal Obturation in Primary Molars: A Pilot SEM and MicroCT Assessment. *Children* **2021**, *8*, 60. [CrossRef]
22. Segato, R.A.B.; Pucinelli, C.M.; Ferreira, D.C.A.; Daldegan, A.D.R.; da Silva, R.S.; Nelson-Filho, P.; da Silva, L.A.B. Physicochemical Properties of Root Canal Filling Materials for Primary Teeth. *Braz. Dent. J.* **2016**, *27*, 196–201. [CrossRef]
23. Pedrotti, D.; Bottezini, P.A.; Casagrande, L.; Braga, M.M.; Lenzi, T.L. Root Canal Filling Materials for Endodontic Treatment of Necrotic Primary Teeth: A Network Meta-Analysis. *Eur. Arch. Paediatr. Dent.* **2022**, *24*, 151–166. [CrossRef] [PubMed]
24. Irzooqee, A.F.; Al Haidar, A.H.M.J.; Abdul-Kareem, M. The Effect of Different Obturation Techniques in Primary Teeth on the Apical Microleakage Using Endoflas: A Comparative In Vitro Study. *Int. J. Dent.* **2023**, *2023*, 4982980. [CrossRef] [PubMed]
25. Coll, J.A.; Vargas, K.; Marghalani, A.A.; Chen, C.-Y.; AlShamali, S.; Dhar, V.; Crystal, Y.O. A Systematic Review and Meta-Analysis of Nonvital Pulp Therapy for Primary Teeth. *Pediatr. Dent.* **2020**, *42*, 256–461. [PubMed]
26. Gharib, S.R.; Tordik, P.A.; Imamura, G.M.; Baginski, T.A.; Goodell, G.G. A Confocal Laser Scanning Microscope Investigation of the Epiphany Obturation System. *J. Endod.* **2007**, *33*, 957–961. [CrossRef]
27. Kikinis, R.; Pieper, S.D.; Vosburgh, K.G. 3D Slicer: A Platform for Subject-Specific Image Analysis, Visualization, and Clinical Support. In *Intraoperative Imaging and Image-Guided Therapy*; Jolesz, F.A., Ed.; Springer: New York, NY, USA, 2014; pp. 277–289. ISBN 978-1-4614-7657-3.
28. Kaloustian, M.K.; Hachem, C.E.; Zogheib, C.; Nehme, W.; Hardan, L.; Rached, P.; Kharouf, N.; Haikel, Y.; Mancino, D. Effectiveness of the REvision System and Sonic Irrigation in the Removal of Root Canal Filling Material from Oval Canals: An In Vitro Study. *Bioengineering* **2022**, *9*, 260. [CrossRef]
29. Kharouf, N.; Eid, A.; Hardan, L.; Bourgi, R.; Arntz, Y.; Jmal, H.; Foschi, F.; Sauro, S.; Ball, V.; Haikel, Y.; et al. Antibacterial and Bonding Properties of Universal Adhesive Dental Polymers Doped with Pyrogallol. *Polymers* **2021**, *13*, 1538. [CrossRef]
30. Kharouf, N.; Pedullà, E.; La Rosa, G.R.M.; Bukiet, F.; Sauro, S.; Haikel, Y.; Mancino, D. In Vitro Evaluation of Different Irrigation Protocols on Intracanal Smear Layer Removal in Teeth with or without Pre-Endodontic Proximal Wall Restoration. *J. Clin. Med.* **2020**, *9*, 3325. [CrossRef]
31. Kharouf, N.; Arntz, Y.; Eid, A.; Zghal, J.; Sauro, S.; Haikel, Y.; Mancino, D. Physicochemical and Antibacterial Properties of Novel, Premixed Calcium Silicate-Based Sealer Compared to Powder–Liquid Bioceramic Sealer. *J. Clin. Med.* **2020**, *9*, 3096. [CrossRef]
32. El Hachem, C.; Kaloustian, M.K.; Nehme, W.; Ghosn, N.; Abou Chedid, J.C. Three-Dimensional Modeling and Measurements of Root Canal Anatomy in Second Primary Mandibular Molars: A Case Series Micro CT Study. *Eur. Arch. Paediatr. Dent.* **2019**, *20*, 457–465. [CrossRef] [PubMed]
33. Aksoy, U.; Küçük, M.; Versiani, M.A.; Orhan, K. Publication Trends in Micro-CT Endodontic Research: A Bibliometric Analysis over a 25-Year Period. *Int. Endod. J.* **2021**, *54*, 343–353. [CrossRef] [PubMed]
34. Bernardes, R.A.; Duarte, M.a.H.; Vivan, R.R.; Alcalde, M.P.; Vasconcelos, B.C.; Bramante, C.M. Comparison of Three Retreatment Techniques with Ultrasonic Activation in Flattened Canals Using Micro-Computed Tomography and Scanning Electron Microscopy. *Int. Endod. J.* **2016**, *49*, 890–897. [CrossRef]
35. Jung, M.; Lommel, D.; Klimek, J. The Imaging of Root Canal Obturation Using Micro-CT. *Int. Endod. J.* **2005**, *38*, 617–626. [CrossRef] [PubMed]

36. Celikten, B.; Uzuntas, C.F.; Orhan, A.I.; Orhan, K.; Tufenkci, P.; Kursun, S.; Demiralp, K.Ö. Evaluation of Root Canal Sealer Filling Quality Using a Single-Cone Technique in Oval Shaped Canals: An In Vitro Micro-CT Study. *Scanning* **2016**, *38*, 133–140. [CrossRef]
37. Migliau, G.; Palaia, G.; Pergolini, D.; Guglielmelli, T.; Fascetti, R.; Sofan, A.; Del Vecchio, A.; Romeo, U. Comparison of Two Root Canal Filling Techniques: Obturation with Guttacore Carrier Based System and Obturation with Guttaflow2 Fluid Gutta-Percha. *Dent. J.* **2022**, *10*, 71. [CrossRef]
38. Subramaniam, P.; Gilhotra, K. Endoflas, Zinc Oxide Eugenol and Metapex as Root Canal Filling Materials in Primary Molars—A Comparative Clinical Study. *J. Clin. Pediatr. Dent.* **2011**, *35*, 365–370. [CrossRef] [PubMed]
39. Orhan, A.I.; Tatli, E.C. Evaluation of Root Canal Obturation Quality in Deciduous Molars with Different Obturation Materials: An In Vitro Micro-Computed Tomography Study. *Biomed. Res. Int.* **2021**, *2021*, 6567161. [CrossRef]
40. Siqueira, J.F.; Favieri, A.; Gahyva, S.M.M.; Moraes, S.R.; Lima, K.C.; Lopes, H.P. Antimicrobial Activity and Flow Rate of Newer and Established Root Canal Sealers. *J. Endod.* **2000**, *26*, 274–277. [CrossRef]
41. Kim, Y.; Kim, B.-S.; Kim, Y.-M.; Lee, D.; Kim, S.-Y. The Penetration Ability of Calcium Silicate Root Canal Sealers into Dentinal Tubules Compared to Conventional Resin-Based Sealer: A Confocal Laser Scanning Microscopy Study. *Materials* **2019**, *12*, 531. [CrossRef]
42. Caceres, C.; Larrain, M.R.; Monsalve, M.; Peña-Bengoa, F. Dentinal Tubule Penetration and Adaptation of Bio-C Sealer and AH-Plus: A Comparative SEM Evaluation. *Eur. Endod. J.* **2021**, *6*, 216–220. [CrossRef] [PubMed]
43. Furtado, T.C.; de Bem, I.A.; Machado, L.S.; Pereira, J.R.; Só, M.V.R.; da Rosa, R.A. Intratubular Penetration of Endodontic Sealers Depends on the Fluorophore Used for CLSM Assessment. *Microsc. Res. Tech.* **2021**, *84*, 305–312. [CrossRef] [PubMed]
44. Van Der Sluis, L.W.M.; Wu, M.-K.; Wesselink, P.R. The Efficacy of Ultrasonic Irrigation to Remove Artificially Placed Dentine Debris from Human Root Canals Prepared Using Instruments of Varying Taper. *Int. Endod. J.* **2005**, *38*, 764–768. [CrossRef] [PubMed]
45. Resende, L.M.; Rached-Junior, F.J.A.; Versiani, M.A.; Souza-Gabriel, A.E.; Miranda, C.E.S.; Silva-Sousa, Y.T.C.; Sousa Neto, M.D. A Comparative Study of Physicochemical Properties of AH Plus, Epiphany, and Epiphany SE Root Canal Sealers. *Int. Endod. J.* **2009**, *42*, 785–793. [CrossRef] [PubMed]
46. Mirfendereski, M.; Roth, K.; Fan, B.; Dubrowski, A.; Carnahan, H.; Azarpazhooh, A.; Basrani, B.; Torneck, C.D.; Friedman, S. Technique Acquisition in the Use of Two Thermoplasticized Root Filling Methods by Inexperienced Dental Students: A Microcomputed Tomography Analysis. *J. Endod.* **2009**, *35*, 1512–1517. [CrossRef] [PubMed]
47. Cancio, V.; de Carvalho Ferreira, D.; Cavalcante, F.S.; Rosado, A.S.; Teixeira, L.M.; Braga Oliveira, Q.; Barcelos, R.; Gleiser, R.; Santos, H.F.; dos Santos, K.R.N.; et al. Can the Enterococcus Faecalis Identified in the Root Canals of Primary Teeth Be a Cause of Failure of Endodontic Treatment? *Acta Odontol. Scand.* **2017**, *75*, 423–428. [CrossRef]
48. Huang, T.-H.; Hung, C.-J.; Chen, Y.-J.; Chien, H.-C.; Kao, C.-T. Cytologic Effects of Primary Tooth Endodontic Filling Materials. *J. Dent. Sci.* **2009**, *4*, 18–24. [CrossRef]
49. Tannure, P.N.; Azevedo, C.P.; Barcelos, R.; Gleiser, R.; Primo, L.G. Long-Term Outcomes of Primary Tooth Pulpectomy with and without Smear Layer Removal: A Randomized Split-Mouth Clinical Trial. *Pediatr. Dent.* **2011**, *33*, 316–320.

Disclaimer/Publisher's Note: The statements, opinions and data contained in all publications are solely those of the individual author(s) and contributor(s) and not of MDPI and/or the editor(s). MDPI and/or the editor(s) disclaim responsibility for any injury to people or property resulting from any ideas, methods, instructions or products referred to in the content.

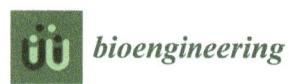

Article

Porcelain Veneers in Vital vs. Non-Vital Teeth: A Retrospective Clinical Evaluation

Maciej Zarow [1], Louis Hardan [2], Katarzyna Szczeklik [3], Rim Bourgi [2,4], Carlos Enrique Cuevas-Suárez [5,*], Natalia Jakubowicz [1], Marco Nicastro [6], Walter Devoto [7], Marzena Dominiak [8], Jolanta Pytko-Polończyk [3], Wioletta Bereziewicz [3] and Monika Lukomska-Szymanska [9,*]

1 "NZOZ SPS Dentist" Dental Clinic and Postgraduate Course Centre, 30-033 Cracow, Poland
2 Department of Restorative Dentistry, School of Dentistry, Saint-Joseph University, Beirut 1107 2180, Lebanon
3 Department of Integrated Dentistry, Institute of Dentistry, Faculty of Medicine, Jagiellonian University Medical College, Montelupich 4, 31-155 Krakow, Poland
4 Department of Biomaterials and Bioengineering, INSERM UMR_S 1121, Biomaterials and Bioengineering, 67000 Strasbourg, France
5 Dental Materials Laboratory, Academic Area of Dentistry, Autonomous University of Hidalgo State, Circuito Ex Hacienda La Concepción S/N, San Agustín Tlaxiaca 42160, Mexico
6 "Studio Nicastro" Dental Clinic, Corso Trieste 142, 00198 Roma, Italy
7 Independent Researcher, 16030 Sestri Levante, Italy
8 Department of Dental Surgery, Silesian Piast Medical University, ul. Krakowska 26, 50-425 Wrocław, Poland
9 Department of General Dentistry, Medical University of Lodz, 251 Pomorska St., 92-213 Lodz, Poland
* Correspondence: cecuevas@uaeh.edu.mx (C.E.C.-S.); monika.lukomska-szymanska@umed.lodz.pl (M.L.-S.); Tel.: +52-(771)-72000 (C.E.C.-S.); +48-605-721-200 or +48-426-757-429 (M.L.-S.)

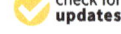

Citation: Zarow, M.; Hardan, L.; Szczeklik, K.; Bourgi, R.; Cuevas-Suárez, C.E.; Jakubowicz, N.; Nicastro, M.; Devoto, W.; Dominiak, M.; Pytko-Polończyk, J.; et al. Porcelain Veneers in Vital vs. Non-Vital Teeth: A Retrospective Clinical Evaluation. *Bioengineering* 2023, 10, 168. https://doi.org/10.3390/bioengineering10020168

Academic Editor: Angelo Michele Inchingolo

Received: 19 December 2022
Revised: 21 January 2023
Accepted: 26 January 2023
Published: 28 January 2023

Copyright: © 2023 by the authors. Licensee MDPI, Basel, Switzerland. This article is an open access article distributed under the terms and conditions of the Creative Commons Attribution (CC BY) license (https://creativecommons.org/licenses/by/4.0/).

Abstract: Nowadays, the ceramic veneer approach can be considered more predictable than direct composite veneer. To date, there is a lack of studies comparing the clinical performance of anterior veneers cemented on vital teeth (VT) and non-vital teeth (NVT). This longitudinal clinical study investigated the performance of ceramic veneers in VT or anterior NVT. A total of 55 patients were evaluated in the study. Two groups were defined based on the vitality status of the teeth (93 teeth—vital and 61 teeth—non-vital). The United States Public Health Service (USPHS) criteria were used to assess the clinical status. The data were evaluated statistically with the Mann–Whitney U test. All restorations were considered acceptable, and only one veneer in VT failed for the criteria of secondary caries. There were no statistically significant differences in any of the criteria evaluated ($p \leq 0.671$). The ceramic veneers evaluated showed a satisfactory clinical performance both in VT and NVT.

Keywords: anterior restorations; ceramic; dental veneers; follow-up; non-vital teeth; porcelain laminate veneers; vital teeth

1. Introduction

Facial and dental aesthetics are currently considered crucial for patients aiming to boost their self-confidence [1,2]. Displeasure with tooth color and shape has amplified the request for aesthetic dental approaches. There are two frequently applied and non-invasive options available to resolve aesthetic problems in contemporary dentistry, namely, direct composites and porcelain veneers [3].

On the one hand, direct composite veneers can be a perfect, minimally invasive, and long-lasting treatment to enhance the color, shape, and incisal embrasures of the teeth [4,5]. The tooth preparation can often be avoided, and direct non-preparation composite veneers can be performed. This solution is especially indicated for adolescent and young patients. Moreover, composite veneers can be easily repaired and corrected if color or shape alterations are needed. Additionally, the hardness and wear resistance of composites are more similar to enamel than porcelain, and accordingly, this material may be preferred to restore mandibular anterior teeth. The anatomical stratification of resin composite along with the application of tints and/or opaquers helps to mimic tooth color, providing an aesthetic appearance [4]. This could be possible in one visit, and the key conditions to attain these cases are to understand dental morphology and to master the diverse layers of resin composite [4]. It should be emphasized that there are some drawbacks associated with the application of resin composite, namely, marginal leakage, low wear resistance, inferior color stability, susceptibility to discoloration, or difficulty in the removal of excess material [6–8]. However, composite veneers are an excellent choice in cases of small tooth repairs, including small chips, minor misalignment, slight discoloration, tooth shape correction, and diastema closure [4,8]. As a relative contraindication, severe discoloration can be considered when opaque materials are applied to mask the discolored tooth structure; thus, the final aesthetic outcome can be compromised. Additionally, occlusal risk factors (occlusal dysfunction, constricted chewing pattern, bruxism, parafunctions, etc.) and severely structurally compromised teeth may also be regarded as contraindications [9]. Moreover, the long-term success of direct composites may depend on patient selection, cavity location and size, material choice, and operative technique [5,7,8].

On the other hand, ceramic veneers have become the primary choice for patients when color alteration (i.e., tetracycline discoloration, non-vital tooth), space closure, shape correction, and the reconstruction of worn, misaligned, malformed, or fractured teeth are needed [3,10–12]. Nowadays, the ceramic veneer approach can be considered more predictable than direct composite veneers in the case of discolored teeth due to laboratory manufacturing and enhanced ceramic properties. Moreover, comprehensive treatment including numerous teeth and complex smile correction (inclination of the axis of individual teeth, relationship of the central incisors to the lateral incisors, etc.) can be meticulously planned and executed in cooperation with the dental technician to achieve perfect final restorations. These restorations can absolutely imitate the characteristics of the tooth structure [3,13], providing good mechanical properties, high aesthetics, biocompatibility, and long-term clinical performance [14–19]. Additionally, minimally invasive preparation and the easy removal of cement excesses along with the ceramic material exhibiting enhanced properties turn this treatment option into a preferred solution. In contrast, it requires more appointments and is more expensive and difficult to repair in the case of ceramic chipping or breakage.

In turn, resin composite veneers can be used as an alternative choice for ceramic veneers in the anterior area; however, limited longevity can affect the final aesthetic outcome of the restoration [20,21]. On the contrary, ceramic veneers (especially felspathic porcelain veneers) offer a durable aesthetic result due to the ability to reproduce the luster of natural teeth and the life-like appearance of the patient [14,22]. The selection of indirect ceramic restoration provides aesthetic reconstructions with higher abrasion resistance, biocompatibility, color stability, appropriate translucency, exceptional marginal integrity, and contour stability. Further, one should state that the preparation is not subgingival in most of the veneer cases, and considering this, porcelain veneers are associated with a low risk of gingival irritation owing to a hindered plaque accumulation on the restoration surface and at the interface [23].

To date, there is a lack of studies comparing the clinical performance of anterior veneers cemented on vital teeth (VT) and non-vital teeth (NVT). Therefore, the aim of this retrospective study was to investigate the clinical behavior of indirect porcelain ceramic veneers cemented on vital and non-vital anterior teeth.

2. Materials and Methods

2.1. Study Characteristics, Participants, and Design

The study was designed as a retrospective evaluation of indirect porcelain veneers cemented on VT and NVT. Informed consent was obtained from all individuals. The recall took place between January 2019 and July 2022. The inclusion criteria were as follows: veneers made from feldspathic porcelain by one dental technician and cemented by one restorative dentist, stable occlusion, full dentition, anterior teeth without occlusal overloading (no sensation of fremitus), VT with confirmed vitality status, NVT with acceptable root canal filling, the absence of periapical lesion, and the presence or lack of fiber post. The exclusion criteria included: subgingival class V restoration beyond cemento–enamel junction, patient under the age of 25 years, and composite restorations exceeding 50% of the adhesive surface. The study obtained the permission of the ethical commission of Jagiellonian University (no. 122.6120.60.2016).

The study population consisted of 55 patients restored with anterior porcelain veneer restorations. Two groups were defined based on the vitality status of the teeth. The VT group consisted of 25 patients (18 females, 7 males) with a mean age of 51.03 years. In total, 93 VT (38 central incisors including only one mandibular incisor, 37 lateral incisors, and 18 canines) were evaluated after a mean observation period of 8.3 years. The NVT group consisted of 30 patients (24 females, 6 males) with a mean age of 46.2 years. In this group, a total of 61 teeth (43 central incisors, 16 lateral incisors, and 2 canines) were evaluated after a mean observation period of 7 years. The distribution according to patient-related factors is shown in Table 1.

Table 1. Distribution of porcelain veneer restorations.

Independent Variable	n	%
Sex		
Male	13	23.6
Female	42	76.3
Total	55	100
Tooth type		
Central incisor	81	52.6
Lateral incisor	53	34.4
Canine	20	13.0
Total	154	100
Follow-up time (years)		
0.5–2	3	1.9
2–3.9	1	0.7
4–5.9	43	27.9
6–7.9	22	14.3
More than 8	85	55.2
Total	154	100
Tooth vitality		
Vital	93	60.4
Non-vital	61	39.6
Total	154	100

2.2. Pre-Treatment Procedures

All restorations were changed to new ones according to indications. In all cases, the color was evaluated by both the dental technician and clinician before starting the porcelain veneer preparation. Additionally, photographs of the tooth before and after preparation were obtained.

The shape of the new porcelain veneers was tested by the mock-up procedure. Transferring the shape of the tooth from the wax-up was performed by means of a silicone index I (Zeta Plus L, Zhermack, Badia Polesine, Italy). The silicone excess was cut away with a surgical scalpel or a straight handpiece carbide bur, and then a composite temporization material (Protemp, 3M ESPE, St. Paul, MN, USA) was applied to the index and was introduced on the teeth. After the composite resin had fully set (about 5 min), the silicone index was gently removed and the excess material on the palatal side and the proximal surfaces was discarded.

Additionally, the silicon index II (Zeta Labor, Zhermack, Italy) was performed based on the diagnostic wax-up and cut with a scalpel no 10 (Swann Morton, Sheffield, England) into two parts in order to control the tooth reduction.

2.3. Tooth Preparation Procedure

The porcelain veneer preparation was made from the temporary mock-up and used additional index II as a control. All of the preparation procedures were performed under local anesthesia (Ubistesin™ Forte Local, 3M ESPE, St. Paul, MN, USA). Horizontal grooves were created on the labial surface and vertical ones on the incisal edge of the mock-up using burs no. 868B018 and 68016 (Komet Brasseler, Lemgo, Germany) on an electric red ring 1:5 increasing contra-angle handpiece with copious water cooling. After the removal of the mock-up under loupe magnification (Zeiss 4.3, Oberkochen, Germany), the minimal invasive outline of the preparation (less than 0.2 mm) was performed using a round ball diamond bur (bur no. 801012, Komet Brasseler, Lemgo, Germany). Then, the incisal edge was reduced by 1.5 to 2 mm in relation to the planned final length of the porcelain veneer (based on the index II and the vertical grooves). The leveling of the labial surface was performed in three different planes: the cervical, the middle, and the incisal. The preparation on the incisal edge was finished with a butt joint. In the case of a sound proximal tooth structure, no interproximal preparation was conducted. Otherwise, in the case of existing composite restorations on the interproximal area, a "wrap around" veneer was performed. Next, the retractive cord #000 (Ultradent, Indaiatuba, Brazil) (without hemostatic agent) was delicately placed using a dental explorer (DG 16 mg 6, HU FRIEDY, USA) into the gingival sulcus for a minimal gingival retraction. The margin of the preparation was brought closer to the gingiva and the outline was clearly marked (bur no. 6844014, Komet Brasseler, Lemgo, Germany). Finally, the surface was smoothed with a silicon polisher no. 9608 (Brownie Point, Komet Dental, Lemgo, Germany) on a contra-angle handpiece with copious water cooling (speed of 5000 rpm). After polishing, all clearly visible imperfections such as sharp edges and unrounded angles were corrected with a gentle motion of the red ring contra-angle handpiece (Synea, WK-99L; W&H, Austria) and fine diamond bur (no. 8868 314 016, Komet Dental, Lemgo, Germany).

2.4. Impression Procedure and Occlusion Registration

Next, a second retraction cord was soaked with a hemostatic agent (cord #0, Ultradent, Indaiatuba, Brazil) and gently placed in the gingival sulcus as described above, and left for 5 to 10 min. Just before the impression, the second retraction cord was removed from the gingival sulcus and the medium body silicon material (Variotime Medium Flow, Heraeus Kulzer, Hanau, Germany) was syringed directly from an Automix system along the gingival margin and on all surfaces of the prepared teeth. The metal impression tray selected based on the width of the dental arch was filled with Automix Heavy Tray a-silicon (Variotime Tray, Heraeus Kulzer GmbH, Germany) and placed on the dental arch and stabilized.

Occlusion was registered with Aluwax bite wax in the maximum intercuspation position (MIP). The impression of the opposing arch was made with alginate impression material and immediately poured with stone.

2.5. Temporalization

The temporary veneers were obtained with the temporary resin (Protemp, 3MESPE, USA) using previously fabricated silicon index I. Provisional veneers remained seated on the teeth thanks to material retention in the interproximal areas; part of the material was left in this area for adequate maintenance until the next visit. Any excess of the material around the gingival papilla was meticulously removed using scalpel no.12 or an Excesso instrument (LM Dental, Turku, Finland). The remaining excess was gently removed with a bur no. 889540009 to avoid bleeding.

2.6. Laboratory Procedure

All porcelain veneers were fabricated in the dental laboratory (by a skilled dental technician) by means of a traditional approach used for the feldspathic porcelain.

2.7. Clinical Try-In and Luting Procedure

The temporary veneers were carefully removed with a solid curette. Next, the veneers were positioned on the teeth and the fit was examined. The interproximal contacts and color were evaluated.

The teeth were isolated with a rubber dam (Nic Tone Dental Dam, thick, mint, MDC dental, Zapopan, Mexico) using the Hygienic B5, B6, or Brinker clamps (Hygienic, Coltene Whaledent, Germany) and the porcelain veneers were again tried in to check for any interferences with the clamps.

The porcelain veneers were cleaned with 70% alcohol and etched with 9% hydrofluoric acid (Ultradent™ Porcelain Etch, USA) for 90 s. Next, the hydrofluoric acid was rinsed from the inner surface of the porcelain veneer with a water spray for 30 s, placed for 5 min in an ultrasound bath, air-dried and silanized with a minimum of three layers of silane (Ultradent Products, South Jordan, UT, USA) for 60 s. Then, the adhesive system EnaBond Seal (Micerium, Genova, Italy) was applied as one layer spread on the inner surface of the porcelain veneer, very thoroughly blown with air-spray to the thin layer, and was protected from strong sources of light to avoid the accidental activation of polymerization.

The prepared tooth was sandblasted with an abrasive unit (27 μm aluminum oxide powder; 40 PSI) in order to remove contaminations such as blood, dental plaque, or materials used for the provisional veneers. Then, orthophosphoric acid (Conditioner36, Dentsply DeTrey, Gmbh, Konstanz, Germany) with the consistency of a gel was applied over the entire preparation surface and actively spread for 20 s and meticulously rinsed with water for 10–20 s and dried. The adhesive system (Ena Bond, Micerium, Genova, Italy) was applied precisely to the entire preparation surface by rubbing in successive layers, and then very thoroughly blown to the thin and homogenous layer before polymerization. The adhesive system was polymerized for 20 s using an LED curing unit (Elipar, 3M ESPE St Paul, MN, USA). Conventional resin composite Enamel Plus (Micerium, Genova, Italy) material (UD3) was heated in a composite heating conditioner (ENA Heat, Micerium, Genova, Italy) up to 55 °C. Next, a thin layer of the heated composite was applied on the entire inner surface of the porcelain veneer. The porcelain veneers were placed on the corresponding teeth and pressed with fingers to reach the desired position (the porcelain veneer–tooth margin was meticulosity inspected). The excess of luting composite was removed from the buccal and palatal surface using a dental probe wetted in unfilled resin (ENA Seal Bond, Micerium, Genova, Italy). On the interproximal surfaces, the excess material was removed with dental floss (Oral B Satin floss, Procter & Gamble, Cincinnati, OH, USA). Next, the porcelain veneers were polymerized for 3 s on the labial surface and the procedure of removing the excess material was repeated. All of the margins were covered with glycerin gel and the final polymerization was carried out for 60 s on each surface (labial side gingivally, the incisal edge, and palatal surface close to the incisal edge). After the final polymerization, the excess composite resin was removed with scalpel no. 12 (Swann Morton, Sheffield, England).

2.8. Occlusal Adjustment and Polishing

Any premature contacts were removed from the porcelain veneer. The patient was seated to assure the upper body position at the inclination of 45°. Then, the fingertips of the operator were placed on the teeth with the porcelain veneers and the patient was asked to bite repeatedly in the MIP. If finger vibrations (fremitus) were detected, the dentist corrected the premature contacts immediately with a diamond bur Komet # 368-016 Bud FG coupled to a W&H contra-angle. A 200 μm horseshoe articulating paper was used to detect premature contacts in order to provide a "base" for the thin and more accurate 16 μm red articulation foil. The premature contact points marked on the front teeth with red and blue articulating paper were eliminated. Then, the patient was seated in the upright position (90°), a 200 μm horseshoe articulating paper was positioned between the teeth, and the patient was asked to simulate chewing a piece of gum. This test was supposed to mimic real chewing while eating [24]. Any extensive blue surfaces (representing an overload between the maxillary and mandibular anterior teeth) that appeared on the front teeth, especially on the palatal surfaces of the porcelain veneers were eliminated. Restoration margins were polished with silicone polishers (Astropol FP, HP, Ivoclar Vivadent, Schaan, Liechtenstein) and interproximal polishing strips (Soft-Lex Finishing Strips, 3M ESPE, Seefeld, Germany).

All patients received written hygiene recommendations in order to avoid using hard toothbrushes or abrasive toothpastes.

2.9. Evaluation Procedures

An independent and blinded calibrated operator performed follow-up examinations. The patients were examined clinically and with intraoral periapical X-ray. The clinical evaluation included: secondary caries, marginal adaptation, marginal discoloration, color match, restoration integrity, and surface roughness according to modified United States Public Health Service (USPHS) criteria (Table 2).

Table 2. Modified United States Public Health Service criteria used for restoration assessment.

Category	Criterion	Definition
Secondary Caries	ALPHA	No evidence of caries
	CHARLIE	Caries is evident, contiguous with the margin of the restoration
Marginal Adaptation	ALPHA	Restoration is contiguous with existing anatomical form, explorer does not catch
	BRAVO	Explorer catches, no crevice is visible into which explorer will penetrate
	CHARLIE	Obvious crevice at margin, dentine or base exposed
	DELTA	Restoration mobile, fractured partially or totally
Marginal Discoloration	ALPHA	No discoloration evident
	BRAVO	Slight staining: can be polished away
	CHARLIE	Obvious staining: cannot be polished away
	DELTA	Gross staining
Color Match	ALPHA	Very good color match
	BRAVO	Slight mismatch in color, shade, or translucency
	CHARLIE	Obvious mismatch, outside the normal range
	DELTA	Gross mismatch
Restoration Integrity	ALPHA	No material defect, no crack
	BRAVO	Two or more cracks not compromising marginal integrity or contacts
	CHARLIE	Restorative fractures compromising marginal integrity or contacts
	DELTA	Partial or complete restorative loss
Surface Roughness	ALPHA	Smooth surface
	BRAVO	Slightly rough or pitted
	CHARLIE	Rough, cannot be refinished
	DELTA	Surface deeply pitted, irregular grooves

Figures 1 and 2 show a case of the veneer preparation of two upper incisors.

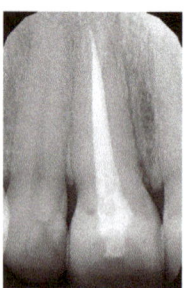

Figure 1. RVG image showing the endo-treated teeth.

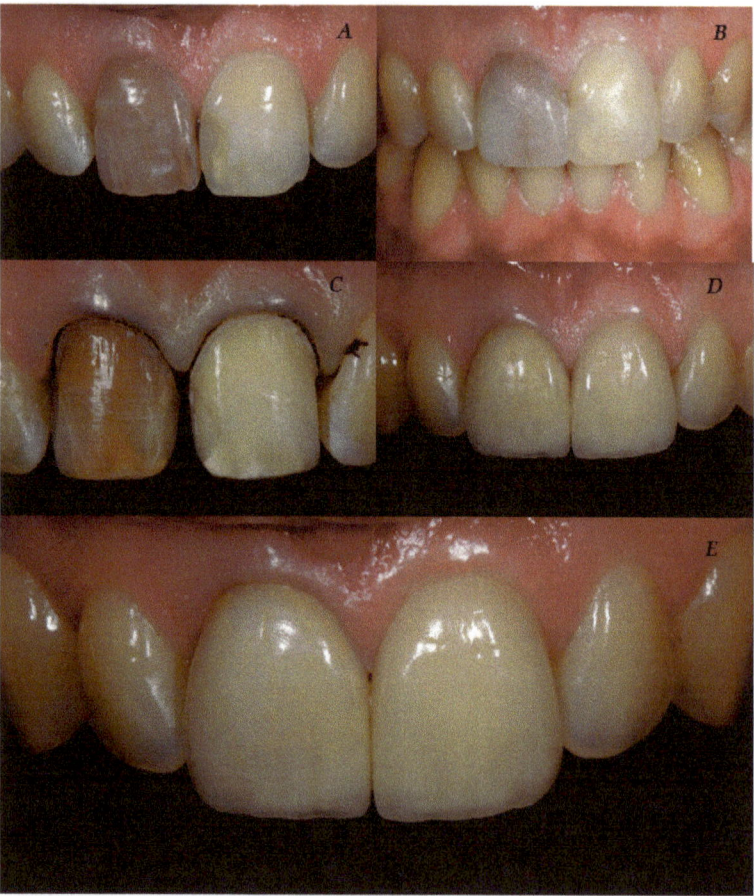

Figure 2. Description of the veneer preparation of two upper central incisors. (**A**) Preoperative situation; (**B**) mock-up; (**C**) tooth preparation procedure; (**D**) immediately after cementation; and (**E**) 6 years follow-up.

2.10. Statistical Analysis

The performance of the restorations was assessed using the Mann–Whitney non-parametric statistical analysis. The level of significance was set at $p < 0.05$. The statistical analyses were conducted using the SigmaPlot software (SigmaPlot 12.0, SPSS Inc., Chicago, IL, USA).

3. Results

The qualitative evaluation using USPHS criteria for the restorations evaluated is shown in Table 3. All restorations were considered acceptable; however, one porcelain veneer cemented on a VT failed due to secondary caries. Despite this, there were no statistically significant differences in any of the criteria evaluated ($p \leq 0.671$).

Table 3. Clinical evaluation of anterior porcelain veneers: comparison between vital and non-vital teeth, according to the United States Public Health Service criteria.

	Vital Teeth		Non-Vital Teeth		Mann–Whitney p
	Restoration Scores (A/B/C/D)	Restorations Clinically Acceptable	Restoration Scores (A/B/C/D)	Restorations Clinically Acceptable	
Secondary Caries	92/1/-/-	98.9%	61/0/-/-	100%	0.188
Marginal Adaptation	66/27/0/0	100%	52/9/0/0	100%	0.635
Marginal Discoloration	66/27/0/0	100%	46/15/0/0	100%	0.871
Color Match	93/0/0/0	100%	59/2/0/0	100%	0.648
Restoration Integrity	91/2/0/0	100%	60/1/0/0	100%	0.867
Surface Roughness	92/1/0/0	100%	60/1/0/0	100%	0.893

4. Discussion

A longitudinal study was conducted evaluating the clinical behavior of indirect porcelain veneers performed in VT and NVT. USPHS Evaluation System criteria were used, as suggested in the literature [25–27]. The qualitative evaluation showed acceptable results for all of the restorations evaluated, although one porcelain veneer cemented on a VT failed due to secondary caries. All in all, the survival rate of these restorations and all of the characteristics were satisfactory after 8-year clinical performance.

Previous longitudinal clinical reports have assessed the performance of dental ceramic veneer restorations and have proven good clinical performance, outstanding aesthetics, and patient fulfilment [16,18,19,21]. In the present study, the porcelain veneers exhibited a higher survival rate of 97.9%–100% after 8 years of performance, which is supported by others reporting survival rate of 91% to 100% [28,29]. A survival rate varying from 80.1 to 100% was found after a follow-up of less than 5 years [30] and of 47 to 100% after 5 to 7 years of clinical service [31–33]. In addition, studies with a follow-up of 10 to 12 years presented a survival rate of 53 to 94.4% [22,29,34].

Indirect veneers can be used as an alternative to full-coverage restorations, since they prevent the aggressive preparation and removal of the palatal tooth structure, therefore preserving dental structure [35]. However, there are many possible well-known failures that can occur to the ceramic veneers including debonding, chipping, fracture, margin discoloration, or secondary caries. Secondary caries was also known as a lesion at the margin level of an existing restoration [33]. In this study, this was only found in the case of one restoration. This particular porcelain veneer was cemented onto the tooth with both mesial and distal composite restorations (class IIIMD). This particular case belongs to a female patient who went through a stressful period in her life and did not perform her mouth care in a proper manner. Both factors—the stress, which can be a cause of xerostomia, and the improper hygiene—could be the reasons for the secondary caries [36].

In addition, the presence of secondary caries at the veneer–tooth interface could be explained by various other factors. Poor oral hygiene, caries susceptibility, and saliva or blood contamination due to the lack of rubber dam isolation during the cementation procedure were described as possible reasons [37]. In this retrospective study, the rubber dam was placed in all cases and the patients were monitored by means of professional hygiene. It was shown that the restorations performed under rubber dam isolation developed a lower failure rate than restorations completed with saliva ejectors and cotton rolls only [37]. In summary, patient- and operator-related factors influence the success rate. Low-risk patients under controlled settings might be a reason for the lower level of secondary caries lesions [38–40]. This supports the findings of this study, as secondary caries lesions developed in only one case.

It is worth emphasizing that, in terms of the clinical success of ceramic restorations, a marginal fit was considered an important factor [41–43]. The external marginal adaptation of ceramic veneers, which is expressed as the vertical distance between the margins of the fabricated veneers and the finish line of the prepared tooth, significantly influences the success rate of the restoration [43]. Since this parameter was acceptable both for VT and NVT, the restorations exhibited good marginal adaptation, therefore minimizing the contact surface of the cement with the oral environment [41]. On the other hand, the internal marginal adaptation is defined by a measurement of the cement film thickness under the dental restoration and is notably prejudiced by the accuracy of the fabrication procedure used [44]. In case of poor internal marginal adaptation, a negative correlation can occur between the thickness of the luting cement and the stress distribution on the inner and outer surfaces of the veneer, which could lead to crack propagation within the restoration [45]. It seems that all of the porcelain veneer restorations were accurate in terms of the fabrication process, which could support the finding of the present study.

For the restoration integrity, the combination of minimal preparation through mock-up provided the maximal conservative approach [46]. A butt joint design was used in this study, as suggested by Castelnuovo et al., who proved the best performance of this preparation modality [47]. It provides the enhanced bonding between the tooth structure and the ceramic material as a consequence of keeping the peripheral enamel layer around the margins and preventing microleakage formation, especially at the interface on the palatal surface, owing to an improved shear stress distribution [47]. Moreover, the literature revealed that significantly better marginal adaptation is observed when etch-and-rinse method along with primer and adhesive were applied [48].

The differences in the marginal discoloration between VT and NVT were not statistically significant in this study. A previous retrospective study with a follow-up of 10 years yielded a survival rate of 93.5%, and 82.8% after 20 years [49]. Beier et al. [49] considered the marginal discoloration as a minor complication since it occurred in 21.3% of cases, predominantly in smokers. This observation is not supported by the present study, where no discoloration with deep penetration of the restoration margins was perceived, and the survival rate was higher. However, both studies cannot be compared due to the different restoration geometry and diverse inclusion and exclusion criteria.

Additionally, all restorations exhibited satisfactory stable color behavior. The color of the veneer restoration matched the color of the VT and endodontically treated teeth. It is important to emphasize that due to the close cooperation between the laboratory and the dentist, the color of the restoration was evaluated individually. The shade, thickness, and type of ceramic materials affected the final color of the ceramic veneer restorations since a target color of the veneer and tooth cannot often be chosen by the practitioner [50–52]. Diverse resin cement shades could be selected to modify the final color outcome of the ceramic veneer restoration [50–52]. In all cases, the same shade was applied, thus no difference in color match was observed. In addition, the thickness of a ceramic veneer restoration is restricted by the minimal amount of tooth preparation and target restorative space.

One should bear in mind that the color of endodontically treated teeth is frequently compromised [53]. Diverse restorative approaches can be considered for discolored teeth starting from NVT bleaching, direct composite restorations, direct composite veneers, indirect veneers, and ending with ceramic crowns [54]. In the past, more invasive treatment alternatives such as crowns were frequently applied; however, recently, more conservative options are preferred in order to predictably restore the endodontically treated anterior tooth. However, there are still controversies among practitioners as to whether a porcelain veneer on a NVT is a reliable option and whether it can be widely recommended [55].

The composition and the surface structure of a dental restorative material impacts the initial bacterial adhesion. A rough material surface will promote more plaque formation [56]. During the evaluations with the follow-up approaches of the restorations presented in this study, no signs of porosity, defect, scratching, or disintegration on the surface were observed. These outcomes might be the reason for the highly polished feldspathic porcelain material used in this study both for treating VT or NVT [57,58]. Additionally, the patients were educated by a dental hygienist to avoid brushing with hard toothbrushes or abrasive toothpaste.

Some limitations could be found in the present study, including that only one adhesive technique, using the same adhesive system and resin cement, was used. The other limitations represent the relatively low number of restorations, the need for multi-center studies, the presence of pre-existing composite restorations, adhesive surface, the inhomogeneous status of the teeth within the study group, the difference between subjects regarding the occlusal relationship, and relatively different occlusal conditions that are difficult to calibrate ideally in the clinical studies. Moreover, different types of ceramics could be evaluated in further research including computer-aided design–computer-aided manufacturing (CAD-CAM)-based materials. Finally, a longer follow-up period is necessary to establish more conclusive findings.

5. Conclusions

Within the limitations of the current study, it can be concluded that the ceramic veneers showed a satisfactory clinical performance both on VT and NVT.

Author Contributions: Conceptualization, M.Z.; methodology, M.Z.; software, L.H., R.B., W.D., N.J. and C.E.C.-S.; validation, M.D., W.B., J.P.-P., M.L.-S. and K.S.; formal analysis, L.H., R.B., W.D., N.J., M.L.-S. and C.E.C.-S.; investigation, M.Z., M.D., M.N., W.B., J.P.-P., M.L.-S. and K.S.; resources, L.H., R.B., W.D., M.N., N.J. and C.E.C.-S.; data curation, M.Z.; writing—original draft preparation, M.Z., L.H., R.B., W.D., M.N., N.J. and C.E.C.-S.; writing—review and editing, M.Z., M.D., W.B., J.P.-P., M.L.-S., M.N., L.H. and K.S.; visualization, M.N., N.J., L.H., R.B. and C.E.C.-S.; supervision, L.H. and M.L.-S.; project administration, M.Z. All authors have read and agreed to the published version of the manuscript.

Funding: This research received no external funding.

Institutional Review Board Statement: The study obtained the permission of the ethical commission of Jagiellonian University (no. 122.6120.60.2016).

Informed Consent Statement: Not applicable.

Data Availability Statement: Not applicable.

Conflicts of Interest: The authors declare no conflict of interest.

References

1. Alshehri, K.A.; Alhejazi, M.A.; Almutairi, S.M.; Alshareef, A.H.; Alothman, K.J.; Alqarni, A.N.; Almutairi, M.S.; Matrood, M.A.; Noorsaeed, A.S. Overview on Dental Veneer Placement. *J. Pharm. Res. Int.* **2021**, *33*, 494–501.
2. Van Wezel, N.A.; Bos, A.; Prahl, C. Expectations of Treatment and Satisfaction with Dentofacial Appearance in Patients Applying for Orthodontic Treatment. *Am. J. Orthod. Dentofacial Orthop.* **2015**, *147*, 698–703. [CrossRef] [PubMed]
3. Monaraks, R.; Leevailoj, C. The Longevity of Ceramic Veneers: Clinical Evaluation of Mechanical, Biologic and Aesthetic Performances of Ceramic Veneers, a 7-Year Retrospective Study. *J. Dent. Assoc. Thai.* **2018**, *68*, 288–301.
4. Fahl, N., Jr.; Ritter, A.V. Composite Veneers: The Direct–Indirect Technique Revisited. *J. Esthet. Restor. Dent.* **2021**, *33*, 7–19. [CrossRef] [PubMed]
5. Korkut, B.; Yanıkoğlu, F.; Günday, M. Direct Composite Laminate Veneers: Three Case Reports. *J. Dent. Res. Dent. Clin. Dent. Prospects* **2013**, *7*, 105.
6. Nalbandian, S.; Millar, B. The Effect of Veneers on Cosmetic Improvement. *Br. Dent. J.* **2009**, *207*, E3. [CrossRef]
7. Alonso, V.; Caserio, M. A Clinical Study of Direct Composite Full-Coverage Crowns: Long-Term Results. *Oper. Dent.* **2012**, *37*, 432–441. [CrossRef]

8. Demarco, F.F.; Collares, K.; Coelho-de-Souza, F.H.; Correa, M.B.; Cenci, M.S.; Moraes, R.R.; Opdam, N.J. Anterior Composite Restorations: A Systematic Review on Long-Term Survival and Reasons for Failure. *Dent. Mater.* **2015**, *31*, 1214–1224. [CrossRef]
9. Pini, N.P.; Aguiar, F.H.B.; Lima, D.A.N.L.; Lovadino, J.R.; Terada, R.S.S.; Pascotto, R.C. Advances in Dental Veneers: Materials, Applications, and Techniques. *Clin. Cosmet. Investig. Dent.* **2012**, *4*, 9.
10. Peumans, M.; De Munck, J.; Fieuws, S.; Lambrechts, P.; Vanherle, G.; Van Meerbeek, B. A Prospective Ten-Year Clinical Trial of Porcelain Veneers. *J. Adhes. Dent.* **2004**, *6*, 65–76.
11. Freire, A.; Regina Archegas, L. Porcelain Laminate Veneer on a Highly Discoloured Tooth: A Case Report. *J. Can. Dent. Assoc.* **2010**, *76*, 305.
12. Walter, R.D.; Raigrodski, A.J.; Swift, J.; Edward, J. Clinical Considerations for Restoring Mandibular Incisors with Porcelain Laminate Veneers. *J. Esthet. Restor. Dent.* **2008**, *20*, 276–281. [CrossRef] [PubMed]
13. Chen, J.; Shi, C.; Wang, M.; Zhao, S.; Wang, H. Clinical Evaluation of 546 Tetracycline-Stained Teeth Treated with Porcelain Laminate Veneers. *J. Dent.* **2005**, *33*, 3–8. [CrossRef]
14. Zarow, M.; Ramirez-Sebastia, A.; Paolone, G.; de Ribot Porta, J.; Mora, J.; Espona, J.; Durán-Sindreu, F.; Roig, M. A New Classification System for the Restoration of Root Filled Teeth. *Int. Endod. J.* **2018**, *51*, 318–334. [CrossRef]
15. Fons Font, A.; Solá Ruiz, M.F.; Granell Ruiz, M.; Labaig Rueda, C.; Martínez González, A. Choice of Ceramic for Use in Treatments with Porcelain Laminate Veneers. *Chem. Dent.* **2006**, *11*, 297–302.
16. Gresnigt, M.; Cune, M.; Jansen, K.; Van der Made, S.; Özcan, M. Randomized Clinical Trial on Indirect Resin Composite and Ceramic Laminate Veneers: Up to 10-Year Findings. *J. Dent.* **2019**, *86*, 102–109. [CrossRef] [PubMed]
17. Soares-Rusu, I.B.; Villavicencio-Espinoza, C.A.; de Oliveira, N.A.; Wang, L.; Honório, H.M.; Rubo, J.H.; Borges, A.F. Using Digital Photographs as a Tool to Assess the Clinical Color Stability of Lithium Disilicate Veneers: A Clinical Trial. *J. Prosthet. Dent.* **2022**, *in press*. [CrossRef]
18. Gresnigt, M.M.M.; Cune, M.S.; Schuitemaker, J.; van der Made, S.A.M.; Meisberger, E.W.; Magne, P.; Özcan, M. Performance of Ceramic Laminate Veneers with Immediate Dentine Sealing: An 11 Year Prospective Clinical Trial. *Dent. Mater.* **2019**, *35*, 1042–1052. [CrossRef] [PubMed]
19. Schlichting, L.H.; Resende, T.H.; Reis, K.R.; Raybolt Dos Santos, A.; Correa, I.C.; Magne, P. Ultrathin CAD-CAM Glass Ceramic and Composite Resin Occlusal Veneers for the Treatment of Severe Dental Erosion: An up to 3-Year Randomized Clinical Trial. *J. Prosthet. Dent.* **2022**, *128*, 158.E1–158.E12. [CrossRef]
20. Abdulateef, O.F.; ÇOBANOĞLU, N. 12-Months Color Stability of Direct Resin Composite Veneers in Anterior Teeth: Clinical Trial. *J. Baghdad Coll. Dent.* **2022**, *34*, 42–49. [CrossRef]
21. Mazzetti, T.; Collares, K.; Rodolfo, B.; da Rosa Rodolpho, P.A.; van de Sande, F.H.; Cenci, M.S. 10-Year Practice-Based Evaluation of Ceramic and Direct Composite Veneers. *Dent. Mater.* **2022**, *38*, 898–906. [CrossRef]
22. Burke, F.T. Survival Rates for Porcelain Laminate Veneers with Special Reference to the Effect of Preparation in Dentin: A Literature Review. *J. Esthet. Restor. Dent.* **2012**, *24*, 257–265. [CrossRef] [PubMed]
23. Pereira, S.; Anami, L.; Pereira, C.; Souza, R.; Kantorski, K.; Bottino, M.; Jorge, A.; Valandro, L. Bacterial Colonization in the Marginal Region of Ceramic Restorations: Effects of Different Cement Removal Methods and Polishing. *Oper. Dent.* **2016**, *41*, 642–654. [CrossRef]
24. Kois, J.; Hartrick, N. Functional Occlusion: Science-Driven Management. *J. Cosmet. Dent.* **2007**, *23*, 54–55.
25. Hardan, L.; Mancino, D.; Bourgi, R.; Cuevas-Suárez, C.E.; Lukomska-Szymanska, M.; Zarow, M.; Jakubowicz, N.; Zamarripa-Calderón, J.E.; Kafa, L.; Etienne, O. Treatment of Tooth Wear Using Direct or Indirect Restorations: A Systematic Review of Clinical Studies. *Bioengineering* **2022**, *9*, 346. [CrossRef] [PubMed]
26. Cerutti, A.; Barabanti, N.; Özcan, M. Clinical Performance of Posterior Microhybrid Resin Composite Restorations Applied Using Regular and High-Power Mode Polymerization Protocols According to USPHS and SQUACE Criteria: 10-Year Randomized Controlled Split-Mouth Trial. *J. Adhes. Dent.* **2020**, *22*, 343–351.
27. Matos, T.P.; Hanzen, T.A.; Almeida, R.; Tardem, C.; Bandeca, M.C.; Barceleiro, M.O.; Loguercio, A.D.; Reis, A. Five-Year Randomized Clinical Trial on the Performance of Two Etch-and-Rinse Adhesives in Noncarious Cervical Lesions. *Oper. Dent.* **2022**, *47*, 31–42. [CrossRef]
28. Friedman, M. A 15-Year Review of Porcelain Veneer Failure—A Clinician's Observations. *Compend. Contin. Educ. Dent.* **1998**, *19*, 625–628.
29. Dumfahrt, H.; Schäffer, H. Porcelain Laminate Veneers. A Retrospective Evaluation after 1 to 10 Years of Service: Part II—Clinical Results. *Int. J. Prosthodont.* **2000**, *13*, 9–18. [PubMed]
30. Gresnigt, M.M.; Kalk, W.; Ozcan, M. Randomized Clinical Trial of Indirect Resin Composite and Ceramic Veneers: Up to 3-Year Follow-Up. *J. Adhes. Dent.* **2013**, *15*, 181–190. [PubMed]
31. Layton, D.; Walton, T. An up to 16-Year Prospective Study of 304 Porcelain Veneers. *Int. J. Prosthodont.* **2007**, *20*, 389.
32. Carvalho, A.A.; Leite, M.M.; Zago, J.K.M.; Nunes, C.A.B.C.M.; Barata, T.D.J.E.; de Freitas, G.C.; de Torres, É.M.; Lopes, L.G. Influence of Different Application Protocols of Universal Adhesive System on the Clinical Behavior of Class I and II Restorations of Composite Resin–a Randomized and Double-Blind Controlled Clinical Trial. *BMC Oral Health* **2019**, *19*, 252. [CrossRef] [PubMed]

33. Machiulskiene, V.; Campus, G.; Carvalho, J.C.; Dige, I.; Ekstrand, K.R.; Jablonski-Momeni, A.; Maltz, M.; Manton, D.J.; Martignon, S.; Martinez-Mier, E.A. Terminology of Dental Caries and Dental Caries Management: Consensus Report of a Workshop Organized by ORCA and Cariology Research Group of IADR. *Caries. Res.* **2020**, *54*, 7–14. [CrossRef] [PubMed]
34. Gurel, G.; Sesma, N.; Calamita, M.A.; Coachman, C.; Morimoto, S. Influence of Enamel Preservation on Failure Rates of Porcelain Laminate Veneers. *Int. J. Periodontics Restor. Dent.* **2013**, *33*, 31–39. [CrossRef] [PubMed]
35. Fradeani, M. Six-Year Follow-up with Empress Veneers. *Int. J. Periodontics Restor. Dent.* **1998**, *18*, 216–225.
36. Mehrabi, F.; Shanahan, D.; Davis, G. Xerostomia. Part 1: Aetiology and Oral Manifestations. *Dent. Update* **2022**, *49*, 840–846. [CrossRef]
37. Wang, Y.; Li, C.; Yuan, H.; Wong, M.C.; Zou, J.; Shi, Z.; Zhou, X. Rubber Dam Isolation for Restorative Treatment in Dental Patients. *Cochrane Database Syst. Rev.* **2016**, *20*, CD009858. [CrossRef]
38. Laske, M.; Opdam, N.J.; Bronkhorst, E.M.; Braspenning, J.C.; Huysmans, M. Ten-Year Survival of Class II Restorations Placed by General Practitioners. *JDR Clin. Transl. Res.* **2016**, *1*, 292–299. [CrossRef]
39. Opdam, N.; Bronkhorst, E.; Loomans, B.; Huysmans, M.-C. 12-Year Survival of Composite vs. Amalgam Restorations. *J. Dent. Res.* **2010**, *89*, 1063–1067. [CrossRef]
40. Askar, H.; Krois, J.; Göstemeyer, G.; Bottenberg, P.; Zero, D.; Banerjee, A.; Schwendicke, F. Secondary Caries: What Is It, and How It Can Be Controlled, Detected, and Managed? *Clin. Oral Investig.* **2020**, *24*, 1869–1876. [CrossRef]
41. Ghaffari, T.; Hamedi-Rad, F.; Fakhrzadeh, V. Marginal Adaptation of Spinell InCeram and Feldspathic Porcelain Laminate Veneers. *Dent. Res. J.* **2016**, *13*, 239. [CrossRef] [PubMed]
42. Baig, M.R.; Akbar, A.A.; Sabti, M.Y.; Behbehani, Z. Evaluation of Marginal and Internal Fit of a CAD/CAM Monolithic Zirconia-Reinforced Lithium Silicate Porcelain Laminate Veneer System. *J. Prosthodont.* **2022**, *31*, 502–511. [CrossRef] [PubMed]
43. Beuer, F.; Aggstaller, H.; Edelhoff, D.; Gernet, W.; Sorensen, J. Marginal and Internal Fits of Fixed Dental Prostheses Zirconia Retainers. *Dent. Mater.* **2009**, *25*, 94–102. [CrossRef] [PubMed]
44. Peumans, M.; Van Meerbeek, B.; Lambrechts, P.; Vanherle, G. Porcelain Veneers: A Review of the Literature. *J. Dent.* **2000**, *28*, 163–177. [CrossRef]
45. Tosco, V.; Monterubbianesi, R.; Orilisi, G.; Sabbatini, S.; Conti, C.; Özcan, M.; Putignano, A.; Orsini, G. Comparison of Two Curing Protocols during Adhesive Cementation: Can the Step Luting Technique Supersede the Traditional One? *Odontology* **2021**, *109*, 433–439. [CrossRef]
46. Mihali, S.G.; Lolos, D.; Popa, G.; Tudor, A.; Bratu, D.C. Retrospective Long-Term Clinical Outcome of Feldspathic Ceramic Veneers. *Materials* **2022**, *15*, 2150. [CrossRef]
47. Castelnuovo, J.; Tjan, A.H.; Phillips, K.; Nicholls, J.I.; Kois, J.C.; University of Washington, School of Dentistry. Fracture Load and Mode of Failure of Ceramic Veneers with Different Preparations. *J. Prosthet. Dent.* **2000**, *83*, 171–180. [CrossRef]
48. Frankenberger, R.; Krämer, N.; Lohbauer, U.; Nikolaenko, S.A.; Reich, S.M. Marginal Integrity: Is the Clinical Performance of Bonded Restorations Predictable in Vitro? *J. Adhes. Dent.* **2007**, *9*, 107–116.
49. Beier, U.S.; Kapferer, I.; Burtscher, D.; Dumfahrt, H. Clinical Performance of Porcelain Laminate Veneers for up to 20 Years. *Int. J. Prosthodont.* **2012**, *25*, 79–85.
50. Hardan, L.; Bourgi, R.; Cuevas-Suárez, C.E.; Lukomska-Szymanska, M.; Monjarás-Ávila, A.J.; Zarow, M.; Jakubowicz, N.; Jorquera, G.; Ashi, T.; Mancino, D.; et al. Novel Trends in Dental Color Match Using Different Shade Selection Methods: A Systematic Review and Meta-Analysis. *Materials* **2022**, *15*, 468. [CrossRef]
51. Sari, T.; Ural, C.; Yüzbasioglu, E.; Duran, I.; Cengiz, S.; Kavut, I. Color Match of a Feldspathic Ceramic CAD-CAM Material for Ultrathin Laminate Veneers as a Function of Substrate Shade, Restoration Color, and Thickness. *J. Prosthet. Dent.* **2018**, *119*, 455–460. [CrossRef] [PubMed]
52. Turgut, S.; Bagis, B.; Ayaz, E.A. Achieving the Desired Colour in Discoloured Teeth, Using Leucite-Based CAD-CAM Laminate Systems. *J. Dent.* **2014**, *42*, 68–74. [CrossRef] [PubMed]
53. Zarow, M. Nonvital Tooth Bleaching: A Case Discussion for the Clinical Practice. *Compend. Contin. Educ. Dent.* **2016**, *37*, 268–276.
54. Calamita, M.; Coachman, C.; Sesma, N.; Kois, J. Occlusal Vertical Dimension: Treatment Planning Decisions and Management Considerations. *Int. J. Esthet. Dent.* **2019**, *14*, 166–181. [PubMed]
55. Mannocci, F.; Cowie, J. Restoration of Endodontically Treated Teeth. *Br. Dent. J.* **2014**, *216*, 341–346. [CrossRef]
56. Rashid, H. The Effect of Surface Roughness on Ceramics Used in Dentistry: A Review of Literature. *Eur. J. Dent.* **2014**, *8*, 571–579. [CrossRef] [PubMed]
57. Rosentritt, M.; Sawaljanow, A.; Behr, M.; Kolbeck, C.; Preis, V. Effect of Tooth Brush Abrasion and Thermo-Mechanical Loading on Direct and Indirect Veneer Restorations. *Clin. Oral Investig.* **2015**, *19*, 53–60. [CrossRef] [PubMed]
58. El Sayed, S.M.; Basheer, R.R.; Bahgat, S.F.A. Color Stability and Fracture Resistance of Laminate Veneers Using Different Restorative Materials and Techniques. *Egypt. Dent. J.* **2016**, *62*, 1–15.

Disclaimer/Publisher's Note: The statements, opinions and data contained in all publications are solely those of the individual author(s) and contributor(s) and not of MDPI and/or the editor(s). MDPI and/or the editor(s) disclaim responsibility for any injury to people or property resulting from any ideas, methods, instructions or products referred to in the content.

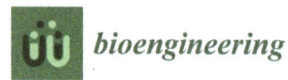

Review

The Effectiveness of Calcium Phosphates in the Treatment of Dentinal Hypersensitivity: A Systematic Review

Mélanie Maillard [1,†], Octave Nadile Bandiaky [2,†], Suzanne Maunoury [1], Charles Alliot [3], Brigitte Alliot-Licht [1], Samuel Serisier [2,3] and Emmanuelle Renard [2,3,*]

1. Faculté de Chirurgie Dentaire, CHU Nantes, Service Odontologie Conser-Vatrice et Pediatrique, Nantes Université, F-44000 Nantes, France
2. Oniris, CHU Nantes, INSERM, Regenerative Medicine and Skeleton, RMeS, Nantes Université, UMR 1229, F-44000 Nantes, France
3. Faculté de Chirurgie Dentaire, CHU Nantes, Service Odontologie Restauratrice et Chirurgicale, Nantes Université, F-44000 Nantes, France
* Correspondence: emmanuelle.renard@univ-nantes.fr
† These authors contribute equally to this work.

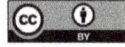

Abstract: Dentin hypersensitivity (DH) pain is a persistent clinical problem, which is a common condition known to affect patients' quality of life (QoL), but no treatment has ever been agreed upon. Calcium phosphates, available in different forms, have properties that allow sealing the dentinal tubules, which may relieve dentin hypersensitivity. The aim of this systematic review is to evaluate the ability of different formulations of calcium phosphate to reduce dentin hypersensitivity pain level in clinical studies. The inclusion criterion was as follows: clinical randomized controlled studies using calcium phosphates in treating dentin hypersensitivity. In December 2022, three electronic databases (Pubmed, Cochrane and Embase) were searched. The search strategy was performed according to Preferred Reporting Items for Systematic Reviews and Meta-Analyses (PRISMA) guidelines. The bias assessment risks results were carried out using the Cochrane Collaboration tool. A total of 20 articles were included and analyzed in this systematic review. The results show that calcium phosphates have properties that reduce DH-associated pain. Data compilation showed a statistically significant difference in DH pain level between T0 and 4 weeks. This VAS level reduction is estimated at about −2.5 compared to the initial level. The biomimetic and non-toxic characteristics of these materials make them a major asset in treating dentin hypersensitivity.

Keywords: dentin hypersensitivity; desensitizing agents; calcium phosphate; hydroxyapatite; nano-hydroxyapatite

1. Introduction

Dentin hypersensitivity (DH) is an oral complaint frequently reported in clinical dental practice. It is characterized by a short, sharp pain arising from exposed dentin in response to thermal, evaporative, tactile, osmotic, or chemical stimuli that cannot be ascribed to any other form of dental defect or pathology [1,2]. A review outlined a prevalence of DH ranging from 1 to 34% after clinical examination; the highest level has been reported to be on the cervical surface of the canine as well as first premolar permanent teeth and also in patients with periodontal alterations [3]. In their daily life, patients with dentin hypersensitivity complain of discomfort and pain while consuming hot or cold foods and beverages (coffee and ice cream) while toothbrushing or sometimes even while breathing. These symptoms and problems may be highly relevant, leading to restrictions on everyday activities and be a determinant of the individual's oral-health-related quality of life (OHRQoL) [4].

Several theories have been proposed in order to explain the biological mechanism of dentin hypersensitivity [3,5,6]. To date, the most widely accepted theory of DH is the hydrodynamic theory of Brännström [7–9]. This theory is based on a rapid movement of the dentinal fluid after external stimuli, which indirectly activates the nociceptors contained in the interface of the pulp and dentine, triggering painful sensations [9]. This would explain why treatments that occlude dentinal tubules and reduce intratubular fluids movement showed beneficial effects with high to moderate certainty [10].

Many active principles have been tested for the treatment of dentin hypersensitivity, including desensitizing toothpastes, gels, varnishes, and mouth rinses. Numerous systematic reviews exist on this topic, and the results are sometimes conflicting. These products typically contain one or more active ingredients that work by modifying the nervous response, preventing or reducing the transmission of pain signals, and/or occluding the permeable dentinal tubules [11]. Water-soluble potassium salts such as potassium fluoride, potassium chloride, and, the most commonly used, potassium nitrate are active ingredients that reduce dentin hypersensitivity pain by decreasing the nervous excitability by depolarizing nervous cells in the dentin tubules [12], resulting in a decrease in the nerve excitability. Another active principle tested for dentin hypersensitivity is fluoride under different molecule forms: sodium fluoride, silver diamine fluoride, tin fluoride, and amine fluoride. These fluorides work by creating a physical barrier by precipitating in the dentin surface and making it more resistant to acid erosion and other types of damage [13]. The oxalates are esters of oxalic acid, which can lead to the formation of calcium oxalate crystals by reacting to calcium ions from the oral cavity and occluding the dentinal tubules [14]. Arginine is an amino acid naturally found in saliva, able to blend with calcium carbonate and precipitate in dentinal tubules, resulting in the creation of a barrier resistant to acid dissolution [13]. Strontium also acts through the precipitation of particles on the exposed dentin and forming a protective barrier [15]. Other active ingredients such as sodium calcium phosphosilicate amorphous [16,17] promote the formation of apatite hydroxycarbonate on the dentin surface, occluding the dentinal tubules. Calcium phosphate, including nano-hydroxyapatite, can help to rebuild and strengthen the tooth structure by providing essential minerals that are lost during the demineralization process [18]. Physical agents such as glass ionomer, resins, and sealants are used in order to seal dentinal tubules and prevent the hydrodynamic dental pulp stimulation [19]. Glutaraldehyde is a molecule that reacts with serum albumin contained in dentinal fluid and is able to reduce the diameter of dentin tubules [19]. High-intensity lasers such as Nd:YAG, Er:YAG, Er, Cr:YSGG, and CO_2 have been tested to reduce DH pain through the obliteration of dentinal tubules, whereas low-intensity lasers such as GaAIA or He-Ne may reduce DH pain symptoms by interfering with the Na^+K^+ ion pump in the cell membrane, in blocking the transmission of nerve stimulation [20,21]. Overall, the active principle being tested in dentin hypersensitivity depends on the specific product being used and the mechanism of action of the active ingredient. However, the goal of all these active principles is to provide relief from the discomfort associated with DH by reducing nerve sensitivity, remineralizing the tooth surface, and providing a protective barrier over the exposed dentin. All these procedures are considered as therapeutic treatments and can be delivered either in-home or in-office. A systematic review comparing the effectiveness of DH treatment showed that dentinal tubules occlusion as well as nerve desensitisation in the at-home or in-office conditions of delivery had similar effects [22]. This multitude of treatments is able to decrease the patient's DH, but none of them constituted a gold-standard agent.

Since the 1950s, ceramic hydroxyapatite (HA) granules for bone defect repair have been reported [23], and in late 1980s, the first self-hardening calcium phosphate cements (CPC) were developed [24]. Indeed, as explained by Chow, 2009 [24], calcium phosphate cement containing an adequate concentration of tetracalcium phosphate and dicalcium phosphate anhydrous has a very high solubility, which enables precipitation in HA, a molecule whose general formula is $Ca_{10}(PO_4)6(OH)_2$, which is highly biocompatible and has low solubility. HA is widely applied in medicine and dentistry as a bone substitute [24–26].

Hydroxyapatite is already used as a DH desensitizer [27]. Other molecules similar to HA, such as synthetic nano-Hydroxyapatite (n-HA) or soluble molecules able to self-set to a hard mass under HA form, such as Tetracalcium phosphate (TTCP) and dicalcium phosphate dihydrate (DCPD) [28], have already been tested in clinical conditions in the treatment of DH. These studies show encouraging results. However, no systematic reviews evaluated the effects of these molecules on the DH pain level.

This systemic review aims to evaluate the effect of various calcium phosphate molecules such as hydroxyapatite, nano-hydroxyapatite, TTCP, DCPD, dicalcium phosphate anhydrous (DCPA), or/and amorphous calcium phosphate (ACP) on the reduction in DH pain level.

2. Materials and Methods

The study protocol was registered in the International Prospective Register of Systematic Reviews (PROSPERO) under ID = CRD42022336712. The present systematic review was conducted per the Preferred Reporting Items for Systematic Reviews and Meta-Analyses (PRISMA 2020) 2020 guidelines [29]. Population, Intervention, Comparison, Outcomes, and Study design components of this systematic review are as follows: Participants (P) were adult patients suffering from dentin hypersensitivity due to non-carious cervical lesions and not associated with post-bleaching hypersensitivity and periodontal therapy. Interventions (I) were in-office or in-home treatments of dentin hypersensitivity with products containing calcium phosphate. For Comparison (C), the comparison with other molecules is not applicable, but we looked at the variation in the level of pain felt by the patients before and after treatment with calcium phosphates. Outcome (O) was the reduction in pain associated with dentin hypersensitivity after treatment with calcium phosphate molecules. The study design (S) selected was a randomized controlled trial (RCT). Case reports, in vitro studies, in situ studies, systematic reviews, meta-analysis, letters to editors, and non-randomized trials, as well as studies on tooth decay or studies with no good molecule tested, were excluded. The research question was as follows: Are calcium phosphate able to reduce the DH pain?

2.1. Search Strategy

Three databases (PubMed/Medline, Cochrane Library, and EMBASE) were searched using relevant keywords to identify articles published until December 2022, with no language restriction, as shown in Table 1. Additionally, bibliographies of all selected articles, specialized journals, and other related publications, including reviews and meta-analyses, were also searched to identify further relevant articles. The records obtained from this extensive literature search were transferred to an EndNote® library, and duplicates were removed.

Table 1. Database and search terms.

Pubmed (filters applied: Randomized Control Trial, Human)	("Dentin Sensitivity" [Mesh] OR Sensitivities, Dentin OR Sensitivity, Dentin OR Dentine Hypersensitivity OR Dentine Hypersensitivities OR Hypersensitivities, Dentine OR Hypersensitivity, Dentine OR Dentine Sensitivity OR Dentine Sensitivities OR Sensitivities, Dentine OR Sensitivity, Dentine OR Tooth Sensitivity OR Sensitivities, Tooth OR Sensitivity, Tooth OR Tooth Sensitivities OR Dentin Hypersensitivity OR Dentin Hypersensitivities OR Hypersensitivities, Dentin OR Hypersensitivity, Dentin) AND ("Dentin Desensitizing Agents" [Mesh] OR Agents, Dentin Desensitizing OR Desensitizing Agents, Dentin OR "Tooth Remineralization" [Mesh]) AND ("Calcium Phosphates" [Mesh] OR dicalcium phosphate OR calcium monohydrogen phosphate dihydrate OR dicalcium phosphate dihydrate OR dibasic calcium phosphate dihydrate OR calcium phosphate, dihydrate OR calcium phosphate, dibasic OR dicalcium phosphate anhydrous OR brushite OR morphous calcium phosphate OR nHAC composite OR "Hydroxyapatites" [MeSH Terms] OR Hydroxyapatite Derivatives)

Table 1. *Cont.*

Cochrane library (All text)	Dentine Hypersensitivity OR Tooth Sensitivities OR Agents Dentin Desensitizing OR Remineralization tooth AND dicalcium phosphate OR calcium monohydrogen phosphate dihydrate OR dicalcium phosphate dihydrate OR dibasic calcium phosphate dihydrate OR calcium phosphates OR dihydrate calcium phosphate OR brushite OR Hydroxyapatite Derivatives OR Amorphous calcium phosphate OR nHAC composite
Embase (filters applied: Human, controlled study)	('dentine hypersensitivity'/exp OR 'dentine hypersensitivity' OR (('dentine'/exp OR dentine) AND ('hypersensitivity'/exp OR hypersensitivity)) OR 'tooth sensitivities' OR ((('tooth'/exp OR tooth) AND sensitivities) OR 'agents dentin desensitizing' OR (agents AND ('dentin'/exp OR dentin) AND desensitizing) OR 'remineralization tooth and dicalcium phosphate or calcium monohydrogen phosphate dihydrate' OR (('remineralization'/exp OR remineralization) AND tooth and dicalcium AND phosphate or AND calcium AND monohydrogen AND ('phosphate'/exp OR phosphate) AND dihydrate) OR 'dicalcium phosphate dihydrate' OR (dicalcium AND ('phosphate'/exp OR phosphate) AND dihydrate) OR 'dibasic calcium phosphate dihydrate' OR (dibasic AND ('calcium'/exp OR calcium) AND ('phosphate'/exp OR phosphate) AND dihydrate) OR 'calcium phosphates'/exp OR 'calcium phosphates' OR (('calcium'/exp OR calcium) AND ('phosphates'/exp OR phosphates)) OR 'dihydrate calcium phosphate ' OR (dihydrate AND ('calcium'/exp OR calcium) AND phosphate) OR 'brushite'/exp OR brushite OR 'hydroxyapatite derivatives' OR (('hydroxyapatite'/exp OR hydroxyapatite) AND derivatives) OR 'amorphous calcium phosphate' OR (amorphous AND ('calcium'/exp OR calcium) AND phosphate) OR 'nhac composite' OR (nhac AND ('composite'/exp OR composite))) AND ([controlled clinical trial]/lim OR [randomized controlled trial]/lim)

2.2. Screening and Study Selection

The research and selection process articles were carried out independently by two authors (M.M. and S.M.). First, the retrieved articles were imported into a bibliographic reference management software program (EndNote), where duplicates were removed. Then, the records' titles and abstracts obtained were screened, based on determined eligibility criteria. Finally, the full texts of the remaining studies were assessed by the same authors. Discrepancies were resolved, and consensus was built by engaging a third author (E.R.). Only randomized controlled trials that assessed the dentinal desensitized effect of calcium phosphate were included.

2.3. Data Extraction

When available, the data of included studies were extracted by both reviewers (M.M and S.M) and verified and confirmed by two other authors (O.N.B. and E.R). An Excel file was previously established to provide support for collecting demographic data (name of first author, year and country of publication, number of participants, and mean age), study methodology (study design, number and characteristics of the participating groups, number of follow-up visits, method of measuring dentin hypersensitivity, composition, concentration and use of calcium phosphate as a desensitizing agent for dentine hypersensitivity), and main results. All these extracted data were listed in Table 2.

Table 2. Studies included in quantitative synthesis.

Author, Year, Country	Participants (ST)	Age Range Mean Age (SD)	Study Design	Study Group (n)	Evaluation Method	Results
Poliakova et al., 2022, Russia [30]	30 (NR)	35–45 years 37.5 (2)	RCT, DB	G1 (n = 10): 20% n-HA paste; G2 (n = 10): nZnMgHA paste; G3 (n = 10): nFAP paste Toothbrushes twice daily for a month	Schiff Index values of CAS at baseline (T0) and after 2 (T1) and 4 (T2) weeks	At 4 weeks the Schiff Index score of 20% n-HA decreased significantly compared to baseline.
Alharith et al., 2021, Saudi Arabie [31]	63 (126)	18–60 years 39 (NR)	RCT, DB	G1 (n = 21): 15% n-HA paste; G2 (n = 21): fluoride paste; G3 (n = 21): placebo Single application of the paste at the baseline visit and 1 week follow up visit	VAS scores of TS and CAS evaluated at baseline (T0), immediately after paste application (T1), and after 1 week (T2)	A statistically significant reduction in VAS scores of TS and CAS tests from T0–T1 and T0–T2. Single application of n-HA paste significantly reduces DH.
Amaechi et al., 2021, USA [32]	85 (NR)	18–80 years 50.8 (11.4)	RCT, DB	G1 (n = 22): 10% n-HA; G2 (n = 19): 15% n-HA; G3 (n = 24): 10% n-HA + 5% Potassium Nitrate; G4 (n = 20): 15% SCPS Toothbrush during 2 min twice a day for 8 weeks	VAS scores of CAS and cold test at baseline (T0), 2 weeks (T1), 4 weeks (T2), 6 weeks (T3), and 8 weeks (T4).	All concentrations of n-HA showed a significant decrease in VAS scores at each time point.
Eyuboglu et al., 2020, Turkey [33]	40 (121)	18–65 years 41.35 (NR)	RCT, DB	G1 (n = 10, n* = 21): TTCP/DCPA; G2 (n = 10; n* = 36): Sodium Fluoride 5%, TCP Xylitol; G3 (n = 10; n* = 33): SR Monomer Matrix + 2-hydroxyethyl methacrylate; G4 (n = 10; n* = 31): 2-hydroxyethyl methacrylate + glutaraldehyde. One application according to manufacturer's instruction	VAS score of TS and CAS evaluated at baseline (T0), immediately after application (T1), after 1 day (T2), after 2 weeks (T3) and after 4 weeks (T4)	TTCP/DCPA showed a significant difference between T0 and T1 and a significantly lower CAS score at T4 than T2 and T3.
Usai et al., 2019, Italy [34]	105 (210–420)	20–50 years 43–50 (NR)	RCT, DB	G1 (n = 35): TTCP/DCPA 30 s application; G2 (n = 35): DD (premixed n-HAP alcohol-based gel) 45 s application; G3 (n = 35): BWE (premixed n-HAP water-based gel) 10 min application	VAS scores of TS and CAS were recorded at baseline (T1), at 1 week (T2), 4 weeks (T2), 12 weeks (T3) and 24 weeks (T4).	TTCP/DCPA paste showed a statistically significant decrease in DH after 24 weeks in comparison to T0.
Amaechi et al., 2018, USA [35]	50 (NR)	18–80 years 45.47 (13)	RCT, DB	G1 (n = 25): 20%n-HA; G2 (n = 25): 20% Silica. One application during 5 min after the 2 min before-bed brushing teeth and water rinsing.	VAS scores of CAS and cold stimulation at baseline (T0), 2 weeks (T1), 4 weeks (T2), 6 weeks (T3) and 8 weeks (T4)	VAS score of CAS indicated significant reduction in DH at each time point with either n-HAP.
Ameen et al., 2018, Egypt [36]	10 (40)	20–45 years (NR)	RCT, DB	G1 (n* = 10): 15%n-HA + 1%NaF; G2 (n* = 10): 15%n-HA; G3 (n* = 10): 25%n-HA + 1%NaF; G4 (n* = 10): 25%n-HA. Four applications during 1 min at T0, 1 day, 1 week, 2 weeks and 4 weeks	Schiff index values for TS, CAS and Cold stimulation were evaluated at baseline (T0), 1 day (T1), 1 week (T2), 2 weeks (T3) and 4 weeks (T4)	n-HA molecules showed significant effects on DH at T1 compared to T0. The level of the Schiff index was back to 0 for all groups after 2 weeks.
Anand et al., 2018, India [37]	60 (60)	18–50 years 42.33 (7.58)	RCT, DB	G1 (n = 30): 8% arginine paste; G2 (n = 30): 1% n-HA paste. One application of 1 cm of toothpaste directly to the sensitive site of the selected tooth, then brushing for two minutes twice a day for 4 weeks	Amperage values were recorded at baseline, 5 min, 1 and 4 weeks with Digitest II (PARKELL, Inc., New York, NY. USA)	n-HA containing toothpastes provided a statistically significant reduction in DH, 5 min, 1 and 4 weeks after application.
Vano et al., 2017, Italy [38]	105 (NR)	20–70 years (NR)	RCT, DB	G1 (n = 35): 2% n-HA gel paste; G2 (n = 35): fluoride gel paste; G3 (n = 35): placebo, 10 min application twice a day during 4 weeks	VAS scores for TS and CAS were evaluated at baseline (T0) and after 2(T1) and 4(T2) weeks	n-HA in gel toothpaste significantly reduced the DH between baseline and 4 weeks

Table 2. Cont.

Author, Year, Country	Participants (ST)	Age Range Mean Age (SD)	Study Design	Study Group (n)	Evaluation Method	Results
De Oliveira et al., 2016, Brazil [39]	8 (138)	22–48 years 29.5 (NR)	RCT, DB	G1 (n * = 33): Strontium acetate/calcium carbonate 60 s application; G2 (n * = 31): Calcium Carbonate/8% Arginine 3 s application by repeating 1 time the procedure; G3 (n * = 39): n-HA 10 s application with rest of 5 min; G4 (n * = 35): toothpaste without fluoride, 60 s application	VAS scores of CAS and cold stimulus with tetrafluoroethane were evaluated at baseline (T0), immediately after paste application (T1), after 24 h (T2) and after 30 days (T3).	n-HA showed significant difference for CAS and cold test between T0 and T3 days.
Wang et al., 2016, Brazil [40]	28 (137)	18–60 years (NR)	RCT, DB	G1 (n * = 31): 20%n-HA paste + NaF; 9000 ppm F; G2 (n * = 22): 20%n-HA + home-care pastes (10% HA, potassium nitrate, and NaF; 900 ppm F); G3 (n * = 28): 8% arginine + home-care toothpaste (8% arginine, sodium monofluorophosphate, 1450 ppm F); G4 (n * = 45): Duraphat. One application twice a day after toot brushing for 3 months	VAS scores of CAS was evaluated at baseline (T0) and after 1 (T1) month and 3(T2) months	n-HA toothpaste was effective treatment for reducing DH over three months.
Gopinath et al., 2015, India [41]	36 (NR)	18–60 years (NR)	RCT, DB	G1 (n = 18): n-HA paste; G2 (n = 18): 5% SCPS. Brushing for two minutes and no more than twice a day in total during 4 weeks	VAS scores of TS, CAS and cold water tests were recorded at baseline (T0) and after 4 weeks (T1).	n-HA paste showed significant reduction in DH after 4 weeks
Jena et al., 2015, India [42]	45 (122)	18–50 years (NR	RCT, DB	G1 (n * = 40): 5% Novamin paste; G2 (n * = 40): 8% arginine paste; G3 (n * = 42): 15% n-HA paste, 60 s application	VAS scores of TS and CAS at baseline (T0) immediately after (T1), 1 (T2) and 4 (T3) weeks after treatment	n-HA showed significant reduction in VAS immediately, after 1 and 4 weeks.
Mehta et al., 2015, India [43]	35 (70)	18–42 years 33.2 (NR)	RCT, DB	G1 (n * = 35): TTCP/DCPA; G2 (n * = 35): Placebo, 30 s application	VAS scores to TS and CAS at baseline T0, 15 min after treatment (T1), 1 day (T2), 1 week (T3), 3 (T4) and 6 (T5) months	TTCP/DCPA toothpaste show a decrease in DH progressively from (T1) to (T5).
Naoum et al., 2015, Australia [44]	71 (NR)	39–45 years (NF)	RCT, DB	G1 (n = 20): Colgate Cavity Protection (1000 ppmF-MFP); G2 (n = 17): Sensodyne Total Care (1000 ppmF-NaF + 19,300 ppmK+ KNO3); G3 (n = 16): Clinpro Tooth Creme (950 ppmF-NaF + f TCP); G4 (n = 18): Clinpro Tooth Creme (brushing + additional topical application). Toothbrush twice daily for 10 weeks	NRS-11 pain rating scale of TS, CAS and hypertonic solution were assessed at baseline (T0), 6 weeks (T1), and 10 weeks (T2)	fTCP (brushing + additional topical application) showed a significant reduction in DH.
Mehta et al., 2014, India [45]	49 (200)	18–50 years (NR)	RCT, DB	G1 (n * = 50): MSC 30 s application; G2 (n * = 50): NAN 20 s application; G3 (n * = 50): TTCP/DCPA (TMD) 30 s application; G4 (n * = 50): GLU, 60 s application	VAS scores to TS and CAS were recorded at baseline (T0) and immediately after application (T1), 1 week (T2), and after 1 (T3), 3 (T4) and 6 (T5) months	TTCP/DCPA showed a significant reduction in DH immediately and after 6 months
Porciani et al., 2014, Italy [46]	100 (NR)	18–65 years 41.35 (NR)	RCT, DB	G1 (n = 50): calcium HA/DCPD; G1 (n = 50): Placebo. Two pieces of gum to chew together, three times per day, for 2 weeks	Schiff index value for TS, CAS and cold water at baseline (T0), and after 1 (T1) and 2 (T2) weeks	Chewing gum containing HA/DCPD had a statistically significant reduction in DH after one and two weeks.
Vano et al., 2014, Italy [47]	105 (NR)	20–70 years (N3)	RCT, DB	G1 (n = 35): 15% n-HA paste; G2 (n = 35): fluoride paste; G3 (n = 35): placebo. Toothbrush during 2 min twice a day for 4 weeks	VAS scores for TS, and CAS were evaluated at baseline (T0) and after 2 (T1) and 4 (T2) weeks	n-HA toothpaste significantly reduced DH between baseline and 4 weeks.

93

Table 2. *Cont.*

Author, Year, Country	Participants (ST)	Age Range Mean Age (SD)	Study Design	Study Group (n)	Evaluation Method	Results
Ghassemi et al., 2009, USA, Canada [48]	208 (NR)	20–64 years 42.22 (NR)	RCT, DB	G1 (n = 106): Single phase ACP + 0.24% NaF paste; G2 (n = 102): Placebo (0.24% NaF). Toothbrush for 1 min twice a day for 8 weeks	VAS score of CAS was evaluated at baseline (T0), 4 weeks (T1) and 8 weeks (T2)	The toothpaste containing ACP showed a significant reduction in CAS VAS score compared to T0.
Geiger et al., 2003, Israel [49]	30 (NR)	NR	RCT, DB	G1 (n = 15): ACP; G2 (n = 15): Placebo 60 s application	VAS scores of TS and CAS were evaluated at baseline (T0), after one week (T1), after four weeks (T2) and after six months (T3)	ACP showed immediate relief of sensibility after application, with CAS and TS stimulation.

ST, Sensitive Teeth; NR, not reported; RCT, randomized clinical trial; DB, double blind; G, group; n-HA, nano-hydroxyapatite; DH, dentin hypersensitivity; TS, tactile sensitivity; CAS, cold air sensitivity; VAS, visual analog scale; SSS, Schiff sensitivity scale; TMD, Teethmate Desensitizer; TTCP, tetracalcium phosphate; DCPD, dicalcium phosphate dihydrate; DD, dentin desensitizer; BWE, Bite & White ExSense; HAP, hydroxyapatite; nZnMgHAP, nano-Zn-Mg-hydroxyapatite; nFAP, nano-fluoroapatite; FTCP, fluoride tricalcium phosphate; NRS, numbered rating scale; NaF, fluoride ions; VRS, verbal ratin scale; SrCl2, strontium chloride; GLU, Gluma Desensitizer Power Gel; MSC, MS Coat One F; NAN, NanoSeal; DCPA, dicalcium phosphate anhydrous; ACP, amorphus calcium phosphate; SCPS, calcium sodium phosphosilicate.

2.4. Quality Assessment

The same two authors (M.M. and S.M.) assessed the risk of bias in the included studies using Cochrane's Collaboration tool for assessing the risk of bias in randomized controlled trials [50]. Disagreements were resolved via discussion, and a third researcher (E.R.) was approached when necessary. This evaluation concerned the generation of the randomization sequence (selection bias), concealment of the allocation (reporting bias), blinding of the investigator and the participant (confusion bias), blind evaluation of the results (performance bias), management of missing data (attrition bias), selection of the reporter, and other types of bias. From these criteria, the bias risk level was determined to be low, unclear, or high.

2.5. Synthesis of Results

A qualitative and quantitative synthesis of the results of the included studies, structured around different outcomes, was performed. The data from these different studies were extracted, and the results are summarized in Table 3. For studies in which the authors reported results as medians and interquartile ranges, the values were converted to means and SDs using the formula (q1 + median + q3)/3, where q1 indicates the 25th percentile and q3 the 75th percentile. An approximation of the standard deviation was obtained by applying this formula (q3 − q1)/1.35. Analysis groups between baseline and 4 weeks of follow-up were formed according to the method of assessment of dental hypersensitivity to determine whether calcium phosphates are effective in reducing pain associated with dental hypersensitivity associated pain. Data from these different groups were pooled to determine the mean pain reduction value. When studies used the same type of intervention and comparison groups with the same outcome measure, the results were pooled with mean differences for continuous outcomes.

3. Results

3.1. Study Selection

The initial search of all sources yielded 10,019 records. Of these, 2435 duplicated studies were removed using the reference manager EndNote®. A total of 7515 articles were excluded after reading titles and/or abstracts, 12 records were excluded since reports were not retrieved, 57 records from database registers and 18 identified through other methods were read and analyzed in their full-text, and 55 records were excluded for reasons such as not good drugs tested ($n = 34$), in vitro studies ($n = 11$), or study on tooth decay ($n = 10$), as shown in Figure 1. Twenty records met the inclusion criteria and were included in the systematic review: Poliakova et al., 2022 [30], Alharith et al., 2021 [31], Amaechi et al., 2021 [32], Eyuboglu et al., 2020 [33], Usai et al., 2019 [34], Amaechi et al., 2018 [35], Ameen et al., 2018 [36], Anand et al., 2018 [37], Vano et al., 2017 [38], De Oliveira et al., 2016 [39], Wang et al., 2016 [40], Gopinath et al., 2015 [41], Jena et al., 2015 [42], Mehta et al., 2015 [43], Naoum et al., 2015 [44], Mehta et al., 2014 [45], Porciani et al., 2014 [46], Vano et al., 2014 [47], Ghassemi et al., 2009 [48], and Geiger et al., 2003 [49]. The selection process has been detailed in the attached PRISMA flowchart (Figure 1).

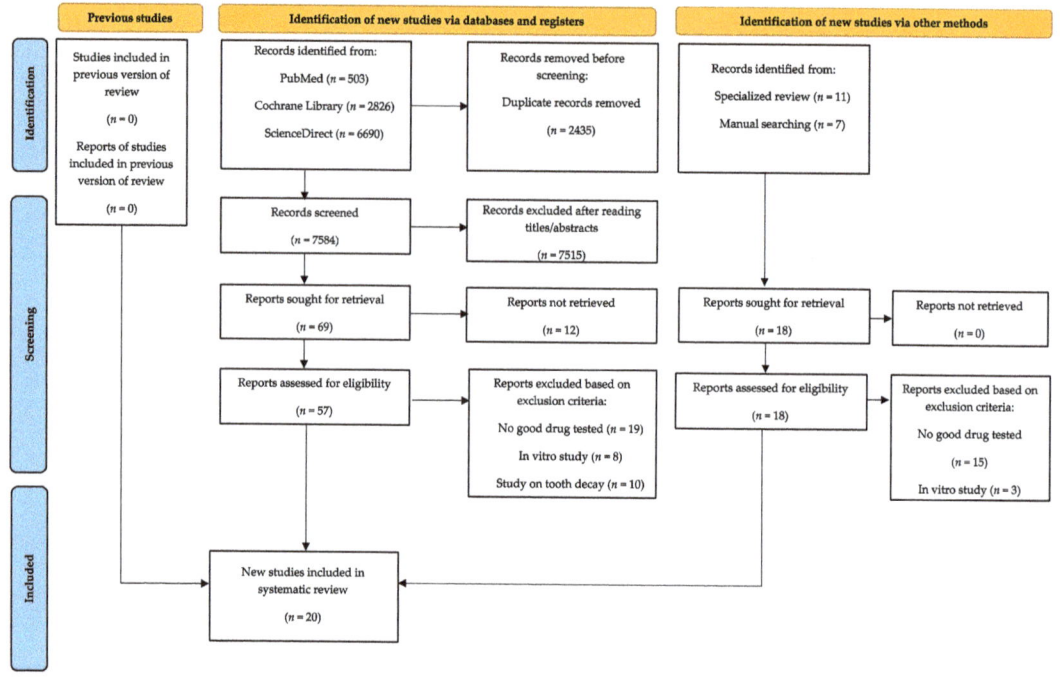

Figure 1. PRISMA flow diagram.

Table 3. Mean difference and standard deviations (SD) of visual analogic scale scores between 4 weeks follow-up and baseline after calcium phosphates application (subgroup analysis according to the test realized).

	Study Reference	Dentin Desensitizing Agents	Manufacturer	No. of Participants (Teeth)	Baseline Mean ± SD	4 Weeks Follow-up Mean ± SD	Mean Difference Random, 95% CI	p-Value
Air blast test	Poliakova et al., 2022, Russia [30]	Toothpaste (20% n−HAP)	NR	10	2.5 ± 0.53	1.3 ± 0.48	−1.20 ± 0.22 (−1.67 to −0.72)	<0.05
	Eyuboglu et al., 2020, Turkey [33]	Teethmate™ Desensitizer (TTCP/DCPA)	Kuraray Noritake Osaka, Japan	10 (21)	5.52 ± 1.66	2.14 ± 0.22	−3.38 ± 0.36 (−4.11 to −2.64)	<0.05
	Usai et al., 20.9, Italy [34]	Teethmate™ Desensitizer (TTCP/DCPA)	Kuraray Noritake Dental Inc., Tokyo, Japan	35	4 ± 2.96	0.66 ± 1.51	−3.34 ± 0.56 (−4.46 to −2.21)	<0.05
	Usai et al., 20.9, Italy [34]	Denfin Desensitizer (gel phase of n−HAP)	Ghimas, Casalecchio di Reno, Bologna, Italy	35	5.33 ± 2.22	1.66 ± 2.22	−3.67 ± 0.53 (−4.72 to −2.61)	<0.05
	Usai et al., 2019, Italy [34]	Bite&White ExSense (gel phase of n−HAP in a water)	Cavex Holland, Haarlem, Netherlands	35	4.33 ± 2.96	1.0 ± 0.01	−3.33 ± 0.50 (−4.32 to −2.33)	<0.05
	Ameen et al., 2018, Egypt [36]	15% nHAP	NR	(10)	3.01 ± 0.01	0 ± 0	−3.01 ± 0.00 (−3.00 to −2.99)	<0.05
	Ameen et al., 2018, Egypt [36]	15% nHAP + 1%NaF	NR	(10)	2.6 ± 0.52	0 ± 0	−2.59 ± 0.16 (−2.93 to −2.24)	<0.05
	Ameen et al., 2018, Egypt [36]	25% nHAP	NR	(10)	3.01 ± 0.01	0 ± 0	−3.01 ± 0.00 (−3.00 to −2.99)	<0.05
	Ameen et al., 2018, Egypt [36]	25%nHAP +1%NaF	NR	(10)	2.6 ± 0.52	0 ± 0	−2.59 ± 0.16 (−2.93 to −2.24)	<0.05
	Vano et al., 2017, Italy [38]	B.te&White ExSense (Gel, 15% n−HA)	Cavex Holland, Haarlem, Netherlands	35	2.97 ± 0.42	1.64 ± 0.43	−1.33 ± 0.10 (−1.53 to −1.12)	<0.05
	De Oliveira et al. 2016, Brazil [39]	Nano P® (hydroxyapatite)	FGM Ltd.a, Brazil	(39)	6.23 ± 2.72	3.54 ± 3.72	−2.69 ± 0.73 (−4.15 to −1.22	<0.05
	Wang et al., 2016, Brazil [40]	Desensibilize Nano−P (20% hydroxyapatite)	FGM−Dentscare, Joinville, Brazil	(31)	7.04 ± 1.62	4.10 ± 3.50	−2.94 ± 0.69 (−4.32 to −1.55)	<0.05
	Wang et al., 2016, Brazil [40]	Desensibilize Nano−P (20% hydroxyapatite) + 10% HA	FGM−Dentscare, Joinville, Brazil	(22)	7.04 ± 1.62	4.48 ± 2.57	−2.56 ± 0.64 (−3.86 to −1.25)	<0.05
	Gopinath et al. 2015, India [41]	Aclaim™ (Nano−HAP)	Group Pharmaceuticals, Bangalore, India	18	7.06 ± 1.55	5.39 ± 1.33	−1.67 ± 0.48 (−2.64 to −0.69)	<0.05
	Mehta et al., 2014, India [45]	Teethmate™ Desensitizer (TTCP/DCPA)	Kuraray Noritake Osaka, Japan	(50)	6.4 ± 0.5	2.2 ± 0.2	−4.20 ± 0.07 (−4.35 to −4.04)	<0.05
	Vano et al., 2014, Italy [47]	PrevDent® toothpaste (15% n−HA)	NR	35	2.82 ± 0.35	1.2 ± 0.49	−1.62 ± 0.10 (−1.82 to −1.41)	<.05
	Ghassemi et al. 2009, USA, Canada [48]	Enamel Care (n−HAP)	NR	106	6.34 ± 1.11	3.47 ± 2.25	−2.87 ± 0.24 (−3.35 to −2.38)	<0.05
	Total N			319 (203)				
	Total mean score (SD)				4.63 ± 1.01	1.92 ± 1.28	−2.71 ± 0.07 (−2.85 to −2.57)	<0.05

Table 3. Cont.

	Study Reference	Dentin Desensitizing Agents	Manufacturer	No. of Participants (Teeth)	Baseline Mean ± SD	4 Weeks Follow-up Mean ± SD	Mean Difference Random, 95% CI	p-Value
Tactile sensitivity test	Eyuboglu et al., 2020, Turkey [33]	Teethmate Desensitizer (TTCP/DCPA)	Kuraray Noritake Osaka, Japan	10 (21)	2.85 ± 1.19	1.04 ± 1.20	−1.81 ± 0.36 (−2.55 to −1.06)	<0.05
	Usai et al., 2019, Italy [34]	Teethmate™ Desensitizer (TTCP/DCPA)	Kuraray Noritake Dental Inc., Tokyo, Japan	35	4.01 ± 2.96	0.66 ± 1.48	−3.35 ± 0.56 (−4.46 to −2.23)	<0.05
	Usai et al., 2019, Italy [34]	Dentin Desensitizer (gel phase of n−HAP)	Ghimas, Casalecchio di Reno, Bologna, Italy	35	5.33 ± 2.22	1.33 ± 2.22	−4.00 ± 0.53 (−5.05 to −2.94)	<0.05
	Usai et al., 2019, Italy [34]	Bite&White ExSense (gel phase of n−HAP in a water)	Cavex Holland, Haarlem, Netherlands	35	4.33 ± 2.96	0.01 ± 0.02	−4.32 ± 0.38 (−5.08 to −3.55)	<0.05
	Ameen et al., 2018, Egypt [36]	15% nHAP	NR	(10)	2.4 ± 1.03	0 ± 0	−2.39 ± 0.32 (−3.07 to −1.70)	<0.05
	Ameen et al., 2018, Egypt [36]	15% nHAP + 1%NaF	NR	(10)	2.2 ± 0.52	0 ± 0	−2.19 ± 0.16 (−2.53 to −1.84)	<0.05
	Ameen et al., 2018, Egypt [36]	25% nHAP	NR	(10)	2.8 ± 1.03	0 ± 0	−2.79 ± 0.32 (−3.47 to −2.10)	<0.05
	Ameen et al., 2018, Egypt [36]	25%nHAP +1%NaF	NR	(10)	2.3 ± 0.52	0 ± 0	−2.29 ± 0.16 (−2.63 to −1.94)	<0.05
	Vano et al., 2017, Italy [38]	Bite&White ExSense (Gel, 15% n−HA)	Cavex Bite&White ExSense, Cavex Holland BV	35	3.17 ± 0.49	1.83 ± 0.63	−1.34 ± 0.14 (−1.60 to −1.07)	<0.05
	Gopinath et al., 2015, India [41]	Aclaim™ (Nano−HAP)	Group Pharmaceuticals, Bangalore, India	18	4.67 ± 1.08	3.78 ± 0.94	−0.89 ± 0.33 (−1.57 to −0.20)	>0.05
	Mehta et al., 2014, India [43]	Teethmate Desensitizer (TTCP/DCPA)	Kuraray Noritake Osaka, Japan	(50)	6.21 ± 1.82	2.81 ± 1.06	−3.4 ± 0.29 (−3.99 to −2.80)	<0.05
	Vano et al., 2014, Italy [47]	PrevDent® toothpaste (15% n−HA)	NR	35	2.54 ± 0.52	0.95 ± 0.59	−1.59 ± 0.13 (−1.85 to −1.32)	<0.05
	Total N			158 (111)				
	Total mean score (SD)				3.56 ± 0.91	1.03 ± 0.72	−2.53 ± 0.07 (−2.66 to −2.39)	<0.05
Cold water test	Ameen et al., 2018, Egypt [36]	15% nHAP	NR	(10)	3 ± 0	0 ± 0	−2.99 ± 0.01 (−2.99 to −2.98)	<0.05
	Ameen et al., 2018, Egypt [36]	15% nHAP + 1%NaF	NR	(10)	2.6 ± 0.52	0 ± 0	−2.59 ± 0.16 (−2.93 to −2.24)	<0.05
	Ameen et al., 2018, Egypt [36]	25% nHAP	NR	(10)	3 ± 0	0 ± 0	−2.99 ± 0.01 (−2.99 to −2.98)	<0.05
	Ameen et al., 2018, Egypt [36]	25%nHAP +1%NaF	NR	(10)	2.4 ± 0.52	0 ± 0	−2.39 ± 0.16 (−2.73 to −2.04)	<0.05
	De Oliveira et al., 2016, Brazil [39]	Nano P® (hydroxyapatite)	FGM Ltd.a, Brazil	(39)	9.14 ± 1.37	6.51 ± 3.65	−2.63 ± 0.62 (−3.87 to −1.38)	<0.05
	Gopinath et al., 2015, India [41]	Aclaim™ (Nano−HAP)	Group Pharmaceuticals, Bangalore, India	18	6.72 ± 1.01	4.94 ± 1.05	−1.78 ± 0.34 (−2.47 to −1.08)	<0.05
	Total N			18 (79)				
	Total mean score (SD)				4.47 ± 0.72	1.91 ± 1.46	−2.56 ± 0.16 (−2.88 to −2.23)	<0.05

A statistically significant decrease in the level of pain associated with dentin hypersensitivity was observed between 4 weeks of follow-up and baseline according to VAS score of air blast, tactile sensitivity, and cold water tests ($p < 0.05$).

3.2. Description of Included Studies

The characteristics of the 20 included articles are presented in Table 2. The number of subjects included varied from 8 to 208. The age range of patients ranged from 18 to 80 years. The follow-up range varied from immediately to 6 months. Most of the studies performed a 4-week follow-up phase [30,32–42,47–49].

Different formulations of calcium phosphate were used by authors: hydroxyapatite, nano-hydroxyapatite in different concentrations, amorphous calcium phosphate (ACP), tetracalcium phosphate (TTCP), dicalcium phosphate anhydrous (DCPA) and dicalcium phosphate dihydrate (DCPD), and tri-calcium phosphate (TCP). Molecules were tested in the form of toothpaste, gel, or chewing gum and administered through an in-office treatment in 10 studies [31,33–36,39,42,43,45,49]. In the other 10 studies, the treatment was performed by the patients themselves, at home [30,32,37,38,40,41,44,46–48]. Most of the included studies used another desensitizing agent as a control [30–42,44,45,48], and four studies used only a placebo as a control [43,46,47,49].

Dentin hypersensitivity is generally assessed through different tests. In all included studies, dentin hypersensitivity was evaluated with an air blast test, tactile test, or cool water test, in accordance with the guidelines described by Holland et al., 1997 [2]. These guidelines, recommending at least two tests, were respected by most of the studies, except for [30,40,48], which only used an air blast test. The majority of studies realized an air blast assessment (evaporative stimulus) associated with a tactile sensitivity test [31,33,34,36,38,41–47,49]. Three studies [36,41,46] also used cold tests or cold-water tests. Two studies [32,39] associated the air blast test with a cold test. Anand et al. [37] recorded the amperage value of an electric test. The dentin hypersensitivity pain was recorded with a visual analogic scale of 100 mm (VAS) [31–35,38–43,45,47–49] or a Schiff scale (SCASS) with a score from 0 to 3 [30,36,46], except for [37], which used an amperage value, and [44], which used an NRS-11 pain rating scale.

All studies showed significant reductions in VAS or Schiff of dentin. In order to determine the efficacy of calcium phosphate in the reduction in DH pain level, we synthetized data in Table 3 accordingly with the realized test. Data compilation showed a statistically significant difference in DH pain level between T0 and 4 weeks. This reduction is estimated at about -2.5 compared to the initial level of pain.

Nine studies showed a significant decrease in VAS or Schiff at 4 weeks for the air blast stimulation [30,33,34,38–41,45,47]. The total calculated mean difference score of all studies between the baseline T0 and 4 weeks was -2.71 ± 0.07 (-2.85 to -2.57) $p < 0.05$. Desensitized agents used were n-HA [34,39,48], n-HA15% [36,38,47], n-HA20% [30,40], n-HA 25% [36], and TTCP/DCPA [33,34,45]. All data are compiled in Table 3.

Six of seven studies showed a significant decrease in VAS or Schiff at 4 weeks for tactile stimulation [33,34,36,38,45,47]. The decrease was not significant in one study [41]. The total calculated mean difference score of the seven studies was -2.53 ± 0.07 (-2.66 to -2.39) $p < 0.05$. All data are compiled in Table 3.

Three studies showed a significant decrease in VAS at 4 weeks for the cold water test [36,39,41]. The total calculated mean difference score of all studies between the baseline T0 and 4 weeks was -2.56 ± 0.16 (-2.88 to -2.23) $p < 0.05$. Desensitized agents were n-HA. All data are compiled in Table 3.

3.3. Analysis of the Risks of Bias

The results of the risk of bias assessment are presented in Figure 2. This analysis was carried out using the Cochrane Collaboration tool [50]. This assessment involved randomized clinical trials and was carried out on all the studies included in this systematic review. The assessment revealed that seven studies were considered to have a low risk of bias [32,34–36,41,44,48]. Five studies were considered to be at high risk of bias for the following reasons: in the study of Eyuboglu et al. [33], because the randomization was performed after the initial pain assessment; in the study of Gopinath et al. [41], because the randomization method and the description of the sample size were not clearly exposed;

and in the study of Jena et al. [42], because the absence of description of the sample size and of duration and location of the study also constituted a risk of bias.

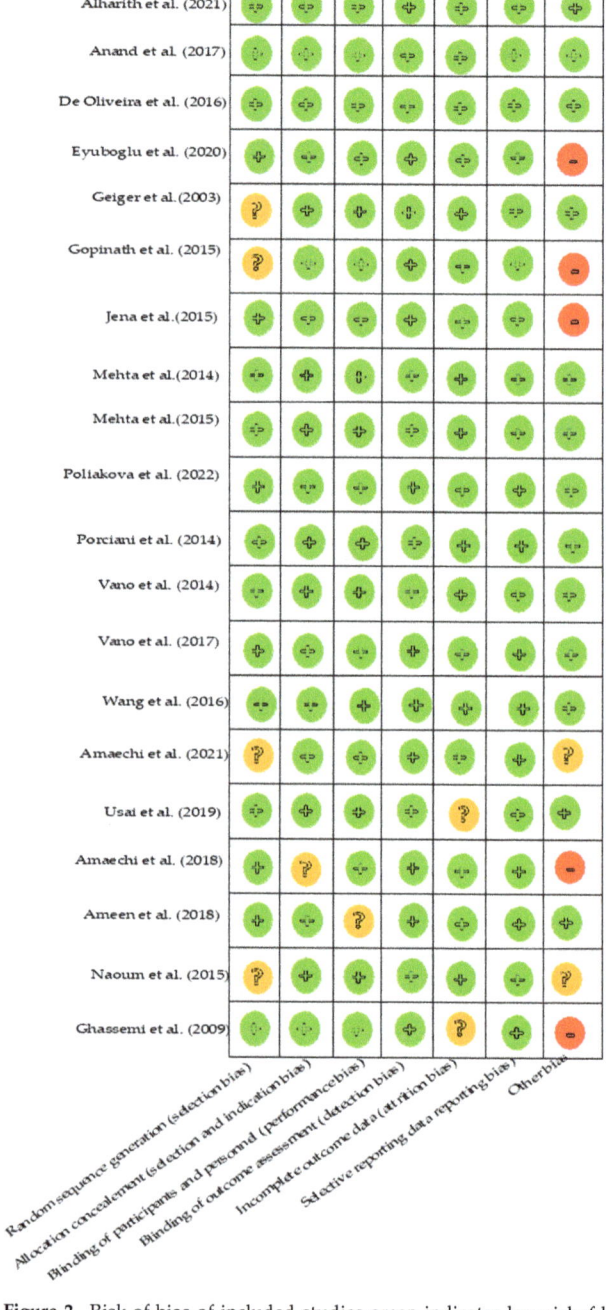

Figure 2. Risk of bias of included studies green indicates low riskof bias [30,31,37–40,43,45–47], orange indicates uncertain or moderate risk of bias [32,34,36,44,49], and red indicates high risk of bias [33,35,41,42,48].

4. Discussion

Recent systematic reviews with meta-analyses have compared the effectiveness of several desensitizing toothpaste formulations, including some containing nano-hydroxyapatite or potassium combined with hydroxyapatite [10,18,19,51–53]. In our review, we focused specifically on the effectiveness of hydroxyapatite and other calcium phosphate materials able to self-set to a hard mass [24], such as tetracalcium phosphate (TTCP) and dicalcium phosphate dihydrate (DCPD) powders, which are able to produce a supersaturated solution and faster hydroxyapatite precipitation due to their high solubility at neutral PH [28]. In this systematic review, we show the beneficial clinical effects of all different calcium phosphate formulations on dentin hypersensitivity. Whatever the test used (air blast, tactile or cold water), calcium phosphate induced a reduction in a mean of 2.5 pain level on the VAS scale after 4 weeks. Additionally, significant beneficial effects appeared immediately after treatment in eight studies [31,33,34,37,39,42,43,45].

These results may be explained by the ability of calcium phosphates to spontaneously form hydroxyapatite at physiological pH and to adhere to the exposed dentine, forming a layer of calcium phosphate components, which may allow them to seal exposed dentinal tubules and consequently be a good candidate for the treatment of dentin hypersensitivity with a VAS drop immediately after the application.

The beneficial effect, as described in our review, is in accordance with the results of a large systematic review and meta-analysis conducted by Marto et al., regarding numerous molecules in the treatment of DH [19]. In this review, hydroxyapatite and other calcium phosphate molecules showed a significant reduction in DH pain at different points in time.

A previous systematic review and meta-analysis conducted by de Melo Alencar et al. in 2019 [18] underlined the effectiveness of nano-hydroxyapatite in the relief of dentin hypersensitivity compared to n-HA free treatment. Indeed, Alencar et al. [18] showed a significant desensitizing effect against evaporative and tactile stimuli but not against cold stimulation. They hypothesized that cold stimulus, the most disturbing test, could involve not only the hydrodynamic theory but also other factors such as TRPM8 channels in odontoblasts. Concerning the air blast test and the tactile test, their results are in accordance with our systematic review, except for the cold water, for which we show a significant reduction in DH pain level after phosphate calcium treatment. De Melo Alencar et al. also compared n-HA to placebo or other desensitizing agents, particularly arginine. This amino acid when combined with calcium carbonate mimics saliva's ability to occlude and seal open dentinal tubules, which renders that tooth surface resistant to acid and thermal attacks. It has been shown by two previous meta-analyses and one systematic review as promising bioactive agent [13,54,55] in DH. In their review, Alencar et al. [18] showed, in the 4-week follow-up, a better result with nano-hydroxyapatite than those presented by arginine in the treatment of dentin hypersensitivity. In our study, we did not compare calcium phosphate with other products or placebo, since this was not our research question.

However, another systematic review and meta-analysis conducted by Hu et al. [56], comparing numerous dentin desensitizing agents, showed a very low level of evidence of nano-hydroxyapatite and amorphous calcium phosphate toothpaste compared with other desensitizing agents. Indeed, this study included fifty-three clinical studies, but only four with calcium phosphate, two with nano-hydroxyapatite and two with amorphous calcium phosphate, which considerably reduces the effect of this evidence [56].

The review by Cunha-Cruz et al. [57] showed a significant effect of n-HA on DH pain levels in two studies but no effects from amorphous calcium phosphate, but this author took into account only results included in previous systematic reviews and meta-analyses [56].

It is worth noting that the hypersensitivity reduction efficacy of nano-hydroxyapatite was increased du to the adjunction of sodium [58] or ionometric sealant [59] or when combined with laser treatment [60].

Furthermore, the concentration of calcium phosphate used is probably an important factor for effectiveness. Shetty et al. [61], in an in vitro study, reported an enhanced desensitizing action with 100% nano-hydroxyapatite over 8 weeks of treatment compared to 25% nano-hydroxyapatite, and the authors concluded that increased concentrations of the molecule increased its penetration into the tubules and probably improved its desensitizing ability. Our study does not allow us to determine the suitable concentration to use to reach the most efficient effect.

Other biomaterials containing calcium such as calcium sodium phosphosilicate seem to have interest in the treatment of dentin hypersensitivity [30,46,47]. Finally, it is important to note that the hypersensitivity was not completely resolved regardless of the treatment applied. According to our results, a level of pain persists after 4 weeks of treatments as shown in Table 3, which could be explained by the fact that the effectiveness of the treatment tends to decrease or disappear over time [34,49].

Alharith et al. [31], De Oliveira et al. [39], Porciani et al. [46], and Geiger et al. [49] showed positive results in the placebo groups, resulting in a significant effect of treatment but no significant reduction compared to the placebo group. In [31,39,46,49], patients felt significant reductions of up to 60% of dentin hypersensitivity following the application of the placebo treatment. These positive effects of placebo treatments are important to consider, since there may be other factors that could explain the effectiveness of desensitizing therapeutics agents in the reduction in dentin hypersensitivity such as desensitizing agents in control groups. Moreover, these lower levels of sensitivity in placebo groups can also be attributed to the well-known Hawthorne effect, which describes the modification of behavior when individuals are aware that they are being observed, which could influence the patient's responses and ca lead to bias in healthcare studies [62]. The placebo effect may also be involved, since positive motivation and emotional stimuli could activate pain inhibitors in the central nervous system [63].

Our systematic review presents limits that required results to be carefully interpreted. Indeed, included studies are still heterogenous in terms of the age of patient from 18 to 80 years, where we do not know if age is an influencing factor of DH level pain. Additionally, different desensitized agents in different concentrations and different application modalities were used by different authors, and the evaluation of the DH realized with three different tests could be different according to the team's research; all these limits did not allow the generalization of results.

5. Conclusions

This systematic review shows a reduction in pain perception after calcium phosphate application immediately and 4 weeks after treatment, making this biomaterial a good candidate for the relief of dentin hypersensitivity.

Author Contributions: M.M., O.N.B. and E.R. contributed to design of the study. M.M., S.M., O.N.B. and E.R. contributed to the data acquisition, analysis and interpretation, and drafting of the manuscript. Data interpretation and manuscript drafting was performed by M.M., O.N.B., E.R., C.A., B.A.-L. and S.S. All authors have read and agreed to the published version of the manuscript.

Funding: This research received no external funding.

Institutional Review Board Statement: Not applicable.

Informed Consent Statement: Not applicable.

Data Availability Statement: Not applicable.

Acknowledgments: The researchers thank Pierre Weiss and Valerie Geoffroy, who are responsible of the REGOS team in the laboratory RMeS, UMR 1229, for their support of publication charges.

Conflicts of Interest: The authors declare no conflict of interest.

References

1. Addy, M. Etiology and clinical implications of dentine hypersensitivity. *Dent. Clin. N. Am.* **1990**, *34*, 503–514. [CrossRef] [PubMed]
2. Holland, G.R.; Narhi, M.N.; Addy, M.; Gangarosa, L.; Orchardson, R. Guidelines for the design and conduct of clinical trials on dentine hypersensitivity. *J. Clin. Periodontol.* **1997**, *24*, 808–813. [CrossRef]

3. Mantzourani, M.; Sharma, D. Dentine sensitivity: Past, present and future. *J. Dent.* **2013**, *41*, S3–S17. [CrossRef]
4. Bekes, K.; Hirsch, C. What is known about the influence of dentine hypersensitivity on oral health-related quality of life? *Clin. Oral Investig.* **2013**, *17* (Suppl. 1), S45–S51. [CrossRef] [PubMed]
5. Rapp, R.; Avery, J.K.; Strachan, D.S. *Possible Role of the Acetylcholinesterase in Neural Conduction within the Dental Pulp*; University of Alabama Press: Birmingham, UK, 1968.
6. West, N.; Lussi, A.; Seong, J.; Hellwig, E. Dentin hypersensitivity: Pain mechanisms and aetiology of exposed cervical dentin. *Clin. Oral Investig.* **2013**, *17*, 9–19. [CrossRef]
7. Brannstrom, M. A hydrodynamic mechanism in the transmission of pain-producing stimuli through the dentin. In *Sensory Mechanisms in Dentine*; Pergamon Press: Oxford, UK, 1963; pp. 73–79.
8. Brannstrom, M. The surface of sensitive dentine. An experimental study using replication. *Odontol. Rev.* **1965**, *16*, 293–299.
9. Brannstrom, M. Sensitivity of dentine. *Oral Surg. Oral Med. Oral Pathol.* **1966**, *21*, 517–526. [CrossRef] [PubMed]
10. Martins, C.C.; Firmino, R.T.; Riva, J.J.; Ge, L.; Carrasco-Labra, A.; Brignardello-Petersen, R.; Colunga-Lozano, L.E.; Granville-Garcia, A.F.; Costa, F.O.; Yepes-Nunez, J.J.; et al. Desensitizing Toothpastes for Dentin Hypersensitivity: A Network Meta-analysis. *J. Dent. Res.* **2020**, *99*, 514–522. [CrossRef]
11. Shiau, H.J. Dentin hypersensitivity. *J. Evid.-Based Dent. Pract.* **2012**, *12*, 220–228. [CrossRef]
12. Karim, B.F.; Gillam, D.G. The efficacy of strontium and potassium toothpastes in treating dentine hypersensitivity: A systematic review. *Int. J. Dent.* **2013**, *2013*, 573258. [CrossRef]
13. Sharif, M.O.; Iram, S.; Brunton, P.A. Effectiveness of arginine-containing toothpastes in treating dentine hypersensitivity: A systematic review. *J. Dent.* **2013**, *41*, 483–492. [CrossRef] [PubMed]
14. Cunha-Cruz, J.; Stout, J.R.; Heaton, L.J.; Wataha, J.C.; Northwest, P. Dentin hypersensitivity and oxalates: A systematic review. *J. Dent. Res.* **2011**, *90*, 304–310. [CrossRef] [PubMed]
15. Magno, M.B.; Nascimento, G.C.R.; Da Penha, N.K.S.; Pessoa, O.F.; Loretto, S.C.; Maia, L.C. Difference in effectiveness between strontium acetate and arginine-based toothpastes to relieve dentin hypersensitivity. A systematic review. *Am. J. Dent.* **2015**, *28*, 40–44. [PubMed]
16. Gendreau, L.; Barlow, A.P.; Mason, S.C. Overview of the clinical evidence for the use of NovaMin in providing relief from the pain of dentin hypersensitivity. *J. Clin. Dent.* **2011**, *22*, 90–95.
17. Zhu, M.; Li, J.; Chen, B.; Mei, L.; Yao, L.; Tian, J.; Li, H. The Effect of Calcium Sodium Phosphosilicate on Dentin Hypersensitivity: A Systematic Review and Meta-Analysis. *PLoS ONE* **2015**, *10*, e0140176. [CrossRef] [PubMed]
18. de Melo Alencar, C.; de Paula, B.L.F.; Guanipa Ortiz, M.I.; Baraúna Magno, M.; Martins Silva, C.; Cople Maia, L. Clinical efficacy of nano-hydroxyapatite in dentin hypersensitivity: A systematic review and meta-analysis. *J. Dent.* **2019**, *82*, 11–21. [CrossRef] [PubMed]
19. Marto, C.M.; Baptista Paula, A.; Nunes, T.; Pimenta, M.; Abrantes, A.M.; Pires, A.S.; Laranjo, M.; Coelho, A.; Donato, H.; Botelho, M.F.; et al. Evaluation of the efficacy of dentin hypersensitivity treatments—A systematic review and follow-up analysis. *J. Oral Rehabil.* **2019**, *46*, 952–990. [CrossRef]
20. Lee, B.S.; Chang, C.W.; Chen, W.P.; Lan, W.H.; Lin, C.P. In vitro study of dentin hypersensitivity treated by Nd:YAP laser and bioglass. *Dent. Mater.* **2005**, *21*, 511–519. [CrossRef]
21. Miglani, S.; Aggarwal, V.; Ahuja, B. Dentin hypersensitivity: Recent trends in management. *J. Conserv. Dent.* **2010**, *13*, 218–224. [CrossRef] [PubMed]
22. Moraschini, V.; da Costa, L.S.; Dos Santos, G.O. Effectiveness for dentin hypersensitivity treatment of non-carious cervical lesions: A meta-analysis. *Clin. Oral Investig.* **2018**, *22*, 617–631. [CrossRef]
23. Ray, R.D.; Ward, A.A., Jr. A preliminary report on studies of basic calcium phosphate in bone replacement. *Surg. Forum* **1951**, 429–434.
24. Chow, L.C. Next generation calcium phosphate-based biomaterials. *Dent. Mater. J.* **2009**, *28*, 1–10. [CrossRef] [PubMed]
25. Daculsi, G.; Laboux, O.; Malard, O.; Weiss, P. Current state of the art of biphasic calcium phosphate bioceramics. *J. Mater. Sci. Mater. Med.* **2003**, *14*, 195–200. [CrossRef] [PubMed]
26. Rajula, M.P.B.; Narayanan, V.; Venkatasubbu, G.D.; Mani, R.C.; Sujana, A. Nano-hydroxyapatite: A Driving Force for Bone Tissue Engineering. *J. Pharm. Bioallied Sci.* **2021**, *13*, S11–S14. [CrossRef]
27. Martins, C.C.; Riva, J.J.; Firmino, R.T.; Schunemann, H.J. Formulations of desensitizing toothpastes for dentin hypersensitivity: A scoping review. *J. Appl. Oral Sci.* **2022**, *30*, e20210410. [CrossRef]
28. Zhou, J.; Chiba, A.; Scheffel, D.L.; Hebling, J.; Agee, K.; Niu, L.N.; Tay, F.R.; Pashley, D.H. Effects of a Dicalcium and Tetracalcium Phosphate-Based Desensitizer on In Vitro Dentin Permeability. *PLoS ONE* **2016**, *11*, e0158400. [CrossRef]
29. Page, M.J.; McKenzie, J.E.; Bossuyt, P.M.; Boutron, I.; Hoffmann, T.C.; Mulrow, C.D.; Shamseer, L.; Tetzlaff, J.M.; Akl, E.A.; Brennan, S.E.; et al. The PRISMA 2020 statement: An updated guideline for reporting systematic reviews. *BMJ* **2021**, *372*, n71. [CrossRef]
30. Polyakova, M.; Sokhova, I.; Doroshina, V.; Arakelyan, M.; Novozhilova, N.; Babina, K. The Effect of Toothpastes Containing Hydroxyapatite, Fluoroapatite, and Zn-Mg-hydroxyapatite Nanocrystals on Dentin Hypersensitivity: A Randomized Clinical Trial. *J. Int. Soc. Prev. Community Dent.* **2022**, *12*, 252–259. [CrossRef]
31. Alharith, D.N.; Al-Omari, M.; Almnea, R.; Basri, R.; Alshehri, A.H.; Al-Nufiee, A.A. Clinical efficacy of single application of plain nano-hydroxyapatite paste in reducing dentine hypersensitivity—A randomized clinical trial. *Saudi Endod. J.* **2021**, *11*, 24.

32. Amaechi, B.T.; Lemke, K.C.; Saha, S.; Luong, M.N.; Gelfond, J. Clinical efficacy of nanohydroxyapatite-containing toothpaste at relieving dentin hypersensitivity: An 8 weeks randomized control trial. *BDJ Open* **2021**, *7*, 23. [CrossRef]
33. Eyüboğlu, G.; Naiboğlu, P. Clinical efficacy of different dentin desensitizers. *Oper. Dent.* **2020**, *45*, E317–E333. [CrossRef]
34. Usai, P.; Campanella, V.; Sotgiu, G.; Spano, G.; Pinna, R.; Eramo, S.; Saderi, L.; Garcia-Godoy, F.; Derchi, G.; Mastandrea, G.; et al. Effectiveness of Calcium Phosphate Desensitising Agents in Dental Hypersensitivity Over 24 Weeks of Clinical Evaluation. *Nanomaterials* **2019**, *9*, 1748. [CrossRef] [PubMed]
35. Amaechi, B.T.; Lemke, K.C.; Saha, S.; Gelfond, J. Clinical Efficacy in Relieving Dentin Hypersensitivity of Nanohydroxyapatite-containing Cream: A Randomized Controlled Trial. *Open Dent. J.* **2018**, *12*, 572–585. [CrossRef]
36. Ameen, S.; Niazy, M.; El-yassaky, M.; Jamil, W.; Attia, M. Clinical Evaluation of Nano-Hydroxyapatite as Dentin Desensitizer. *Al-Azhar Dent. J. Girls* **2018**, *5*, 79–87. [CrossRef]
37. Anand, S.; Rejula, F.; Sam, J.V.G.; Christaline, R.; Nair, M.G.; Dinakaran, S. Comparative Evaluation of Effect of Nano-hydroxyapatite and 8% Arginine Containing Toothpastes in Managing Dentin Hypersensitivity: Double Blind Randomized Clinical Trial. *Acta Med. (Hradec Kral.)* **2017**, *60*, 114–119. [CrossRef]
38. Vano, M.; Derchi, G.; Barone, A.; Pinna, R.; Usai, P.; Covani, U. Reducing dentine hypersensitivity with nano-hydroxyapatite toothpaste: A double-blind randomized controlled trial. *Clin. Oral Investig.* **2018**, *22*, 313–320. [CrossRef]
39. Douglas de Oliveira, D.W.; Oliveira, E.S.; Mota, A.F.; Pereira, V.H.; Bastos, V.O.; Gloria, J.C.; Goncalves, P.F.; Flecha, O.D. Effectiveness of Three Desensitizing Dentifrices on Cervical Dentin Hypersensitivity: A Pilot Clinical Trial. *J. Int. Acad. Periodontol.* **2016**, *18*, 57–65. [PubMed]
40. Wang, L.; Magalhaes, A.C.; Francisconi-Dos-Rios, L.F.; Calabria, M.P.; Araujo, D.; Buzalaf, M.; Lauris, J.; Pereira, J.C. Treatment of Dentin Hypersensitivity Using Nano-Hydroxyapatite Pastes: A Randomized Three-Month Clinical Trial. *Oper. Dent.* **2016**, *41*, E93–E101. [CrossRef] [PubMed]
41. Gopinath, N.M.; John, J.; Nagappan, N.; Prabhu, S.; Kumar, E.S. Evaluation of Dentifrice Containing Nano-hydroxyapatite for Dentinal Hypersensitivity: A Randomized Controlled Trial. *J. Int. Oral Health* **2015**, *7*, 118–122. [PubMed]
42. Jena, A.; Shashirekha, G. Comparison of efficacy of three different desensitizing agents for in-office relief of dentin hypersensitivity: A 4 weeks clinical study. *J. Conserv. Dent.* **2015**, *18*, 389–393. [CrossRef]
43. Mehta, D.; Gowda, V.; Finger, W.J.; Sasaki, K. Randomized, placebo-controlled study of the efficacy of a calcium phosphate containing paste on dentin hypersensitivity. *Dent. Mater.* **2015**, *31*, 1298–1303. [CrossRef] [PubMed]
44. Naoum, S.J.; Lenard, A.; Martin, F.E.; Ellakwa, A. Enhancing Fluoride Mediated Dentine Sensitivity Relief through Functionalised Tricalcium Phosphate Activity. *Int. Sch. Res. Not.* **2015**, *2015*, 905019. [CrossRef]
45. Mehta, D.; Gowda, V.S.; Santosh, A.; Finger, W.J.; Sasaki, K. Randomized controlled clinical trial on the efficacy of dentin desensitizing agents. *Acta Odontol. Scand.* **2014**, *72*, 936–941. [CrossRef]
46. Porciani, P.F.; Chazine, M.; Grandini, S. A clinical study of the efficacy of a new chewing gum containing calcium hydroxyapatite in reducing dentin hypersensitivity. *J. Clin. Dent.* **2014**, *25*, 32–36. [PubMed]
47. Vano, M.; Derchi, G.; Barone, A.; Covani, U. Effectiveness of nano-hydroxyapatite toothpaste in reducing dentin hypersensitivity: A double-blind randomized controlled trial. *Quintessence Int.* **2014**, *45*, 703–711. [CrossRef]
48. Ghassemi, A.; Hooper, W.; Winston, A.E.; Sowinski, J.; Bowman, J.; Sharma, N. Effectiveness of a baking soda toothpaste delivering calcium and phosphate in reducing dentinal hypersensitivity. *J. Clin. Dent.* **2009**, *20*, 203–210.
49. Geiger, S.; Matalon, S.; Blasbalg, J.; Tung, M.; Eichmiller, F.C. The clinical effect of amorphous calcium phosphate (ACP) on root surface hypersensitivity. *Oper. Dent.* **2003**, *28*, 496–500.
50. Higgins, J.P.; Altman, D.G.; Gotzsche, P.C.; Juni, P.; Moher, D.; Oxman, A.D.; Savovic, J.; Schulz, K.F.; Weeks, L.; Sterne, J.A.; et al. The Cochrane Collaboration's tool for assessing risk of bias in randomised trials. *BMJ* **2011**, *343*, d5928. [CrossRef] [PubMed]
51. Behzadi, S.; Mohammadi, Y.; Rezaei-Soufi, L.; Farmany, A. Occlusion effects of bioactive glass and hydroxyapatite on dentinal tubules: A systematic review. *Clin. Oral. Investig.* **2022**, *26*, 6061–6078. [CrossRef]
52. Gul, H.; Ghaffar, M.A.; Kaleem, M.; Khan, A.S. Hydroxyapatite, a potent agent to reduce dentin hypersensitivity. *J. Pak. Med. Assoc.* **2021**, *71*, 2604–2610. [CrossRef]
53. Limeback, H.; Enax, J.; Meyer, F. Clinical Evidence of Biomimetic Hydroxyapatite in Oral Care Products for Reducing Dentin Hypersensitivity: An Updated Systematic Review and Meta-Analysis. *Biomimetics* **2023**, *8*, 23. [CrossRef] [PubMed]
54. Bae, J.H.; Kim, Y.K.; Myung, S.K. Desensitizing toothpaste versus placebo for dentin hypersensitivity: A systematic review and meta-analysis. *J. Clin. Periodontol.* **2015**, *42*, 131–141. [CrossRef]
55. Yang, Z.Y.; Wang, F.; Lu, K.; Li, Y.H.; Zhou, Z. Arginine-containing desensitizing toothpaste for the treatment of dentin hypersensitivity: A meta-analysis. *Clin. Cosmet. Investig. Dent.* **2016**, *8*, 1–14. [CrossRef]
56. Hu, M.L.; Zheng, G.; Zhang, Y.D.; Yan, X.; Li, X.C.; Lin, H. Effect of desensitizing toothpastes on dentine hypersensitivity: A systematic review and meta-analysis. *J. Dent.* **2018**, *75*, 12–21. [CrossRef]
57. Cunha-Cruz, J.; Zeola, L.F. Limited Evidence Suggests That Many Types of Desensitizing Toothpaste May Reduce Dentin Hypersensitivity, but Not the Ones With Strontium or Amorphous Calcium Phosphate. *J. Evid.-Based Dent. Pract.* **2019**, *19*, 101337. [CrossRef] [PubMed]
58. Zang, P.; Parkinson, C.; Hall, C.; Wang, N.; Jiang, H.; Zhang, J.; Du, M. A Randomized Clinical Trial Investigating the Effect of Particle Size of Calcium Sodium Phosphosilicate (CSPS) on the Efficacy of CSPS-containing Dentifrices for the Relief of Dentin Hypersensitivity. *J. Clin. Dent.* **2016**, *27*, 54–60.

59. Machado, A.C.; Maximiano, V.; Yoshida, M.L.; Freitas, J.G.; Mendes, F.M.; Aranha, A.C.C.; Scaramucci, T. Efficacy of a calcium-phosphate/fluoride varnish and ionomeric sealant on cervical dentin hypersensitivity: A randomized, double-blind, placebo-controlled clinical study. *J. Oral Rehabil.* **2022**, *49*, 62–70. [CrossRef] [PubMed]
60. Alencar, C.D.; Ortiz, M.I.; Silva, F.A.; Alves, E.B.; Araujo, J.L.; Silva, C.M. Effect of nanohydroxyapatite associated with photobiomodulation in the control of dentin hypersensitivity: A randomized, double-blind, placebo-controlled clinical trial. *Am. J. Dent.* **2020**, *33*, 138–144.
61. Shetty, S.; Kohad, R.; Yeltiwar, R. Hydroxyapatite as an in-office agent for tooth hypersensitivity: A clinical and scanning electron microscopic study. *J. Periodontol.* **2010**, *81*, 1781–1789. [CrossRef]
62. Demetriou, C.; Hu, L.; Smith, T.O.; Hing, C.B. Hawthorne effect on surgical studies. *ANZ J. Surg.* **2019**, *89*, 1567–1576. [CrossRef]
63. Colloca, L. The Placebo Effect in Pain Therapies. *Ann. Rev. Pharmacol. Toxicol.* **2019**, *59*, 191–211. [CrossRef] [PubMed]

Disclaimer/Publisher's Note: The statements, opinions and data contained in all publications are solely those of the individual author(s) and contributor(s) and not of MDPI and/or the editor(s). MDPI and/or the editor(s) disclaim responsibility for any injury to people or property resulting from any ideas, methods, instructions or products referred to in the content.

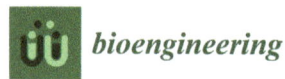

Article

Deep Learning for Dental Diagnosis: A Novel Approach to Furcation Involvement Detection on Periapical Radiographs

Yi-Cheng Mao [1], Yen-Cheng Huang [1], Tsung-Yi Chen [2,†], Kuo-Chen Li [3,*], Yuan-Jin Lin [4], Yu-Lin Liu [2], Hong-Rong Yan [4], Yu-Jie Yang [4], Chiung-An Chen [5,*], Shih-Lun Chen [2,†], Chun-Wei Li [1], Mei-Ling Chan [1,6,†], Yueh Chuo [1] and Patricia Angela R. Abu [7]

[1] Department of General Dentistry, Chang Gung Memorial Hospital, Taoyuan City 33305, Taiwan; lynn202207017@jyu.edu.cn (M.-L.C.)
[2] Department of Electronic Engineering, Chung Yuan Christian University, Taoyuan City 32023, Taiwan; chischen@cycu.edu.tw (S.-L.C.)
[3] Department of Information Management, Chung Yuan Christian University, Taoyuan City 320317, Taiwan
[4] Department of Electrical Engineering and Computer Science, Chung Yuan Christian University, Chung Li City 32023, Taiwan
[5] Department of Electrical Engineering, Ming Chi University of Technology, New Taipei City 243303, Taiwan
[6] School of Physical Educational College, Jiaying University, Meizhou 514000, China
[7] Department of Information Systems and Computer Science, Ateneo de Manila University, Quezon City 1108, Philippines; pabu@ateneo.edu
* Correspondence: kuochen@cycu.edu.tw (K.-C.L.); joannechen@mail.mcut.edu.tw (C.-A.C.)
† These authors contributed equally to this work.

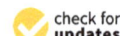

Citation: Mao, Y.-C.; Huang, Y.-C.; Chen, T.-Y.; Li, K.-C.; Lin, Y.-J.; Liu, Y.-L.; Yan, H.-R.; Yang, Y.-J.; Chen, C.-A.; Chen, S.-L.; et al. Deep Learning for Dental Diagnosis: A Novel Approach to Furcation Involvement Detection on Periapical Radiographs. *Bioengineering* **2023**, *10*, 802. https://doi.org/10.3390/bioengineering10070802

Academic Editors: Naji Kharouf and Madhur Upadhyay

Received: 13 April 2023
Revised: 15 June 2023
Accepted: 21 June 2023
Published: 4 July 2023

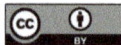

Copyright: © 2023 by the authors. Licensee MDPI, Basel, Switzerland. This article is an open access article distributed under the terms and conditions of the Creative Commons Attribution (CC BY) license (https://creativecommons.org/licenses/by/4.0/).

Abstract: Furcation defects pose a significant challenge in the diagnosis and treatment planning of periodontal diseases. The accurate detection of furcation involvements (FI) on periapical radiographs (PAs) is crucial for the success of periodontal therapy. This research proposes a deep learning-based approach to furcation defect detection using convolutional neural networks (CNN) with an accuracy rate of 95%. This research has undergone a rigorous review by the Institutional Review Board (IRB) and has received accreditation under number 202002030B0C505. A dataset of 300 periapical radiographs of teeth with and without FI were collected and preprocessed to enhance the quality of the images. The efficient and innovative image masking technique used in this research better enhances the contrast between FI symptoms and other areas. Moreover, this technology highlights the region of interest (ROI) for the subsequent CNN models training with a combination of transfer learning and fine-tuning techniques. The proposed segmentation algorithm demonstrates exceptional performance with an overall accuracy up to 94.97%, surpassing other conventional methods. Moreover, in comparison with existing CNN technology for identifying dental problems, this research proposes an improved adaptive threshold preprocessing technique that produces clearer distinctions between teeth and interdental molars. The proposed model achieves impressive results in detecting FI with identification rates ranging from 92.96% to a remarkable 94.97%. These findings suggest that our deep learning approach holds significant potential for improving the accuracy and efficiency of dental diagnosis. Such AI-assisted dental diagnosis has the potential to improve periodontal diagnosis, treatment planning, and patient outcomes. This research demonstrates the feasibility and effectiveness of using deep learning algorithms for furcation defect detection on periapical radiographs and highlights the potential for AI-assisted dental diagnosis. With the improvement of dental abnormality detection, earlier intervention could be enabled and could ultimately lead to improved patient outcomes.

Keywords: deep learning; periapical radiograph; furcation involvement; image segmentation; Gaussian high-pass filtering; image preprocessing; CNN

1. Introduction

With the increasing emphasis on health awareness, people are paying more and more attention to health matters. Seeing a doctor or undergoing health check-ups has become part of daily life. However, this has also led to a shortage of medical resources due to the high demand. This research focuses on one of the most high-demand reasons for check-ups, periodontitis. Periodontitis is a type of periodontal disease [1]. The symptoms of periodontitis can be further classified based on the furcation involvements occurring at the bifurcation or trifurcation of the roots of molars. Traditionally, dentists rely on repeated X-ray examinations, palpation, and mobility tests to confirm the presence of furcation involvements (FI) and take appropriate measures [2,3]. Therefore, the purpose of this research is to train a convolutional neural network (CNN) model to accurately identify FI on PAs. This helps dentists to quickly distinguish and compare the severity of the disease, thereby reducing the consumption of medical resources.

The motivation behind this project is to delegate the task of identifying dental symptoms to artificial intelligence (AI). With the rapid development of AI technology, there have been numerous AI applications in recent years, such as vehicle counting [4], financial field applications [5], medical education [6], chip design field [7], and foreign language teaching [8]. In the current standard process of dental diagnosis and treatment, the use of X-rays can reduce the probability of misjudgment by assisting in the identification of symptoms that are difficult to detect with the naked eye. However, there is still a possibility of misjudgment due to differences in lighting or shooting angles. Additionally, dentists spend a significant amount of time interpreting dental lesions before treating each patient, which accumulates into significant time and physical costs for the practitioner. Therefore, a well-trained model from this project could significantly assist dentists in diagnosis. Dentists can use AI-classified images for pre-screening and comparison and then perform further detailed invasive examinations [9]. The goal of this research is to construct a CNN model [10] that can identify the presence or absence of FI [11] through transfer learning. This disease frequently occurs at the root bifurcation of multi-rooted teeth, particularly in upper and lower molars. The key difference between multi-rooted teeth and single-rooted teeth is the number of roots, with multi-rooted teeth resembling a forked root system where the gap between roots is referred to as furcation. Under normal circumstances, the furcation is filled with alveolar bone. However, when periodontal disease occurs, the alveolar bone is lost. Bacteria can penetrate deeper into the gap, ultimately leading to a decrease in tooth stability or even tooth loss. The prevalence of periodontal disease today is a common occurrence that is also associated with an increased incidence of FI [12]. Since FI usually occurs in narrow and complex-to-clean locations, missing the golden treatment period can quickly escalate the disease to a point where even surgery cannot restore long-term stability [13]. The early detection and repair of bone augmentation can prevent tooth loss.

Radiographic diagnosis is the most widely used and important means of evaluating teeth in dentistry. The use of new X-ray techniques like cone beam-computed tomography (CBCT) and magnetic resonance imaging (MRI) has the potential to enhance the accuracy of diagnosing root canal bifurcations [14]. This means that clinical dentists still mostly rely on traditional X-ray images. Although these new imaging techniques are indeed more precise than traditional 2D X-rays in many areas, they are still not widely used in general clinical practice due to the time and cost required. Additionally, the resources for these techniques are limited and difficult to distribute equitably to patients. Furthermore, high-precision images like those provided by CBCT are only helpful in assisting dentists with initial diagnoses [15,16]. Unless the condition is complex, dentists still rely more on traditional X-rays such as PA, bitewing, and panoramic films. The main goal of this research is to address the shortcomings of traditional X-ray images and improve image quality by reducing noise or improving clarity. Additionally, this research aims to assist or simplify the clinical workflow for dentists by training a CNN transfer learning model to automatically detect and identify periapical lesions on PA images. This will save dentists time and energy in reviewing PA images and reduce the risk of visual fatigue [2,17].

Moreover, the model will better define FI lesions and eliminate the need for the discussion or repeated confirmation of suspicious lesions [18–21]. This helps dentists to reduce patient consultation time and respond more quickly to these elusive conditions. The Innovations of this research are listed as follows:

1. A CNN-based automated recognition system for FI lesions has been developed in this research, and the proposed final model can achieve an accuracy of 94%, which is a 5% increase compared to [19].
2. An adaptive threshold and an adjusted segmentation line operation have been proposed in this research to enhance fault tolerance, which has proven helpful for the research process and final learning results.
3. The model for distinguishing between single-rooted and double-rooted teeth in this research has achieved a high recognition accuracy of 97%, which enables the proper classification of the sample data contained in a single image. Additionally, the proposed model for classifying single and double-rooted teeth can help in the collection and categorization of samples for medical and AI automation applications in the future.

The structure of this research is as follows: Section 2 introduces the CNN model architecture and the automated image data generation methods used for training. Section 3 presents and analyzes the results of various experiments, including comparisons between different models and an examination of factors that may have impacted the outcomes. Section 4 discusses the findings obtained from the experiments. Finally, Section 5 concludes this research and suggests future directions for further explorations.

2. Materials and Methods

In this research, the most important areas are image preprocessing and image masking, which were the main factors affecting CNN training and validation. In the image preprocessing step, the noise in the original PA image is removed. In the meantime, the characteristics of the diseases classified in this research can be enhanced. This step is crucial to the next PA image classification step as it obtains better recognition accuracy. The overall flow chart of this research is shown in Figure 1.

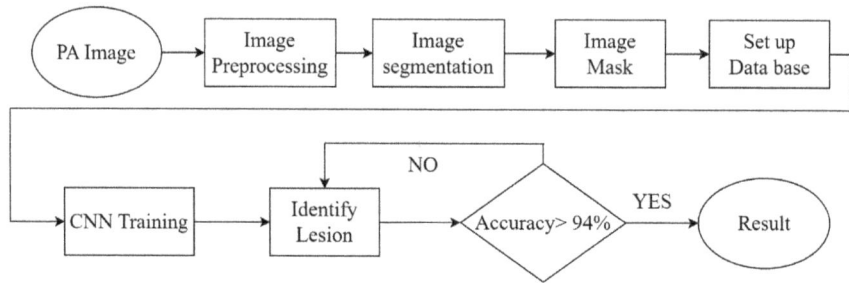

Figure 1. The flowchart of this proposal.

2.1. Image Preprocessing

One of the focuses of this research is to locate FI in the posterior molars from PA images. However, due to issues such as the angle of the X-ray beam or lighting, distinguishing the three targets in PA images (teeth, gingiva, and background) is often challenging. Additionally, PA images frequently contain noise and distortion, which make it tedious and time-consuming for dentists to locate the targets and might cause the possibility of misdiagnosis. Therefore, the aim of this step is to standardize PA images by eliminating interfering confounding variables and enabling the clear differentiation of the three targets. The pre-processing step comprises three parts: gray-level adjustment, Gaussian high-pass filtering, and adaptive thresholding, as shown in Figure 2.

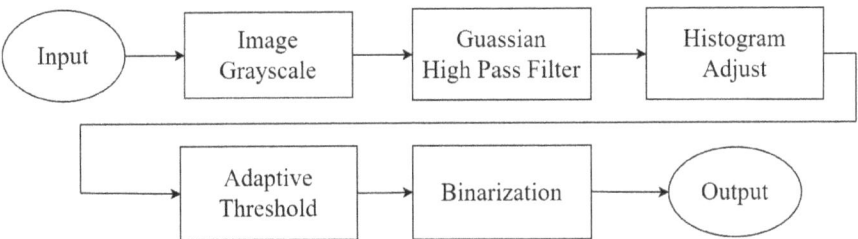

Figure 2. The flowchart of using this system.

2.1.1. Image Grayscale

To improve the image adjustment and the efficiency of CNN training, the original RGB images are converted to grayscale images. While RGB images have three dimensions, grayscale images have only two dimensions and are more suitable for image adjustment. Furthermore, since the colors captured by PA images are grayscale, there is no loss of information in converting to grayscale [22]. This conversion simplifies the representation of the image data and allows the pixel coordinates of the image to be more easily displayed. Grayscaling makes it simpler to detect errors and make adjustments.

2.1.2. Gaussian High-Pass Filtering

The most challenging problems in this research are the image noise on the PA image and the indistinct contours of the target disease. Cui and Zhang [23] used frequency domain filtering to sharpen the image in which the edge features are highlighted. Gaussian filtering is separated into high-pass and low-pass filtering. Low-pass filtering can filter out the noise. It is concentrated in high frequencies and smooths the image edge, but it can also cause the image to become too blurry and lose details. On the other hand, high-pass filtering can suppress the low-frequency parts and focus on highlighting the edge features, effectively extracting noise and interference. Thus, this research subtracts the filtered noise image from the original image, as described in [24]. Equation (1) can decrease the noise and interference on the original image. Figure 3 shows the results of achieving a more pronounced contrast, displaying different gray levels in different areas and clearer tooth contours.

$$H(u, v) = 1 - e^{\frac{-D^2(u, v)}{2D_0^2}} \quad (1)$$

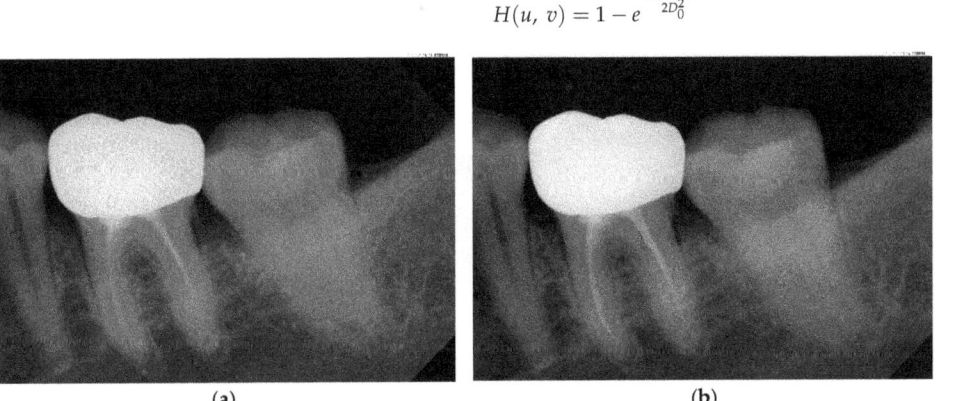

Figure 3. Schematic diagram of the result of Gaussian filtering on the image. (**a**) Original image. (**b**) Using Gaussian high-pass filter.

2.1.3. Adaptive Threshold

After filtering out the noise and highlighting the contours of PA images, the adaptive thresholding is performed. The main goal of this step was to find a suitable threshold for the image to perform binarization, dividing the image into two parts: teeth and gums, background and diseases, and alveolar bone. The accuracy of this step affected the determination of the target object in the later steps. This research tested the fixed threshold using the Otsu algorithm, as mentioned in [25]; the iterative algorithm, as mentioned in [26]; and the adaptive threshold, as mentioned in [27]. However, for the molars' PA, the pixel brightness was a significant factor, which is different from the PA of a single tooth. The variation in the molar area makes it even more challenging to find a pattern. Therefore, this research developed a newly defined adaptive algorithm to find the optimal threshold.

To address the issue of possible extreme values in the images, Chen et al. adjusted the grayscale image to avoid this problem [28]. Based on that, this research improved the process by redistributing extremely bright areas (grayscale > 170) to lower grayscale. After the adjustment, the subsequent algorithms were not affected by external lighting factors during the image capture process. The result is shown in Figure 4.

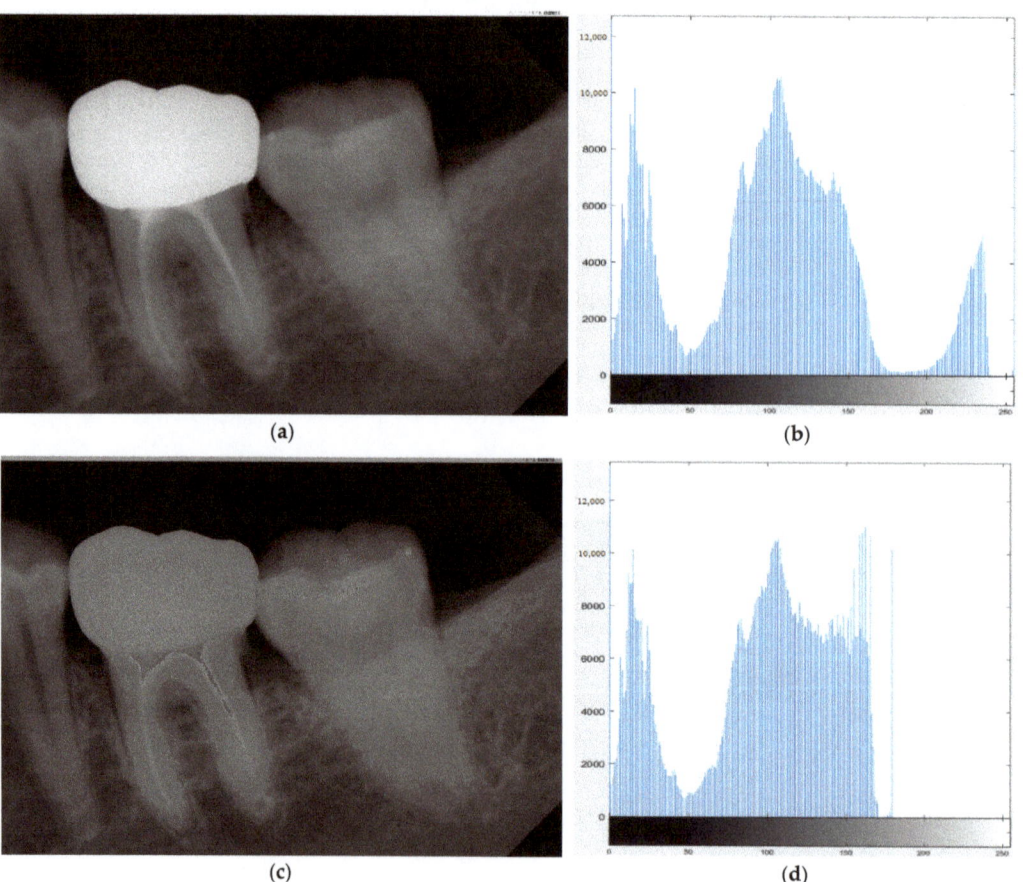

Figure 4. The result of the adaptive threshold. (**a**,**b**) are the original image and histogram. (**c**,**d**) adjust the grayscale and histogram.

After solving the extreme value variations, adaptive threshold values could be calculated. First, the minimum value (Zmin) in the grayscale range of 60 to 120, the maximum value (Lmax) in the grayscale range of 30 to 90, and the maximum value (Rmax) in the grayscale range of 91 to 170 was identified from the preprocessed grayscale image. Second, the midpoint gray value (Zmid) was calculated using Equation (2) and used as the initial binary threshold value (T0). In the next step, the total number of pixels in the image (Ztotal) and the total number of pixels from T0 to 170 (Zcheck) was calculated to obtain all parameters. Finally, three verification methods, namely checking whether the X-distance between two pairs of values (Zmin, Zmid) was less than 15, Equation (3), and Equation (4), were utilized to validate the results. If any of these tests failed, the process entered into an iterative calculation, either by changing the first step to find the second lowest value or by adjusting the threshold value to meet the restrictions.

$$Z_{mid} = \frac{Lmax + Rmax}{2} \qquad (2)$$

$$Z_{check} \leq Z_{total} \times \frac{5}{6} \qquad (3)$$

$$Z_{check} \geq Z_{total} \times \frac{2}{3} \qquad (4)$$

Two situations require the re-finding of the threshold. The first is when multiple T0 values meet the above constraints, and the other is when the suitable threshold within the grayscale range of 80–95 cannot be found. These two situations may cause multiple unsatisfactory segmenting results in the image cropping stage. Therefore, the ideal threshold value is continuously re-found through an iterative method. The ideal threshold value is used for binary thresholding where the pixel value greater than the threshold value is set to 1 (white) and the other pixel values are set to 0 (black). The binary image result was tested to ensure that the total mean of all pixels is greater than 0.6 and less than 0.85. The binary result is shown in Figure 5.

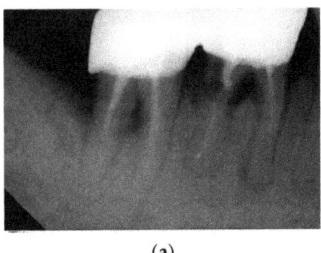
(a)
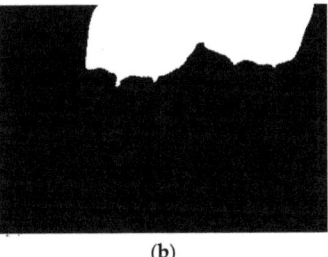
(b)
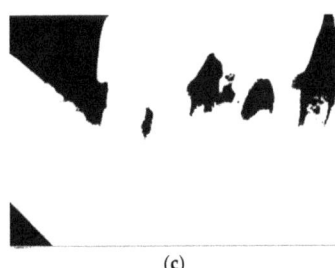
(c)

Figure 5. The result of the preprocessing. (a) Original image. (b) Directly binarized image. (c) Adjusted grayscale image.

2.2. Image Segmentation

The purpose of this step is to separate each tooth in PA image and create a database of images for each tooth. This step can effectively improve the target object recognition and reduce the interference from non-target objects before CNN training.

This research tested the segmentation method proposed in previous research [27]. The result showed that it worked well for front teeth but had difficulty with back teeth due to lighting or imaging conditions. Therefore, this research modified the method based on the other research [29] to automatically locate the segmenting line for back teeth. The masking technique for CNN training was also adjusted. The details of these modifications are described in the following sections.

2.2.1. Vertical Projection

Neighboring teeth segmenting lines inevitably lie on the interdental space, which is black (pixel value 0) in the binary image of PA. In addition, a PA image can have up to five teeth, so this research calculated the vertical pixel sum of each row. According to the algorithm conditions, neighboring interdental spaces must be divided by at least one tooth distance. The result is shown in Figure 6.

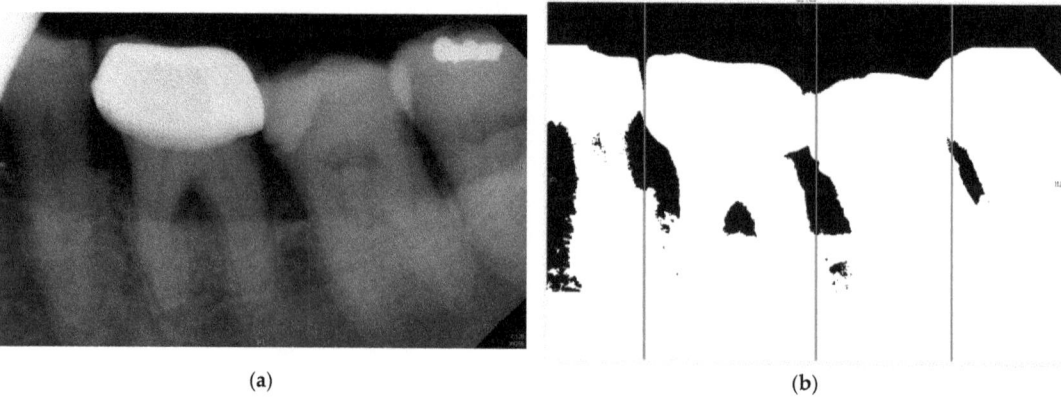

(a) (b)

Figure 6. The segmenting line results for this study. (**a**) Original image (**b**) Preliminary cutting line coordinates. The tangent line is shown as the red line.

2.2.2. Rote Tangent

Unlike the rotation algorithm in other research [29], instead of rotating the image, this research moves the vertical coordinates to rotate the segmenting line and create the marked positions. The positions of the five smallest pixel values are marked from left to right. This operation can avoid encountering complex rotation functions and converting the image coordinate system to or from the original coordinate system. It makes the automated program simpler, more efficient, and more error-tolerant. The segmentation result is shown in Figure 7. After locating the optimal rotation for the segmentation line, the coordinates of the two endpoints of the segmentation line are obtained. Comparing the distances between the two endpoints and the target tooth, the endpoint which is further away from the target tooth is considered to be on the outer side of the tooth. Then, a vertical trimming is performed on the X-coordinate to ensure that the target tooth is included without cutting through the tooth root. Bad segmentation would cause the loss of features. Previous research [27] has proposed using grayscale for segmentation. However, for posterior periapical radiographs (PA), which are sensitive to lighting conditions, the high grayscale values of gingiva can be similar to or even higher than those of the tooth roots. This can lead to misjudgment during the subsequent rotation and segmentation steps, indirectly confirming the importance of the pre-processing step mentioned.

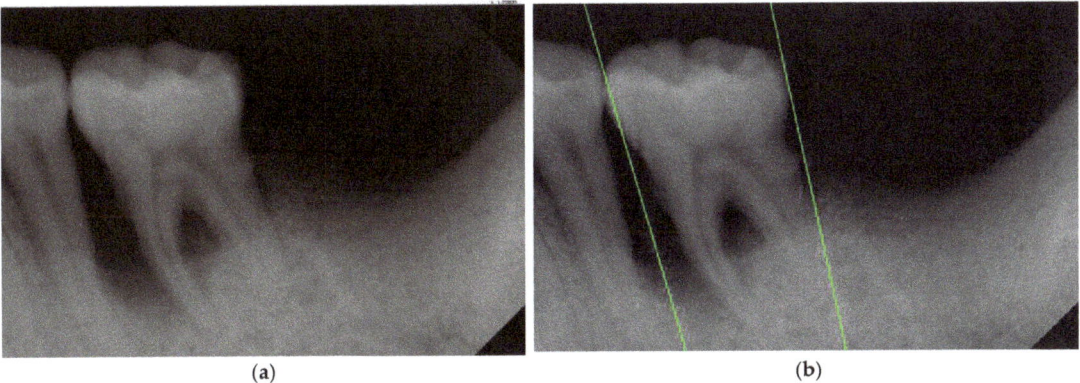

Figure 7. The result image of segmenting lines. (**a**) Original image. (**b**) After rotating segmentation lines. Corrected tangents are shown as green lines.

2.3. Image Mask

After determining the optimal rotation angle and segmentation lines, automated masking was applied to the areas outside the two segmentation lines. This isolates the target object of interest (a single tooth) from external factors that may affect the accuracy of CNN recognition and can improve the learning effectiveness of CNN in recognizing the target object.

This research proposes a method expanding each cutting line outward by 1/30th of the original image width to avoid damaging the target while the misplacement of the segmentation lines occurs. This step provides some error tolerance to the process. In addition, the extended area provides surrounding information of the target object that would help with CNN training. The segmentation result is shown in Figure 8.

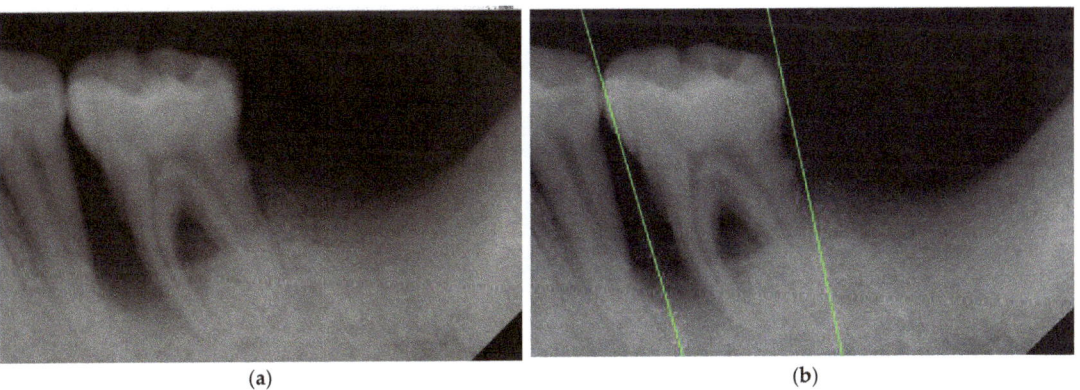

Figure 8. The results of the masking image. (**a**) Original segmentation. (**b**) Retouched segmentation and masking.

2.4. Image Identification

To validate the effectiveness and reliability of the proposed model, this study selected 128 lesion images and 140 normal teeth images from the database, as listed in Table 1. The images are augmented through horizontal, vertical, and reverse flipping to increase the number of images. Based on transfer learning theory, the database was divided into training and validation sets in a ratio of approximately 7:3 and was classified into the database, as shown in Table 2.

Table 1. Data classification of original periapical image from clinical.

Tooth	The Number of Original Images from Clinical		
	Lesion	Normal	total
Quantity	128	140	368

Table 2. Data classification of periapical image after preprocessing.

	Training Set	Validation Set	Total
Lesion	271 (Expanded)	41	312
Normal	245 (Expanded)	106	351

2.4.1. CNN Model

The experimental environment used in this proposal includes hardware and software specifications as shown in Table 3. Several famous transfer learning models in Matlab namely GoogLeNet, AlexNet, Inception v3, and Vgg19 are used for comparison. Taking GoogLeNet, which was performed best in this experiment as an example, the architecture is shown in Table 4. GoogLeNet is composed of Inception modules [30], which allow GoogLeNet to obtain the kernels of different scales during training and learn multiple features. Additionally, the inclusion of 1×1 convolutional layers prevents an excessive number of kernels and increases the non-linearity of the neural network with more comprehensive learning. Moreover, GoogLeNet eliminates connected layers. It reduces the number of parameters by nearly nine times compared to AlexNet [31]. Despite achieving similar or even higher accuracy than other models, the significant reduction in parameters makes GoogLeNet much lighter compared to other models. The remaining two models used for the experiment are Vgg19 [32] and Inception v3 [33]. These two models have shown better performance than other image recognition models in detecting image patterns.

Table 3. The hardware and software detailed specifications.

Hardware Platform	Version
CPU	AMD R5-5600X
GPU	GeForce GTX 1660 SUPER
DRAM	DDR4 3200 32 GB
OS	Windows 10
Software platform	Version
MATLAB	R2022b

Table 4. The input and output of GoogLeNet model.

Layer	Type	Activation
1	Data	$224 \times 224 \times 3$
2	Convolution	$112 \times 112 \times 64$
3	Max Pool	$56 \times 56 \times 64$
4	Convolution	$56 \times 56 \times 192$
5	Max Pool	$28 \times 28 \times 192$
6	Inception (3a)	$28 \times 28 \times 256$

Table 4. *Cont.*

Layer	Type	Activation
7	Inception (3b)	28 × 28 × 480
8	Max Pool	14 × 14 × 480
9	Inception (4a)	14 × 14 × 512
10	Inception (4b)	14 × 14 × 512
11	Inception (4c)	14 × 14 × 512
12	Inception (4d)	14 × 14 × 528
13	Inception (4e)	14 × 14 × 832
14	Max Pool	7 × 7 × 832
15	Inception (5a)	7 × 7 × 832
16	Inception (5b)	7 × 7 × 1024
17	Avg Pool	1 × 1 × 1024
18	Dropout (40%)	1 × 1 × 1024
19	Linear	1 × 1 × 1000
20	Softmax	1 × 1 × 1000

The randomly selected validation dataset is tested for the proposed model after the transfer learning is accomplished. The validation accuracy is then calculated and evaluated. The confusion matrix can be calculated to evaluate the quality of the trained model.

2.4.2. Adjust Hyper-Parameter

The adjustment of hyper-parameters is crucial for deep learning outcomes. The best combination of parameter settings can be slowly found through the appropriate fine tuning for each training process. The most frequently adjusted parameters in this experiment are max epoch, initial learning rate, mini batch size, and learn drop period. The suggested values of hyper-parameters are shown in Table 5.

Table 5. This study uses hyperparameters in the CNN model.

Hyperparameters	Value
Max Epoch	50
Initial Learning Rate	0.0001
Mini Batch Size	32
Learn Drop Period	5
Validation Frequency	3
Learn Rate Drop Factor	0.2000

A. Optimizer

SGDM (stochastic gradient descent with momentum) and Adam (adaptive moment estimation) are two popular optimization algorithms used in deep learning to train neural networks. Although Adam is faster than SGDM in terms of training speed, SGDM exhibits better convergence and more stable training performance. Considering the current number of images in the training set, the advantage of using Adam's fast convergence speed is not significant and may encounter convergence issues.

B. Initial Learning Rate

The rate at which the gradient descends during model training is affected by the initial learning rate. A small value can cause slow convergence and make the model prone to overfitting. Conversely, a large value can cause the model to learn too quickly and fail to converge, leading to divergence. After several trials, a stable learning rate of 1e-4 was determined for GoogLeNet.

C. Mini Batch Size

The mini batch size parameter determines how many data points are used to train the neural network at once. It is essentially a subset of the training set. If the mini batch size is too large, more data need to be considered for training. This leads to a more accurate correction direction, but the training process will take longer. On the other hand, if the mini batch size is too small, the correct direction will be biased because only a small amount of data are used in each iteration. However, this allows for more frequent corrections. For example, if the mini batch size is set to 20, this means that only 20 data points are used for training at a time. The mini batch size and epoch are closely related. If there are 400 data points in total and mini batch size is set to 20, then 20 training instances comprise one epoch.

3. Results

This section provides an overview of the model performance in this research. To monitor the training progress, a validation set was utilized. Table 6 presents the training process of GoogLeNet at intervals of five epochs. Additionally, Figures 9 and 10 offer a detailed representation of the training progress of GoogLeNet, including the final convergence status. The black line in both figures represents the validation results. Finally, the trained model was tested using the test set, and the confusion matrix was calculated. The results of the confusion matrix are presented in Table 7.

Based on the data presented in Table 8, it is evident that using PA images without excessive noise adjustment as a training database leads to an accuracy of over 80%. However, this approach also results in significant loss on the validation set. These findings suggest potential flaws in the database, such as blurred features or excessive noise. The second column demonstrates the results of training with Gaussian high-pass filtered raw images. Correcting image size and enhancing features significantly reduces the loss, resulting in an accuracy of 87.21%. However, these results fall short of the project's standards. Additionally, the loss rebounds after reaching 0.4 during training, indicating the need for further image preprocessing. The third column of Table 8 showcases the results of this project, which involve enhancing image features through masking techniques to exclude non-target regions. This enhancement dramatically improves the model's performance in image classification, achieving a validation set accuracy of 94.97% and reducing the loss to below the threshold of 0.18. Furthermore, Figure 11 illustrates the training process using different image preprocessing techniques. The three curves represent test accuracy on the training set. All curves show an increasing trend in accuracy as the number of iterations increases. The gray curve represents post-training using raw images. The orange curve represents applying high-precision automatic segmentation to raw images, followed by a Gaussian high-pass filter. The blue curve incorporates the previous process with an automatic masking step. The trend of the line graph indicates the significant impact of image preprocessing on the accuracy, further demonstrating that adding image filters and masking processing can significantly improve the model's accuracy, with an improvement rate as high as 10.8%.

Classifying images into molars and non-molar teeth was the first trial in this research, as illustrated in Figure 12, where the molar tooth on the left was the target, and the single-rooted non-molar tooth on the right was used as a comparison. A CNN model was developed for this classification task. The results demonstrated excellent classification accuracy with an average of over 97.5%, as shown in Table 9.

Table 6. The training process of GoogLeNet with every five epochs as the unit period.

Epoch	Iteration	Time Elapsed	Mini-Batch Accuracy	Validation Accuracy	Mini-Batch Loss	Validation Loss
1	1	00:00:02	34.38%	55.28%	1.6001	0.9257
5	60	00:00:37	90.62%	77.89%	0.3410	0.4747
10	130	00:01:15	75.00%	81.91%	0.5390	0.3947
15	200	00:01:53	78.12%	88.44%	0.3817	0.3297
20	280	00:02:40	87.50%	90.45%	0.2633	0.2445
25	350	00:03:17	93.75%	88.94%	0.1366	0.2721
30	420	00:03:55	96.88%	89.95%	0.0668	0.2637
35	480	00:04:28	90.62%	92.46%	0.1284	0.2018
40	550	00:05:07	93.75%	91.96%	0.1689	0.2093
45	620	00:05:44	93.75%	94.47%	0.1187	0.1702
50	700	00:06:30	96.88%	94.97%	0.0486	0.1700

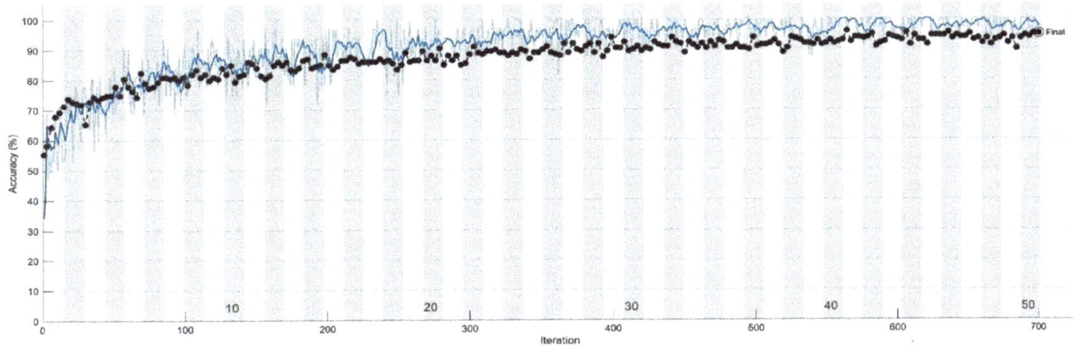

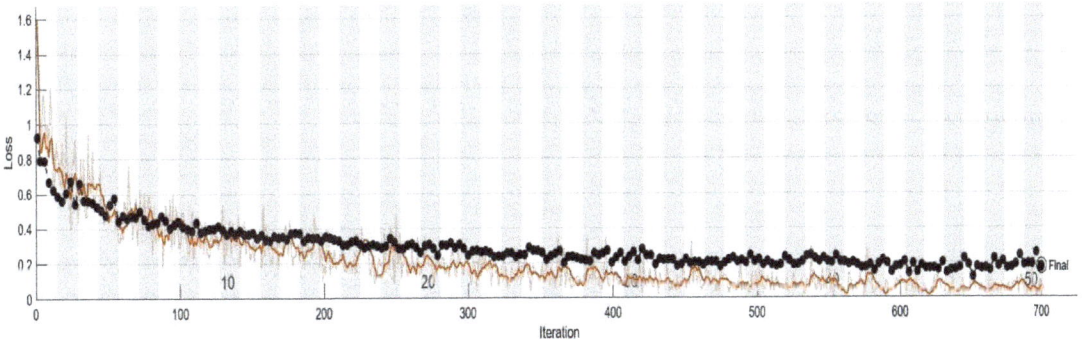

Figure 9. The accuracy of GoogLeNet model during training process. The validation set is the black line and the training set is the blue line.

Figure 10. The loss of GoogLeNet model during training process. The validation set is the black line, and the training set is the orange line.

Table 7. The confusion matrix of the GoogLeNet training result.

		Actual Values	
		Normal	Lesion
Predicted Value	Normal	46.8%	4.3%
	Lesion	2.1%	46.8%

Table 8. Compare the impact of various training sets on training results.

	Original Images	Gaussian High-Pass Filter	Gaussian High-Pass Filter + Mask
Validation Accuracy	84.16%	87.21%	94.97%
Validation Loss	0.7634	0.4578	0.1822
Model	GoogLeNet	GoogLeNet	GoogLeNet
Image			

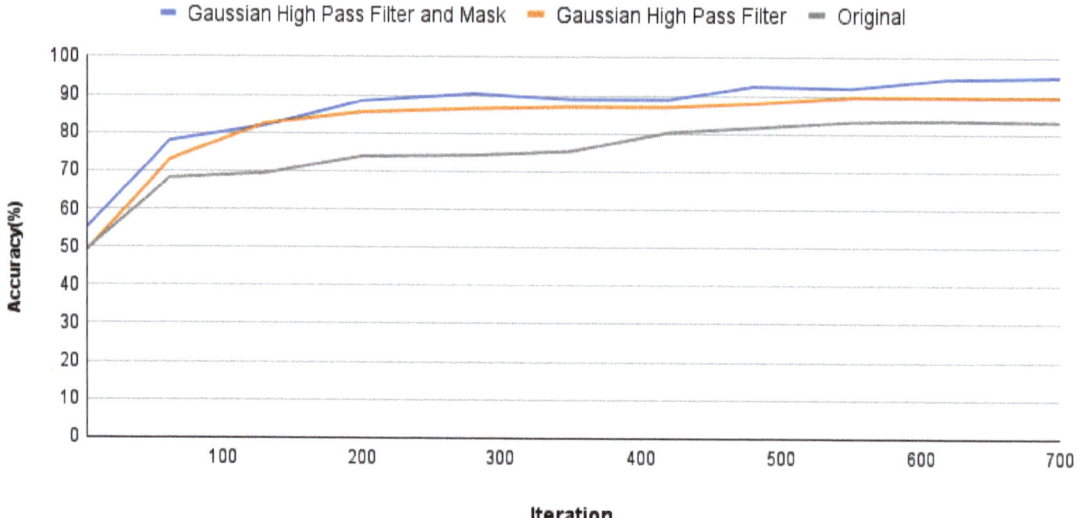

Figure 11. Accuracy comparison of GoogLeNet training process using only Gaussian high-pass filter and additional high-precision masking.

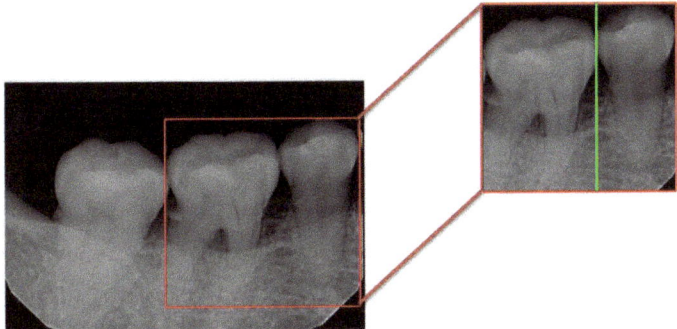

Figure 12. Validation example after image cropping in this study.

Table 9. The clinical data compare to the result.

Tooth Position in Figure 12	Recognition Accuracy	
Clinical Analysis	Molar	Single Tooth
Vgg19	98.01%	97.53%
Inception v3	97.76%	98.01%
Google Net	98.51%	98.42%
AlexNet	98.51%	98.26%

To enhance the recognition accuracy of the model on PA images for FI, the training samples were filtered to focus on the variables that could affect recognition accuracy. This approach made CNN more sensitive to the disease, more focused on the target, and resulted in a higher learning effect. In this study, image screening was performed on the training samples to improve the recognition accuracy. The results in Table 10 indicate that the CNN classification had an impact of 3–4% on the training outcomes. Moreover, in order to assess the model's performance, a set of evaluation metrics was employed, including recall, precision, and F1 score. These metrics provide a comprehensive analysis of the model's ability to accurately classify various cases and identify relevant features. Furthermore, alongside evaluating the model's performance, it is crucial to analyze the computational aspects of the proposed method. This analysis incorporates metrics such as computation time and actual operating time. These metrics facilitate a comparison of the efficiency and scalability of the proposed methods and aid in understanding the practical feasibility and potential computational requirements of the approach. The findings are presented in Table 11.

Table 10. Result of the FI identification accuracy of different models.

Training Process	Directly Identify the Disease	Identify the Disease after Classification
Vgg19	89.21%	92.96%
Inception v3	91.58%	94.23%
Google Net	92.18%	95.48%
AlexNet	91.58%	94.97%

Table 11. Model Efficacy Comparison For FI.

	GoogLeNet	Vgg19	AlexNet	Inceptionv3
Accuracy	94.97%	92.96%	94.92%	94.21%
Recall	95.6%	73.9%	86.9%	86.9%
Precision	91.6%	68%	80.0%	83.3%
F1	93.5%	70.8%	83.3%	85.0%
Elapsed time	25 min 30 s	87 min 47 s	29 min 34 s	76 min 50 s
Runtime	2.5981 s	6.4115 s	2.7535 s	4.2417 s

Table 12 indicates that the automated FI detection results in this research exhibit a significant contrast to the disease identification accuracy obtained using CT images at the apical region in the literature [34]. The symptom judgment accuracy using Vgg19 was nearly 93%, while the judgment accuracy of GoogLeNet and AlexNet was nearly 95% in this research.

Table 12. Comparison results of CNN models in this study and past studies.

Method	Method in [34]	This Research			
		GoogLeNet	AlexNet	Vgg19	Inceptionv3
Accuracy	89%	94.97%	94.92%	92.96%	94.21%

4. Discussion

A preprocessing step for dental images was found to be crucial in the research process. Proper preprocessing is essential for training a CNN, as raw PA images may not provide accurate information without it. However, establishing a standard processing method applicable to all images is challenging due to interference and external factors unique to each image. A lack of preprocessing can make subsequent segmentation difficult and result in lower accuracy due to potential noise in the PA images. In this study, the accuracy of the trained model was significantly improved by segmenting multiple teeth in PA images into individual tooth images before training. The adaptive threshold preprocessing method designed in this study accurately defined the cutting points during image segmentation, leading to improved segmentation accuracy. Preprocessing techniques like Gaussian high-pass filtering also reduced the inclusion of non-target regions. These improvements in segmentation accuracy enhanced symptom enhancement and overall model accuracy, highlighting the importance of preprocessing in this study. Furthermore, an automated process was developed to assist dentists in identifying bifurcations in PA images without causing visual or mental fatigue. During the CNN training phase, several mainstream image recognition models were tested, all achieving judgment accuracies above 90%. Following preprocessing and initial CNN recognition, the model effectively located teeth with potential diseases, with accuracy comparable to visual judgment. Specifically, GoogLeNet and AlexNet achieved judgment accuracies close to 95%. In comparison to the method proposed in [34], this study improved judgment accuracy by nearly 5%. These results demonstrate the efficacy of the proposed technique in detecting FI disease and showcase the success of training a CNN using conventional PA images, surpassing recognition capabilities based on CT images.

The results indicate that the proposed model exhibits mature and successful problem-solving capabilities, producing results highly similar to human judgment. However, there is room for improvement in the model's ability to further classify FI disease locations and enhance existing image enhancement techniques. In the future, this research aims to improve the automated process flow by integrating it within a chip, augmenting databases and developing a GUI interface. This will allow the automated process flow to be successfully integrated into clinical operations for dentists and result in a reduction in their workload and a shortening of patients' treatment time.

5. Conclusions

In general, this research study highlights the importance of preprocessing in improving the accuracy of a CNN model for detecting furcation involvements (FI) in dental images. The findings demonstrate that without proper preprocessing, raw PA images do not provide accurate information for training the model. The study proposes various preprocessing techniques, such as adaptive thresholding and Gaussian high-pass filtering, which significantly enhances the segmentation accuracy and the overall performance of the model. Additionally, an automated process was developed to assist dentists in identifying FI in PA images, offering a reliable and efficient alternative to visual judgment. The trained CNN model, particularly utilizing GoogLeNet and AlexNet architectures, achieved high accuracy in locating teeth with potential diseases, surpassing the performance of previous methods. Overall, this study provides valuable insights into the significance of preprocessing and the potential of CNN models in dental image analysis. The results contribute to the development of a high-accuracy medical assistance system, reducing the workload for dentists and improving the quality of dental care. Further research can build upon these findings to refine the model and explore additional enhancements for accurate FI detection and classification.

Author Contributions: Conceptualization, Y.-C.M., Y.-C.H., Y.C., and C.-W.L.; data curation, Y.-C.M., Y.-C.H., Y.C., and C.-W.L.; formal analysis, K.-C.L. and Y.-J.L.; funding acquisition, S.-L.C.; methodology, T.-Y.C., and M.-L.C.; resources, C.-A.C., S.-L.C., and P.A.R.A.; software, S.-L.C., Y.-L.L., Y.-J.L., H.-R.Y.; supervision, C.-A.C. and S.-L.C.; validation., Y.-J.Y.; visualization, H.-R.Y., K.-C.L., and P.A.R.A.; writing—original draft, T.-Y.C.; writing—review and editing, K.-C.L., M.-L.C., C.-A.C., and P.A.R.A. All authors have read and agreed to the published version of the manuscript.

Funding: This work was supported by the Ministry of Science and Technology (MOST), Taiwan, under grant numbers MOST-112-2410-H-033-014, MOST-111-2221-E-033-041, MOST-111-2823-8-033-001, MOST-111-2622-E-131-001, MOST-110-2223-8-033-002, MOST-110-2221-E-027-044-MY3, MOST-110-2218-E-035-007, MOST-110-2622-E-131-002, MOST-109-2622-E-131-001-CC3, MOST-109-2221-E-131-025, and MOST-109-2410-H-197-002-MY3, as well as by the National Chip Implementation Center, Taiwan.

Institutional Review Board Statement: Institutional Review Board Statement: Chang Gung Medical Foundation Institutional Review Board; IRB number: 02030B0C505; date of approval: 1 December 2020; protocol title: A Convolutional Neural Network Approach for Dental Bite-Wing, Panoramic and Periapical Radiographs Classification; executing institution: Chang-Geng Medical Foundation Taoyuan Chang-Geng Memorial Hospital of Taoyuan; duration of approval: from 1 December 2020 to 30 November 2021. The IRB reviewed this work and determined it to be an expedited review, i.e., case research or cases treated or diagnosed via clinical routines. However, this does not include HIV-positive cases.

Informed Consent Statement: The IRB approves the waiver of the participants' consent.

Conflicts of Interest: The authors declare no conflict of interest.

References

1. Nicholson, J.W. Periodontal Therapy Using Bioactive Glasses: A Review. *Prosthesis* **2022**, *4*, 648–663. [CrossRef]
2. Arslan, H.; Ahmed, H.M.A.; Şahin, Y.; Yıldız, E.D.; Gundoğdu, E.C.; Güven, Y.; Khalilov, R. Regenerative Endodontic Procedures in Necrotic Mature Teeth with Periapical Radiolucencies: A Preliminary Randomized Clinical Study. *J. Endod.* **2019**, *45*, 863–872. [CrossRef]
3. Shaker, Z.M.H.; Parsa, A.; Moharamzadeh, K. Development of a Radiographic Index for Periodontitis. *Dent. J.* **2021**, *9*, 19. [CrossRef]
4. Al-Ariny, Z.; Abdelwahab, M.A.; Fakhry, M.; Hasaneen, E.-S. An Efficient Vehicle Counting Method Using Mask R-CNN. In Proceedings of the 2020 International Conference on Innovative Trends in Communication and Computer Engineering (ITCE), Aswan, Egypt, 8–9 February 2020; pp. 232–237. [CrossRef]

5. Ma, J. Research on the Application of Financial Intelligence Based on Artificial Intelligence Technology. In Proceedings of the 2021 2nd International Conference on Artificial Intelligence and Education (ICAIE), Dali, China, 18–20 June 2021; pp. 72–75. [CrossRef]
6. Chen, J.; Zhan, X.; Wang, Y.; Huang, X. Medical Robots based on Artificial Intelligence in the Medical Education. In Proceedings of the 2021 2nd International Conference on Artificial Intelligence and Education (ICAIE), Dali, China, 18–20 June 2021; pp. 1–4. [CrossRef]
7. Chung, R.-L.; Hsueh, Y.; Chen, S.-L.; Abu, P.A.R. Efficient and Accurate CORDIC Pipelined Architecture Chip Design Based on Binomial Approximation for Biped Robot. *Electronics* 2022, *11*, 1701. [CrossRef]
8. Yanhua, Z. The Application of Artificial Intelligence in Foreign Language Teaching. In Proceedings of the 2020 International Conference on Artificial Intelligence and Education (ICAIE), Tianjin, China, 26–28 June 2020; pp. 40–42. [CrossRef]
9. Chen, S.-L.; Chen, T.-Y.; Lin, T.-L.; Chen, C.-A.; Lin, S.-Y.; Chiang, Y.-L.; Tung, K.-H.; Chiang, W.-Y. Fast Control for Backlight Power-Saving Algorithm Using Motion Vectors from the Decoded Video Stream. *Sensors* 2022, *22*, 7170. [CrossRef]
10. Wang, L.-H.; Yu, Y.-T.; Liu, W.; Xu, L.; Xie, C.-X.; Yang, T.; Kuo, I.-C.; Wang, X.-K.; Gao, J.; Huang, P.-C.; et al. Three-Heartbeat Multilead ECG Recognition Method for Arrhythmia Classification. *IEEE Access* 2022, *10*, 44046–44061. [CrossRef]
11. Huang, H.-L.; Ma, Y.-H.; Tu, C.-C.; Chang, P.-C. Radiographic Evaluation of Regeneration Strategies for the Treatment of Advanced Mandibular Furcation Defects: A Retrospective Study. *Membranes* 2022, *12*, 219. [CrossRef]
12. Pihlstrom, B.L.; Michalowicz, B.S.; Johnson, N.W. Periodontal diseases. *Lancet* 2005, *366*, 1809–1820. [CrossRef]
13. Yanni, P.; Curtis, D.A.; Kao, R.T.; Lin, G.-H. The Pattern of Tooth Loss for Periodontally Favorable Teeth: A Retrospective isd. *Biology* 2022, *11*, 1664. [CrossRef]
14. Alasqah, M.; Alotaibi, F.D.; Gufran, K. The Radiographic Assessment of Furcation Area in Maxillary and Mandibular First Molars while Considering the New Classification of Periodontal Disease. *Healthcare* 2022, *10*, 1464. [CrossRef]
15. ElSheshtawy, A.S.; Nazzal, H.; El Shahawy, O.I.; El Baz, A.A.; Ismail, S.M.; Kang, J.; Ezzat, K.M. The effect of platelet-rich plasma as a scaffold in regeneration/revitalization endodontics of immature permanent teeth assessed using 2-dimensional radiographs and cone beam computed tomography: A randomized controlled trial. *Int. Endod. J.* 2020, *53*, 905–921. [CrossRef]
16. Keerthana, G.; Duhan, J.; Tewari, S.; Sangwan, P.; Gupta, A.; Mittal, S.; Kumar, V.; Arora, M. Patient-centric outcome assessment of endodontic microsurgery using periapical radiography versus cone beam computed tomography: A randomized clinical trial. *Int. Endod. J.* 2023, *56*, 3–16. [CrossRef]
17. Jayalakshmi, G.S.; Kumar, V.S. Performance analysis of Convolutional Neural Network (CNN) based Cancerous Skin Lesion Detection System. In Proceedings of the 2019 International Conference on Computational Intelligence in Data Science (ICCIDS), Chennai, India, 21–23 February 2019; pp. 1–6. [CrossRef]
18. Lam, J.; Yeung, A.W.K.; Acharya, A.; Fok, C.; Fok, M.; Pelekos, G. Comparison between Conventional Modality Versus Cone-Beam Computer Tomography on the Assessment of Vertical Furcation in Molars. *Diagnostics* 2022, *13*, 106. [CrossRef]
19. Yilmaz, E.; Kayikcioglu, T.; Kayipmaz, S. Semi-automatic segmentation of apical lesions in cone beam computed tomography images. In Proceedings of the 2017 25th Signal Processing and Communications Applications Conference (SIU), Antalya, Turkey, 15–18 May 2017; pp. 1–4. [CrossRef]
20. Yusof, N.A.M.; Noor, E.; Reduwan, N.H.; Yusof, M.Y.P.M. Diagnostic accuracy of periapical radiograph, cone beam computed tomography, and intrasurgical linear measurement techniques for assessing furcation defects: A longitudinal randomised controlled trial. *Clin. Oral Investig.* 2021, *25*, 923–932. [CrossRef]
21. Shaikh, M.S.; Shahzad, Z.; Tash, E.A.; Janjua, O.S.; Khan, M.I.; Zafar, M.S. Human Umbilical Cord Mesenchymal Stem Cells: Current Literature and Role in Periodontal Regeneration. *Cells* 2022, *11*, 1168. [CrossRef]
22. Chen, S.-L.; Chen, T.-Y.; Huang, Y.-C.; Chen, C.-A.; Chou, H.-S.; Huang, Y.-Y.; Lin, W.-C.; Li, T.-C.; Yuan, J.-J.; Abu, P.A.R.; et al. Missing Teeth and Restoration Detection Using Dental Panoramic Radiography Based on Transfer Learning With CNNs. *IEEE Access* 2022, *10*, 118654–118664. [CrossRef]
23. Cui, J.; Zhang, M. Time-Domain versus frequency-domain approach for an accurate simulation of phased arrays. In Proceedings of the 2008 International Conference on Microwave and Millimeter Wave Technology, Nanjing, China, 21–24 April 2008; pp. 454–457. [CrossRef]
24. Dogra, A.; Bhalla, P. Image Sharpening By Gaussian And Butterworth High Pass Filter. *Biomed. Pharmacol. J.* 2014, *7*, 707–713. [CrossRef]
25. Devi, M.P.A.; Latha, T.; Sulochana, C.H. Iterative thresholding based image segmentation using 2D improved Otsu algorithm. In Proceedings of the 2015 Global Conference on Communication Technologies (GCCT), Thuckalay, India, 23–24 April 2015; pp. 145–149. [CrossRef]
26. Mao, Y.-C.; Chen, T.-Y.; Chou, H.-S.; Lin, S.-Y.; Liu, S.-Y.; Chen, Y.-A.; Liu, Y.-L.; Chen, C.-A.; Huang, Y.-C.; Chen, S.-L.; et al. Caries and Restoration Detection Using Bitewing Film Based on Transfer Learning with CNNs. *Sensors* 2021, *21*, 4613. [CrossRef]
27. Chuo, Y.; Lin, W.-M.; Chen, T.-Y.; Chan, M.-L.; Chang, Y.-S.; Lin, Y.-R.; Lin, Y.-J.; Shao, Y.-H.; Chen, C.-A.; Chen, S.-L.; et al. A High-Accuracy Detection System: Based on Transfer Learning for Apical Lesions on Periapical Radiograph. *Bioengineering* 2022, *9*, 777. [CrossRef]
28. Chen, S.-L.; Chen, T.-Y.; Mao, Y.-C.; Lin, S.-Y.; Huang, Y.-Y.; Chen, C.-A.; Lin, Y.-J.; Hsu, Y.-M.; Li, C.-A.; Chiang, W.-Y.; et al. Automated Detection System Based on Convolution Neural Networks for Retained Root, Endodontic Treated Teeth, and Implant Recognition on Dental Panoramic Images. *IEEE Sens. J.* 2022, *22*, 23293–23306. [CrossRef]

29. Li, C.-W.; Lin, S.-Y.; Chou, H.-S.; Chen, T.-Y.; Chen, Y.-A.; Liu, S.-Y.; Liu, Y.-L.; Chen, C.-A.; Huang, Y.-C.; Chen, S.-L.; et al. Detection of Dental Apical Lesions Using CNNs on Periapical Radiograph. *Sensors* **2021**, *21*, 7049. [CrossRef]
30. Szegedy, C.; Liu, W.; Jia, Y.; Sermanet, P.; Reed, S.; Anguelov, D.; Erhan, D.; Vanhoucke, V.; Rabinovich, A. Going deeper with convolutions. In Proceedings of the IEEE Conference on Computer Vision and Pattern Recognition, Boston, MA, USA, 7–12 June 2015; pp. 1–9.
31. Krizhevsky, A.; Sutskever, I.; Hinton, G.E. Imagenet classification with deep convolutional neural networks. *Commun. ACM* **2012**, *60*, 84–90.
32. Simonyan, K.; Zisserman, A. Very deep convolutional networks for large-scale image recognition. *arXiv* **2014**, arXiv:1409.1556.
33. Szegedy, C.; Vanhoucke, V.; Ioffe, S.; Shlens, J.; Wojna, Z. Rethinking the inception architecture for computer vision. In Proceedings of the IEEE Conference on Computer Vision and Pattern Recognition, Las Vegas, NV, USA, 27–30 June 2016; pp. 2818–2826.
34. He, K.; Zhang, X.; Ren, S.; Sun, J. Deep Residual Learning for Image Recognition. *arXiv* **2015**, arXiv:1512.03385.

Disclaimer/Publisher's Note: The statements, opinions and data contained in all publications are solely those of the individual author(s) and contributor(s) and not of MDPI and/or the editor(s). MDPI and/or the editor(s) disclaim responsibility for any injury to people or property resulting from any ideas, methods, instructions or products referred to in the content.

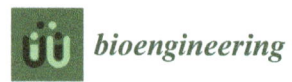

Article

Improving Dental Implant Outcomes: CNN-Based System Accurately Measures Degree of Peri-Implantitis Damage on Periapical Film

Yi-Chieh Chen [1,†], Ming-Yi Chen [2,†], Tsung-Yi Chen [3,†], Mei-Ling Chan [1,4,*,†], Ya-Yun Huang [3], Yu-Lin Liu [3], Pei-Ting Lee [3], Guan-Jhih Lin [3], Tai-Feng Li [3], Chiung-An Chen [5,†], Shih-Lun Chen [3,*], Kuo-Chen Li [6,†] and Patricia Angela R. Abu [7]

1. Department of General Dentistry, Keelung Chang Gung Memorial Hospital, Keelung City 204201, Taiwan
2. Department of General Dentistry, Chang Gung Memorial Hospital, Taoyuan City 33305, Taiwan
3. Department of Electronic Engineering, Chung Yuan Christian University, Taoyuan City 32023, Taiwan; g10976016@cycu.edu.tw (T.-Y.C.)
4. School of Physical Educational College, Jiaying University, Meizhou 514000, China
5. Department of Electrical Engineering, Ming Chi University of Technology, New Taipei City 243303, Taiwan
6. Department of Information Management, Chung Yuan Christian University, Taoyuan City 320317, Taiwan
7. Ateneo Laboratory for Intelligent Visual Environments, Department of Information Systems and Computer Science, Ateneo de Manila University, Quezon City 1108, Philippines
* Correspondence: lynn202207017@jyu.edu.cn (M.-L.C.); chrischen@cycu.edu.tw (S.-L.C.)
† These authors contributed equally to this work.

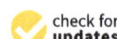

Citation: Chen, Y.-C.; Chen, M.-Y.; Chen, T.-Y.; Chan, M.-L.; Huang, Y.-Y.; Liu, Y.-L.; Lee, P.-T.; Lin, G.-J.; Li, T.-F.; Chen, C.-A.; et al. Improving Dental Implant Outcomes: CNN-Based System Accurately Measures Degree of Peri-Implantitis Damage on Periapical Film. *Bioengineering* 2023, 10, 640. https://doi.org/10.3390/bioengineering10060640

Academic Editors: Naji Kharouf, Davide Mancino, Salvatore Sauro and Louis Hardan

Received: 13 April 2023
Revised: 9 May 2023
Accepted: 19 May 2023
Published: 25 May 2023

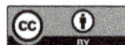

Copyright: © 2023 by the authors. Licensee MDPI, Basel, Switzerland. This article is an open access article distributed under the terms and conditions of the Creative Commons Attribution (CC BY) license (https://creativecommons.org/licenses/by/4.0/).

Abstract: As the popularity of dental implants continues to grow at a rate of about 14% per year, so do the risks associated with the procedure. Complications such as sinusitis and nerve damage are not uncommon, and inadequate cleaning can lead to peri-implantitis around the implant, jeopardizing its stability and potentially necessitating retreatment. To address this issue, this research proposes a new system for evaluating the degree of periodontal damage around implants using Periapical film (PA). The system utilizes two Convolutional Neural Networks (CNN) models to accurately detect the location of the implant and assess the extent of damage caused by peri-implantitis. One of the CNN models is designed to determine the location of the implant in the PA with an accuracy of up to 89.31%, while the other model is responsible for assessing the degree of Peri-implantitis damage around the implant, achieving an accuracy of 90.45%. The system combines image cropping based on position information obtained from the first CNN with image enhancement techniques such as Histogram Equalization and Adaptive Histogram Equalization (AHE) to improve the visibility of the implant and gums. The result is a more accurate assessment of whether peri-implantitis has eroded to the first thread, a critical indicator of implant stability. To ensure the ethical and regulatory standards of our research, this proposal has been certified by the Institutional Review Board (IRB) under number 202102023B0C503. With no existing technology to evaluate Peri-implantitis damage around dental implants, this CNN-based system has the potential to revolutionize implant dentistry and improve patient outcomes.

Keywords: peri-implantitis; periodontitis; periapical radiograph; deep learning; neural networks; image enhancement

1. Introduction

In recent decades, dental implant technology has gained popularity, boasting a success rate of over 90% for artificial dental implant surgery [1]. The human mouth contains 32 permanent teeth, each with an interlocking function. Missing teeth lead to a cascade of oral health issues, causing more significant long-term damage than adjacent natural teeth [2]. Failure to address a missing tooth can lead to tooth decay and peri-implantitis, impairing the original function of the mouth. In more severe cases, adjacent teeth can shift, bone shrinkage can occur, and bite and temporomandibular joint disorder (TMD) can develop [3,4]. Symptoms associated with TMD include Temporomandibular Joint (TMJ) pain, chewing pain, pain around the ear, and facial asymmetry due to uneven force application [5,6]. According to the American Dental Association, around 5 million dental implants are annually implanted in the U.S., and the worldwide market for dental implants is projected to reach USD 4.6 billion by 2022 [7]. Today, dental implants are a common dental procedure, involving the surgical implantation of a titanium root into the alveolar bone where a tooth is missing [8]. After sterile treatment and a secure bond between the root and tissue, an artificial crown is placed to replace the missing tooth [9]. The structure of the implant is similar to that of a natural tooth and will not cause any foreign body sensations when biting [10].

The use of artificial intelligence (AI) has become prevalent across various fields due to technological advancements. In recent years, the integration of AI and medicine has emerged in areas such as Cardiology [11], Pulmonary Medicine [12], and Neurology [13]. Artificial intelligence can help doctors to consolidate data and provide diagnostic methods. It also brings medical resources to rural areas to improve the quality of medical care around the world, which shows that artificial intelligence is extremely helpful to society [14]. The combination of Convolutional Neural Networks (CNN) and dentistry has resulted in a wealth of information. Research in AI has displayed promising results in utilizing the three common X-ray film types used in routine dental exams, including Panoramic radiographs, Periapical films, and Bite-Wing films. In the realm of dental radiology research, two primary areas of focus are tooth localization and identification of disease symptoms. Image enhancement techniques have been proposed to increase the accuracy of cutting and positioning of individual teeth. For instance, some studies have utilized a polynomial function to connect gap chains into a smooth curve, resulting in a 4% improvement and 93.28% accuracy rate [15]. Additionally, Gaussian filtering and edge detection technology have been proposed to enhance the visibility of tooth gaps and facilitate the cutting and positioning of individual teeth [16]. Filters have been helpful in reducing the impact of point creation on cutting technology and recognition in PA [17]. Furthermore, adaptive thresholds have been suggested to improve the application of cropping technology in dental radiology research [18]. Regarding the identification of disease symptoms, the backpropagation neural network has been used to diagnose dental caries with an accuracy rate of 94.1% [19]. Tooth detection and classification have been carried out on panoramic radiographs by training and classifying tooth types into four groups using a quadruple cross-validation method with 93.2% accuracy. Dental status has also been classified into three groups with an accuracy of 98.0% [20]. These findings demonstrate the enormous potential of AI in the dental field, with the ability to provide accurate diagnosis and improve patient care.

The dental implant surgery carries potential complications such as sinus perforation or jaw paralysis due to its location in nerve-ridden gums [21], making focus and attention crucial to avoid medical disputes. Currently, the objective of research in this area focuses on two areas: inspection and pre-operative analysis, thus reducing clinic time for dentists and enabling them to focus on treatment and technique. For example, CNN technology has been used for whole oral cavity analysis and inspection of periapical radiographs during the inspection stage [22,23]. Other studies have proposed an automatic synchronous detection system for two-dimensional grayscale cone beam computed tomography (CBCT) images of alveolar bone (AB) and the mandibular canal (MC) for preoperative treatment planning [24]. Additionally, pain and discomfort during the operation can affect its smoothness, and some research has proposed evaluating and predicting pain [25]. However, there is a limited amount of research conducted on postoperative analysis. Insufficient cleaning by the patient may result in peri-implantitis [26,27], wherein bacteria can gradually erode the tissues surrounding the implant, leading to bone and flesh loss. As a result, the implant may lose support and become loose or dislodged. In view of this, the aim of this study is to assess the extent of periodontal damage surrounding implants and provide accurate and objective evaluation results for postoperative follow-up examinations. The study aims to decrease the workload of dentists, protect the rights and interests of patients, and prevent potential medical disputes. This proposal provides three contributions and innovations:

1. The YOLOv2 model is trained using the manually created ROI database provided by the dentist to detect the implant position and return data for individual implant thread cropping;
2. Histogram equalization, overlapping techniques, and adaptive histogram equalization are employed to enhance the boundary lines. Additionally, the gingival area is colored orange, while the threaded area is green, thereby improving subsequent CNN judgment;
3. The study trains preprocessed data in a CNN model to detect damages, utilizing the AlexNet algorithm, achieving a final accuracy rate of 90.4%. Additionally, this research presents the first medical assistance system for automated thread analysis of implants.

The structure of this paper is as follows: Section 2 introduces the use of deep learning models for implant location labeling, cropping, and anterior processing, and finally, the use of CNN to build a model for arguing whether there is damage; Section 3 mainly integrates the methods used and the research results; Section 4 discusses the experimental results; and Section 5 describes the conclusion and future prospects.

2. Materials and Methods

The database used in this research is collected from relevant cases diagnosed by professional dentists. It can be roughly divided into three parts: implant cropping, image preprocessing, and implant classification. The damages of dental implants are determined by the M(mesial) and the D(distal). Therefore, the step of implant cropping will be divided into cutting out single implants from one to multiple implants in the PA. This part will use a deep learning model to label the implant position and then separate it into M and D by using the linear regression algorithm. Although both implant cropping and implant classification require machine learning, the training methods are very different. Not only are different models used but also different types of databases are introduced. The implant cropping is trained using a manually selected ROI database, while the implant classification is trained using preprocessed images. The major problem encountered in this research is that the validation set cannot converge when the cropped implant images are directly fed into the model for training, which leads to overfitting. To solve this problem the research colors different parts of the implant image, adding reference lines and adjusting the parameters of the CNN model. The flowchart of this research is shown in Figure 1.

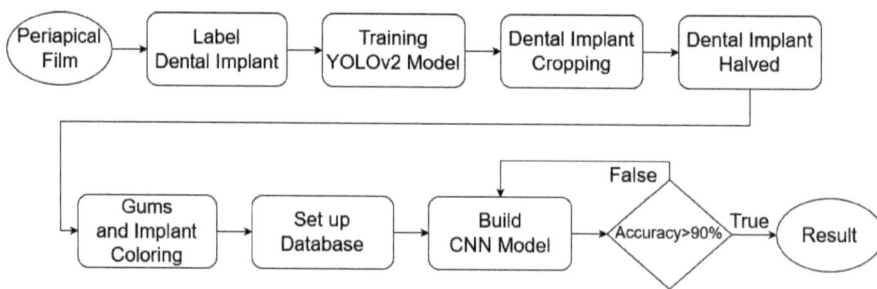

Figure 1. The flowchart of this research.

2.1. Image Cropping

To enable the CNN model to focus specifically on identifying destruction of dental implants on the mesial and distal sides, the PA image needs to be cropped to a single implant. Manual cropping is a time-consuming process. This study utilizes YOLOv2 to detect the position of the implant. Using the position information returned by YOLOv2, the implant can be cropped efficiently. Next, a linear regression algorithm is used to find the central cutting line of the implant. The output image is then named and classified by comparing it with the diagnosis results provided by the hospital, creating a database for the CNN model. To prepare the data for further analysis, image preprocessing is then performed.

2.1.1. Label Dental Implant

The key issue in this step is to determine the Region of Interest (ROI) for training the object detection model. If the ROI encompasses the entire implant, the damage feature of the screw thread may not be classified accurately. This is because the area above the screw thread occupies most of the picture as depicted in Figure 2a, which can also make subsequent cropping steps challenging. Labeling only the screw thread, on the other hand, will not affect the determination process. Hence, the research sets the ROI to the thread instead of the implant body as shown in Figure 2b, to preserve the damage features of the screw thread as much as possible. Additionally, the damage detection also requires the gingival features surrounding the screw thread. Therefore, in the subsequent step of cropping the screw thread, the ROI returns the position that expands horizontally by several pixels to preserve these features for the next step.

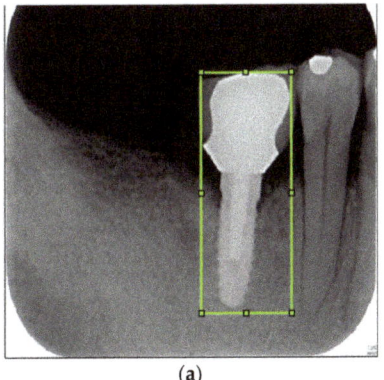
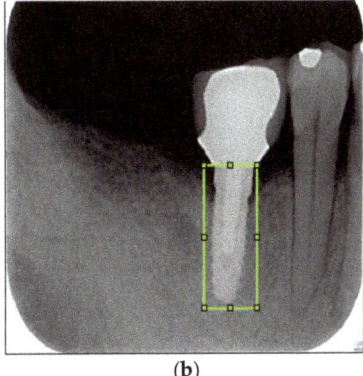

(a)   (b)

Figure 2. Illustrating the marking of the Region of Interest (ROI) in this study. (**a**) The dental implant is depicted, including the area above the screw thread. (**b**) Only dental implants with screw threads are included in the ROI.

2.1.2. YOLOv2 Model

The main purpose of training the object detection model in this study is to improve operational efficiency and reduce the time required for manual image cropping. Therefore, this study uses specific instruments to achieve the best training effect, including hardware equipment, as listed in Table 1; software, i.e., YOLOv2 layer structure model, as listed in Table 2; and training parameter settings, as listed in Table 3.

Table 1. Experimental environment specifications.

Hardware Platform	Version
CPU	Intel i5-12400
GPU	GeForce RTX 3080
DRAM	DDR4 3200 32 GB
Software Platform	**Version**
MATLAB	R2022b

Table 2. The Layers of YOLOv2 model.

	Type	Activations
1	Image Input	416 × 416 × 3
2	2-D Convolution	416 × 416 × 16
3	Batch Normalization	416 × 416 × 16
4	Leaky ReLU	416 × 416 × 16
5	2-D Max Pooling	208 × 208 × 16
6	2-D Convolution	208 × 208 × 32
7	Batch Normalization	208 × 208 × 32
8	Leaky ReLU	208 × 208 × 32
9	2-D Max Pooling	104 × 104 × 32
10	2-D Convolution	104 × 104 × 64
11	Batch Normalization	104 × 104 × 64
12	Leaky ReLU	104 × 104 × 64
13	2-D Max Pooling	52 × 52 × 64
14	2-D Convolution	52 × 52 × 128
15	Batch Normalization	52 × 52 × 128
16	Leaky ReLU	52 × 52 × 128
17	2-D Max Pooling	26 × 26 × 128
18	2-D Convolution	26 × 26 × 256
19	Batch Normalization	26 × 26 × 256
20	Leaky ReLU	26 × 26 × 256
21	2-D Max Pooling	13 × 13 × 256
22	2-D Convolution	13 × 13 × 512
23	Batch Normalization	13 × 13 × 512
24	Leaky ReLU	13 × 13 × 512
25	2-D Max Pooling	13 × 13 × 512
26	2-D Convolution	13 × 13 × 1024
27	Batch Normalization	13 × 13 × 1024
28	Leaky ReLU	13 × 13 × 1024
29	2-D Convolution	13 × 13 × 512
30	Batch Normalization	13 × 13 × 512
31	Leaky ReLU	13 × 13 × 512
32	2-D Convolution	13 × 13 × 30
33	Transform Layer	13 × 13 × 30
34	Output	13 × 13 × 30

Table 3. Hyperparameters for YOLOv2 training.

Hyperparameters	Value
Optimizer	sgdm
Initial Learning Rate	0.001
Max Epoch	24
Mini Batch Size	16

To train the YOLOv2 model to label the position of an implant, this research manually labels a total of 211 photos with 147 used for training and 64 for testing. The remaining 173 images are labeled directly by the YOLOv2 model as indicated in Table 4. Ultimately, the position of an implant is exported to the next step while the confusion matrix is calculated using the results of the following step. By employing this approach, the research can reduce the time required for manual image cropping and achieve accurate labeling of implant positions. This is accomplished by training the YOLOv2 model to identify the position of the implant within the image. The ability of the YOLOv2 model to identify the location of the implant quickly and accurately allows for efficient and accurate cropping of the image, therefore reducing the amount of time required for this process. To ensure the accuracy of the YOLOv2 model, manually labeling a significant portion of the images used for training was conducted in this research. This manual labeling allowed for the evaluation of the performance of the model and made any necessary adjustments to improve its accuracy. The remaining images were labeled by the YOLOv2 model to further improve its accuracy.

Table 4. The distribution of data in the original periapical image obtained from clinical sources.

	The Number of Original Periapical Images			
	Training	Test	The Others	Total
Quantity	147	46	263	456

In conclusion, the object detection of the model training is critical to reducing the time required for manual image cropping in this research. The use of hardware and software configurations was optimized for this purpose along with the manual labeling of images, thus allowing the YOLOv2 model to accurately identify implant positions in the image. By doing so, this proposed study can achieve efficient and accurate image cropping, therefore reducing the amount of time required for this process.

Optimizer

Optimizers play a crucial role in machine learning by helping to minimize the loss function. The choice of optimizer depends on the specific network and the problem at hand. In MATLAB, there are several options for optimizers, including Sgdm, RMSProp, and Adam.

The Sgdm optimizer is a variant of stochastic gradient descent with momentum, which uses the gradients of the current mini-batch and the previous mini-batch to update the model parameters. It has been shown to be effective in improving convergence speed and reducing the likelihood of becoming stuck in local optima. RMSProp optimizer, on the other hand, adjusts the learning rate adaptively for each parameter based on the average of the squares of the gradients. It is known to be useful for training recurrent neural networks. Adam optimizer is another popular algorithm that combines the ideas of momentum and adaptive learning rates. It has been shown to be effective in training large-scale deep learning models.

For this research, the Sgdm optimizer was chosen for the YOLOv2 network. The reason for this choice may be related to its effectiveness in improving convergence speed, reducing the likelihood of becoming stuck in local optima, and its ability to handle large datasets. Ultimately, the choice of optimizer depends on the specific problem being addressed and the characteristics of the data.

Initial Learning Rate

The initial learning rate is a critical hyperparameter that determines the step size at each iteration during model training. It controls the speed of gradient descent and affects the performance of the model. However, choosing an optimal learning rate can be challenging. If the learning rate is set too high, the model may learn too quickly, resulting in convergence problems. Conversely, a learning rate that is too low may lead to slow learning, which is ineffective and can result in overfitting or becoming trapped in a local minimum. Therefore, selecting an appropriate learning rate is essential for achieving global minimum and successfully training the model.

Max Epoch, Mini Batch Size and Iteration

In neural network learning, an epoch refers to a complete iteration over the entire dataset. In MATLAB, the Max Epoch parameter is used to set the total number of epochs before the network training is stopped. However, when the size of each dataset is large, it may not be possible to process all the data at once due to limited memory resources. In such cases, the data are divided into smaller subsets called batches, with each batch containing a certain number of samples. In addition, the number of samples in each batch is referred to as the batch size. It is important to choose an appropriate batch size as it affects the performance of the neural network during training. Using a large batch size may accelerate the training process, but it can also cause overfitting where the network becomes excessively attuned to the training data, resulting in poor performance on new data. On the other hand, a small batch size can lead to slower convergence, but it also makes the training process more robust and generalizable to new data. Thus, choosing the right batch size is crucial in achieving good performance in neural network training.

The concept of Iteration is closely related to batch size. For instance, if a dataset contains 10 samples and the batch size is set to 2, then it would take 5 iterations to complete one epoch of training. During each iteration, the neural network updates its parameters based on the gradients calculated from the samples in the current batch. The relationship between dataset size, batch size, and iterations can be expressed mathematically, as shown in Equation (1):

$$Data\ set\ size = Iteration\ Batch\ size(1\ Epoch) \qquad (1)$$

2.1.3. Cropping Dental Implant by YOLOv2

The detector after training will return the position of the object, including the dot in the upper left corner of the object and the length and width of the ROI. The key point of this step is to use the returned value to crop the required image. In 2.1.1, it is necessary to preserve the features between the implant and the gingiva to the greatest extent possible during cropping. Therefore, the returned data will add several pixels to the horizontal field as shown in Figure 3.

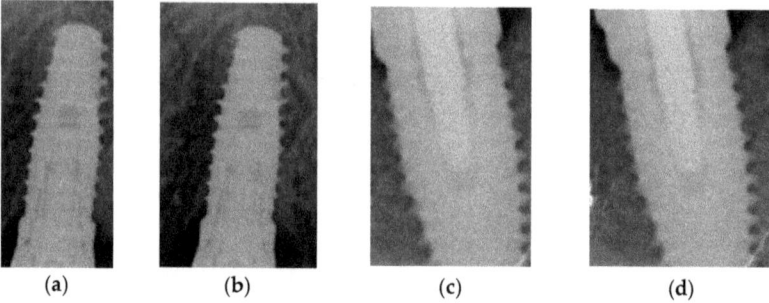

Figure 3. The cropping example with and without extending: (a,c) the image cropped directly; (b,d) the image cropped after extending.

The detection of damages in implant screw threads is not based on a single implant, but rather on a single side. Thus, after cropping the region of interest (ROI) of the implant thread using YOLOv2, further segmentation is necessary. To simplify the classification of items in the CNN model database and enable the model to focus more on damage identification, the cropped image is segmented into the mesial and distal sides. However, cropping poses a challenge as the thread may not be parallel to the Y-axis of the image. Therefore, linear regression analysis [28] is employed to determine the position of the implant in the image for cropping purposes, as shown in Equation (2):

$$y = \beta_0 + \beta_1 x \tag{2}$$

where 0 represents the intercept, and 1 represents the slope. By analyzing the distribution of points on the coordinate axis, a line that represents the overall trend can be obtained. Based on the observation of dental implants in this project, the length of the implant is greater than its width in the photo. Therefore, by placing the implant horizontally on the coordinate axis, a linear equation that passes through the center of the implant can be obtained.

The initial step involves the binarization of the image to extract the implant as illustrated in Figure 4a. The following step entails plotting the extracted implant on the XY plane as depicted in Figure 4b. Due to the closely distributed pixels of the implant, the last step involves utilizing linear regression analysis to determine the cutting line via the centerline of the implant. Padding is applied to maintain the symmetry of the cropped image, therefore resulting in two images each containing only half of the screw thread as demonstrated in Figure 4.

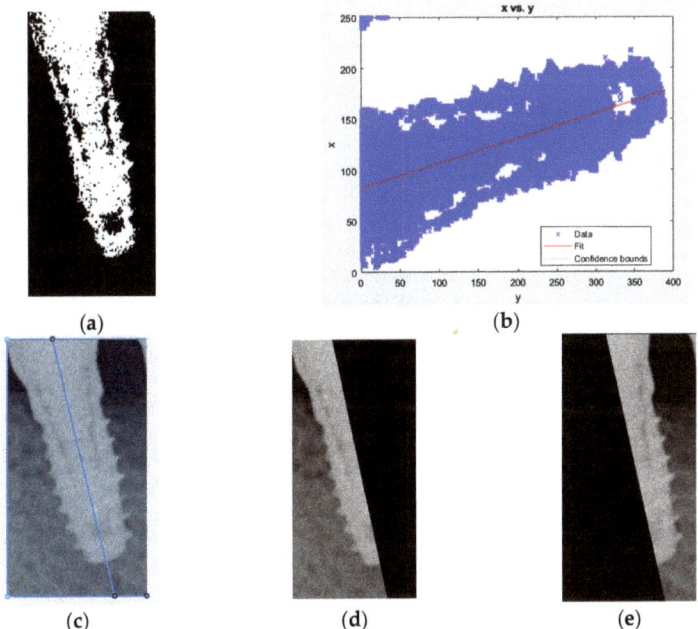

Figure 4. The result of the images: (**a**) image binarization; (**b**) dental implants plot on coordinate axis; (**c**) dental implant midline; (**d**) the left half of the image after cutting; (**e**) the right half of the image after cutting.

2.2. Preprocessing

It is crucial to establish a well-characterized database that can effectively aid the CNN model in identifying the presence of peri-implantitis. In order to achieve this, this research categorized the database into two groups: the control group, consisting of implants without signs of peri-implantitis; and the test group, consisting of implants with signs of peri-implantitis. To classify the database, this research consulted and referred to the assessment of three physicians with at least five years of clinical experience on whether the model has detected peri-implantitis. Although the cropped images can be used as a database for the CNN model, the original images still contain significant amounts of noise. This noise hinders the ability of the CNN model to differentiate between damage and health. To enhance the learning ability of the CNN model, it is necessary to remove the noise and improve the features to make the differences between damaged and healthy more distinct. For instance, in the test group's data, implants with signs of peri-implantitis exhibit obvious black subsidence marks around the alveolar bone on the image, which is not present in the control group's data. Hence, this research proposed the steps for image enhancement to improve efficacy of the CNN model in detecting peri-implantitis.

The first step is to filter out any unnecessary noise. This involves converting the RGB images to grayscale and using histogram equalization and adaptive histogram equalization to accomplish this. The resulting images are overlaid onto the original images to enhance their boundaries. The second step is to enhance the features by examining the differences in color levels between the implant and gingiva. The research plots the values of each pixel in a 3D space and colors them accordingly on the original image. These steps are then combined to produce a pre-processed image. A CNN model training database is created using these pre-processed images which possess the necessary features and sufficiently high recognition accuracy to enable more effective CNN model training.

2.2.1. Histogram Equalization and Adjust Histogram Equalization

The original image in Figure 5a has a color scale that is too similar between the gingival and screw threads; this makes it difficult to distinguish damaged features due to excessive noise. The main objective of this step is to increase the color scale between the gingival and implant while filtering out the unnecessary noise. Histogram equalization [29] (Figure 5b) and adaptive histogram equalization [30] (Figure 5c) are used to achieve this goal. The result in Figure 5d is obtained by subtracting one image from the other. Then, the norm of the horizontal and vertical gradients of the image is calculated and the results are plotted in 3D as shown in Figure 6, capturing the edge features. Finally, the results are combined with the coloring from the next step to complete the preprocessing. In Equation (3), $p_x(i)$ is the probability value of the occurrence of grayscale values from 0 to 255, n_i is the total number of occurrences of grayscale value i in the picture, and n is the total number of pixels in the image and L is 256. Equation (4) presents the cumulative distribution function which calculates the cumulative probability of pixels from 0 to 255 and linearizes the probability of the occurrence of all pixels. Finally, it multiplies 255 by the cumulative distribution function as shown in Equation (5) to scale the cumulative probability of 0 to 1 to 0 to 255.

$$p_x(i) = n_i/n, \ 0 \leq i < L \tag{3}$$

$$cdf_x(i) = \sum_{j=0}^{i} p_x(j) \tag{4}$$

$$cdf_x(i) \times (255 - 0) \tag{5}$$

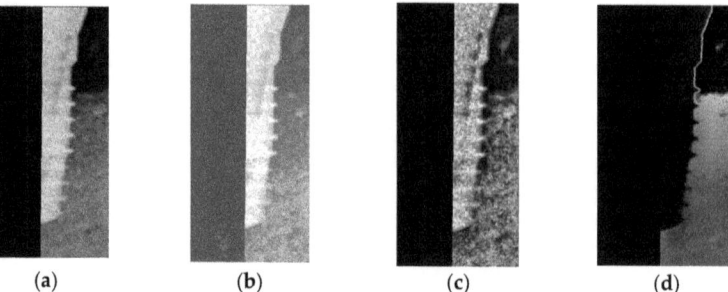

Figure 5. The results of pre-processing: (**a**) original image; (**b**) image after histogram equalization, (**c**) image after adaptive histogram equalization; (**d**) result after subtraction.

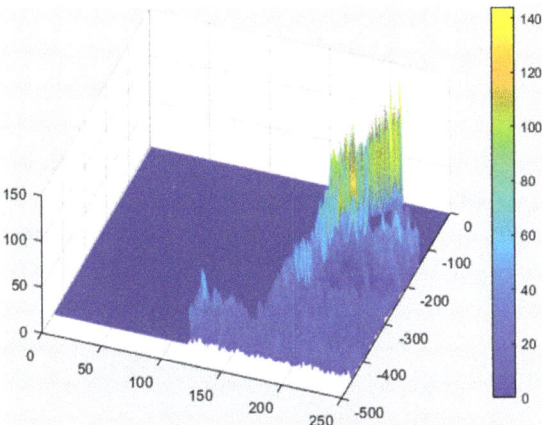

Figure 6. The plot of gradient result in 3D map.

2.2.2. Image Enhanced with 3D Graphics Technology

In the previous step, we were able to identify edge features. However, to further emphasize the differences between damaged and healthy, it is necessary to use the distribution of gingiva on the image to enhance the distinction between the two categories of features. The main challenge in this step is distinguishing between the gum and dental implant regions. To address this issue, the correlation between the 3D map output of the previous step and the 3D map of the original image is utilized as shown in Figure 7a. The range value is used to determine whether a pixel is located on the edge or on the flat surface. When a pixel is on the flat surface, the Z-axis position in the 3D map is used as reference to determine whether it belongs to the dental implant or gum. If the Z-axis position is higher than the threshold between the dental implant and gum, the pixel is considered a dental implant and is colored green. If it is lower, it is considered gum and colored orange. A gate value is also used to separate the gum region from the rest of the original image. Pixels below this gate are set to 0 which appears black. Finally, to enhance the discriminability, a red reference line is added at the position of the damaged platform on each image as shown in Figure 7b.

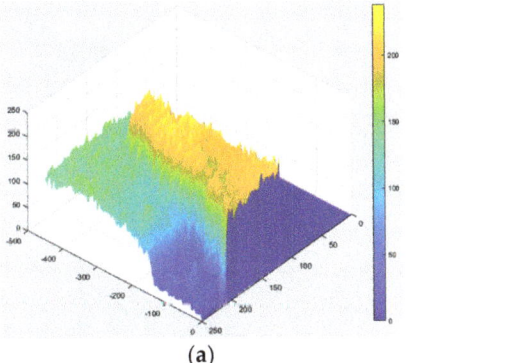
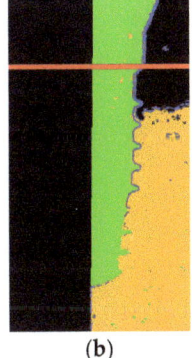

(a)　　　　　　　　　　　　(b)

Figure 7. Enhanced schematics through 3D graphics technology: (**a**) the plot of the original image in a 3D map; (**b**) changing the color of the dental implant and gums in the image with added reference lines.

2.3. Image Classification

To monitor the learning progress of the model during training, the project divides the training data into an 80% training set and a 20% validation set as listed in Table 5. The validation set is used to observe if the model is overly focused on the training data, leading to incorrect predictions of new data, known as "Overfitting". Insufficient data is a factor contributing to model overfitting. This project augments the data by horizontally and vertically flipping images, therefore increasing the data volume by a factor of four. To ensure the accuracy of the training process, the number of damaged and healthy data in the training and validation sets must be adjusted to approximately 1:1 to ensure that each category has a consistent distribution of the probability of correct predictions.

Table 5. Image classification of the periapical image before and after preprocessing.

The Number of Periapical Images before and after Preprocess		
Before	Training Set	Validation Set
Healthy	162	40
Damaged	164	40
Total	326	80
After	Training Set	Validation Set
Healthy	648 (Augmented)	40
Damaged	656 (Augmented)	40
Total	1304	80

2.3.1. CNN Model

The hardware setup used to train the CNN image classification model is the same as described in Table 1 in Section 2.1.2. The CNN model is built using the Deep Network Designer app of MATLAB with AlexNet as the base model. However, the input size is different from the original $227 \times 227 \times 3$ and is set to $450 \times 450 \times 3$ to accommodate the elongated shape of dental implants and avoid distortion caused by stretching rectangular images into squares as shown in Figure 8a. This approach also prevents excessive padding resulting from filling the square as shown in Figure 8b. The final architecture of AlexNet is presented in Table 6. To ensure accuracy in the training process, it is necessary to adjust the quantity of damaged and health data in the training and validation sets to approximately 1:1.

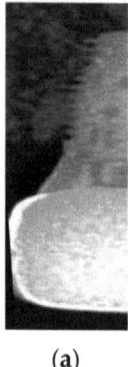
(a)

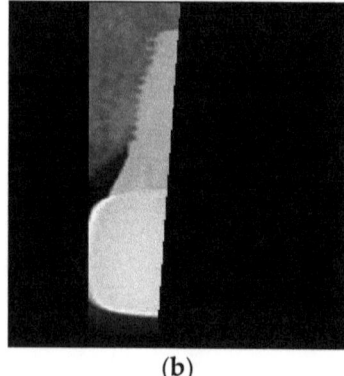
(b)

Figure 8. The image used for training the CNN: (**a**) distortion image; (**b**) over padding image.

Table 6. The model architecture of AlexNet.

	Type	Activations
1	Image Input	$450 \times 250 \times 3$
2	2-D Convolution	$110 \times 60 \times 96$
3	ReLU	$110 \times 60 \times 96$
4	Cross Channel Normalization	$110 \times 60 \times 96$
5	2-D Max Pooling	$54 \times 29 \times 96$
6	2-D Grouped Convolution	$54 \times 29 \times 256$
7	ReLU	$54 \times 29 \times 256$
8	Cross Channel Normalization	$54 \times 29 \times 256$
9	2-D Max Pooling	$26 \times 14 \times 256$
10	2-D Convolution	$26 \times 14 \times 384$
11	ReLU	$26 \times 14 \times 384$
12	2-D Grouped Convolution	$26 \times 14 \times 384$
13	ReLU	$26 \times 14 \times 384$
14	2-D Grouped Convolution	$26 \times 14 \times 256$
15	ReLU	$26 \times 14 \times 256$
16	2-D Max Pooling	$12 \times 6 \times 256$
17	Fully Connected	$1 \times 1 \times 1152$
18	ReLU	$1 \times 1 \times 1152$
19	Dropout	$1 \times 1 \times 1152$
20	Fully Connected	$1 \times 1 \times 144$
21	ReLU	$1 \times 1 \times 144$
22	Dropout	$1 \times 1 \times 144$
23	Fully Connected	$1 \times 1 \times 2$
24	Softmax	$1 \times 1 \times 2$
25	Classification Output	$1 \times 1 \times 2$

2.3.2. Hyperparameter

To train a model effectively, it is crucial to tune the appropriate training parameters according to the data characteristics. The parameters used in the YOLOv2 model trained in Section 2.1.2 differ from those used in the AlexNet model in this step. In this section, we will provide details about the Initial Learning Rate, Mini Batch Size, Max Epoch, and Dropout Factor. Moreover, the parameters used to train AlexNet are presented in Table 7.

Table 7. Hyperparameters in AlexNet model.

Hyperparameters	Value
Optimizer	Sgdm
Initial Learning Rate	0.00006
Max Epoch	50
Mini Batch Size	16
LearnRateDropFactor	0.75
LearnRateDropPeriod	30

Learning Rate Dropout

Machine learning models must be generalized to all types of data within their respective domains to make accurate predictions. Overfitting happens when a model becomes too closely fitted to the training dataset and fails to generalize. Preventing overfitting is crucial for successful model training. Dropout is a regularization technique utilized to address overfitting. It involves assigning a probability of dropping out hidden layer neurons during each iteration or epoch of training. The dropped-out neurons do not transmit any information.

3. Results

This chapter is divided into two sections: the first focuses on the training process and results of the YOLOv2 object detection model; while the second covers the CNN image classification model. Both models will be compared with those proposed in other papers, and the precision and accuracy achieved by this project will be assessed using the confusion matrix.

3.1. YOLOv2 Object Detector

Table 8 presents a comprehensive overview of the YOLOv2 training process employed in this study. In this study, an unvalidated model was utilized to detect dental implants due to the fact that the YOLOv2 training function in MATLAB does not support validation. The results of the detection process are detailed in the confusion matrix provided in Table 9. Moreover, Figure 9 depicts the training process for the YOLOv2 loss function. To evaluate the accuracy of the CNN model, the validation set was utilized as the input for the network in this study. The accuracy of the AlexNet model was evaluated by comparing its predictions with the correct answers obtained from the images.

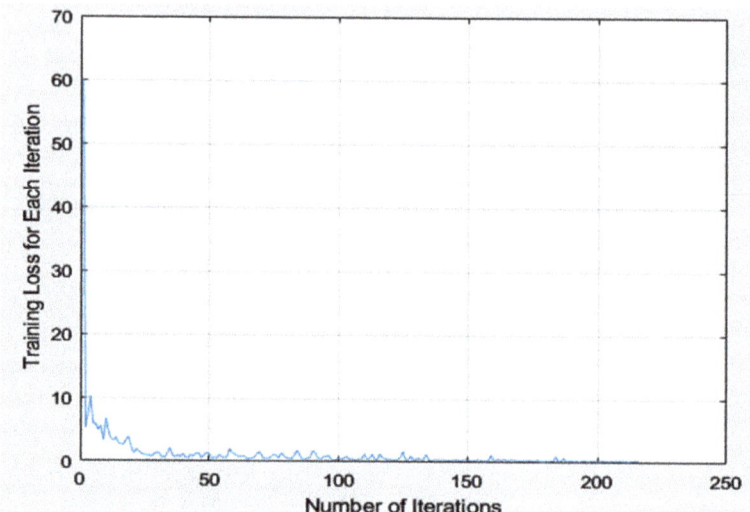

Figure 9. The training process for the YOLOv2 loss function. The blue line represents the change in the loss function over the number of iterations.

Table 8. Training process for YOLOv2.

Epoch	Iteration	Time Elapsed	Mini-Batch RMSE	Mini-Batch Loss
1	1	00:03	7.75	60.0
6	50	00:27	1.13	1.3
12	100	00:51	0.77	0.6
17	150	01:14	0.56	0.3
23	200	01:37	0.44	0.2
24	216	01:43	0.53	0.3

Table 9. The confusion matrix of YOLOv2 test.

Category		Target Class		
		Implant	Tooth	Subtotal
Output Class	Implant	287 (68.2%)	15 (3.6%)	95%
	Tooth	30 (7.1%)	89 (21.1%)	74.8%
	Subtotal	90.5%	78%	89.3%

The appropriate selection of hyperparameters is crucial for the success of any machine learning algorithm. In this study, the hyperparameters of YOLOv2 were carefully selected based on the data characteristics. Zero (0) indicates that the YOLOv2 model correctly predicted 287 implants across all test cases, achieving a recall of 90.5%. Additionally, it correctly predicted 89 cases of normal teeth, resulting in a true negative rate of 78%. The accuracy rate of the model in this study is 89.3%. In addition, the model is 95% accurate. The YOLOv2 model displays lower propensity for erroneously detecting healthy teeth, but another issue was encountered during testing. As depicted in Figure 10, the system tends to repeatedly detect incomplete implants in the same tooth leading to high false negative values. In contrast to literature [31,32] that employ positioning and identification technology, the proposed technology in this study integrates automatic image cropping, resulting in a difference in the accuracy of less than 2%. This proposal has attained high precision and accuracy in dental implant detection and image classification. In general, these outcomes suggest that our proposed models exhibit a potential for clinical applications and could serve as a valuable tool for dental implant planning.

Figure 10. The image of detecting an incomplete implant.

3.2. CNN AlexNet Image Classification

To monitor the training progress of the model, a validation set was employed in this project. The training process is presented in Table 10, while Figures 11 and 12 display the accuracy and loss of training AlexNet, respectively. The black line in both figures represents the validation.

Table 10. The detailed process of AlexNet training.

Epoch	Iteration	Mini-Batch Accuracy	Validation Accuracy	Mini-Batch Loss	Validation Loss
1	1	56.25	50.00	8.3222	3.1206
10	810	81.25	87.50	0.2822	0.2692
20	1620	100.00	95.00	0.0358	0.1354
30	2430	100.00	96.25	0.0376	0.1144
40	3240	100.00	96.25	0.0177	0.0951
50	4050	100.00	96.25	0.0126	0.0676
60	4860	100.00	97.50	0.0070	0.0989
70	5670	100.00	97.50	0.0109	0.0740
80	6480	100.00	97.50	0.0051	0.0672
90	7290	100.00	97.50	0.0035	0.0551
100	8100	100.00	97.50	0.0055	0.0766

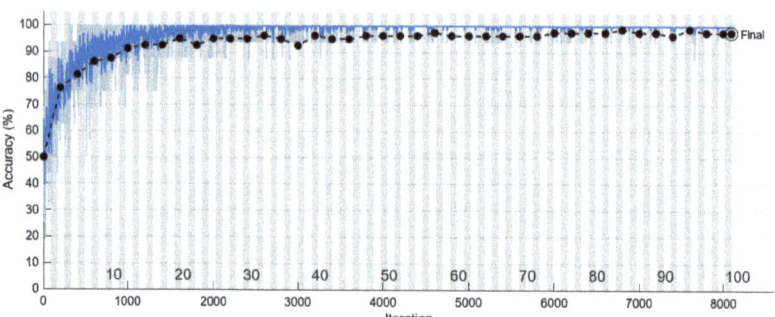

Figure 11. The accuracy of AlexNet model in the validation set (black line) and training set (blue line) during training process.

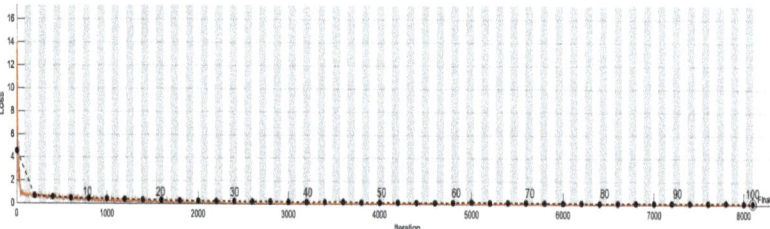

Figure 12. The accuracy of AlexNet model in the validation set (black line) and the training set (orange line) during loss training process.

Based on the data presented in Table 11, it is evident that the use of distorted images, which were not adjusted for relative size, as the training database led to a very high loss of the validation set and an accuracy of less than 50%. These findings suggest that the database may have some fatal flaws such as indistinct features resulting from image stretching or excessive noise in the image. The second column of Table 11 presents the results of training using histogram equalization, the overlaid original image, and adaptive histogram equalization. As a result of correcting image size and enhancing features, the loss decreased significantly, and the accuracy increased to 81.43%. Nonetheless, these results were still below the standards set by this project. Furthermore, during the training process, the loss rebounded after reaching 0.5, indicating the need for further image pre-processing. The third column of Table 11 shows the result of this project which significantly enhances the features of an image by coloring different regions and adding damage reference lines. This enhancement has helped the model to perform better in image classification, achieving a validation set accuracy of 97.5%, and the loss has also dropped below the threshold of 0.5 to 0.08.

Table 11. Comparison of the datasets used in various stages and the validation results.

	Original Images	Adaptive Histogram Equalization	Adaptive Histogram Equalization + Damage Reference Lines
Validation Accuracy	48.64	81.43	97.5
Validation Loss	2.21	0.54	0.08
Net	AlexNet	AlexNet	AlexNet
Image			

The evaluation of prediction results in terms of accuracy and precision was performed by comparing the predicted outcomes with the ground truth using a confusion matrix based on the test set, as presented in Table 12. Initially, the AlexNet model employed original images during the training process, and after continuous adjustments, the accuracy increased from 60% to 80%. However, it reached a bottleneck. Further improvement was achieved with the use of preprocessing. The final training outcomes are depicted in Table 12. Nevertheless, some images in the test data have unclear boundaries such as those without obvious screw threads or gums having similar grayscale values to screw threads which may also lead to misjudgment by the human eye. Consequently, there were approximately 10% errors in the final testing. It is evident that the CNN model performed remarkably well on the test set; it accurately predicted 107 out of all 117 samples, with damages accounting for 91.4% of the total damaged test data; similarly, it accurately predicted 92 out of all 103 healthy samples, accounting for 89.3% of the total healthy test data. The accuracy rate was 90.4% and the precision rate was 90.7%.

Table 12. The confusion matrix of AlexNet test.

Category		Target Class		
		Damaged	Healthy	Subtotal
Output Class	Damaged	107 (48.6%)	11 (5%)	90.7%
	Healthy	10 (4.5%)	92 (41.8%)	90.2%
	Subtotal	91.4%	89.3%	90.4%

The direct classification of dental implant damages has not yet been addressed in the current state of the art. The paper that is closest in technique is [33] which focuses solely on determining the fit between two sides of a dental implant rather than directly detecting damages on one side of the implant using the method employed in this project. Table 13 presents a comparison with this technology, revealing that the image enhancement technology utilized in this study contributes to the final recognition result of the CNN, with an accuracy rate increasing to 90.4%. This marks significant progress, as this research currently represents the highest performance in detecting implant damages in teeth.

Table 13. The comparison table between the prior art and this study.

	This Work	Method in [33]
Method	CNN	Faster R-CNN
Accuracy	90.4%	81%

4. Discussion

The YOLOv2 model achieved an 89.3% accuracy rate in detecting the position of dental implants, surpassing the performance of existing methods [34]. The multiple identification process revealed that the system may repeatedly detect the same tooth when there are incomplete implants, leading to high false negative values. In addition to the positioning and recognition technology used in [31,32], this study introduced automatic image cropping, resulting in less than a 2% accuracy difference. This is a promising direction. Another study [35] used YOLOv3 to identify dental implants, with TP ratios and APs ranging from 0.50 to 0.82 and 0.51 to 0.85 for each implant system, respectively. The resulting mAP and mIoU of the model were 0.71 and 0.72, respectively. This is with a small amount of training data used, which may have compromised the accuracy of the model. For the AlexNet data used in this study, grayscale images were initially used for training, resulting in lower accuracy rates. When distorted images were used, the accuracy rate was even lower. Therefore, this research strengthens the high-precision image preprocessing process, improves the accuracy of the model to detect damages to 90.4%, and innovates and breaks through the latest similar related research.

The most related investigation [33] utilized Faster R-CNN to identify marginal bone loss surrounding implants (the κ value for the bone loss site was 0.547, while the κ value for the bone loss implant was 0.568) and compared the judgments of the AI to those of MD students and resident dentists on the same data. The results showed significant differences in the judgments of human observers. Therefore, training a consistent and accurate model can greatly facilitate healthcare by providing real-time treatment. However, the model is limited in its ability to detect finer levels of bone loss or the number of threads affected. Future research could address this limitation by exploring the use of additional imaging techniques or developing more sophisticated algorithms to detect these features, reducing misjudgment, and avoiding medical disputes.

5. Conclusions

The YOLOv2 model achieved an accuracy rate of 89.3% in capturing the implant position, while the AlexNet damage detection model achieved an accuracy rate of 90.4%. Moving forward, this research will continue to optimize the model and investigate better methods to improve accuracy rates. In terms of capturing dental implants, this study improves the cropping method by cutting through the interdental space to avoid capturing teeth outside the target area. In addition, this study obtained different grayscale ranges and blurred glue and line edges in the image. This automatic image preprocessing method greatly improves on the current manual preprocessing process. This automated approach not only improves efficiency and consistency but also reduces manual operation errors. Moreover, it is advisable to investigate the potential of incorporating advanced imaging techniques or developing more sophisticated algorithms that can accurately detect even subtle levels of bone loss or the number of affected threads. Moreover, creating a user interface can improve user satisfaction and increase the ease of use and efficiency of the system, leading to improved work efficiency and product quality.

Author Contributions: Conceptualization, Y.-C.C. and M.-Y.C.; Data curation, Y.-C.C. and M.-Y.C.; Formal analysis, M.-L.C.; Funding acquisition, S.-L.C. and C.-A.C.; Methodology, T.-Y.C. and M.-L.C.; Resources, C.-A.C., S.-L.C. and P.A.R.A.; Software, S.-L.C., Y.-L.L., P.-T.L., G.-J.L. and T.-F.L.; Supervision, C.-A.C. and S.-L.C.; Validation, P.-T.L., G.-J.L. and T.-F.L.; Visualization, Y.-Y.H., K.-C.L. and P.A.R.A.; Writing—original draft, T.-Y.C.; Writing—review and editing, M.-L.C, K.-C.L., C.-A.C. and P.A.R.A. All authors have read and agreed to the published version of the manuscript.

Funding: This work was supported by the Ministry of Science and Technology (MOST), Taiwan, under grant numbers of MOST-111-2221-E-033-041, MOST-111-2823-8-033-001, MOST-111-2622-E-131-001, MOST-110-2223-8-033-002, MOST-110-2221-E-027-044-MY3, MOST-110-2218-E-035-007, MOST-110-2622-E-131-002, MOST-109-2622-E-131-001-CC3, MOST-109-2221-E-131-025, and MOST-109-2410-H-197-002-MY3.

Institutional Review Board Statement: Chang Gung Medical Foundation Institutional Review Board; IRB number: 02102023B0C503; Date of Approval: 1 December 2020; Protocol Title: A Convolutional Neural Network Approach for Dental Bite-Wing, Panoramic and Periapical Radiographs Classification. Executing Institution: Chang-Geng Medical Foundation Taoyuan Chang-Geng Memorial Hospital of Taoyuan; Duration of Approval: From 1 December 2020 to 30 November 2021. The IRB reviewed and determined that it is an expedited review according to case research or cases treated or diagnosed by clinical routines. However, this does not include HIV-positive cases.

Informed Consent Statement: The IRB approves the waiver of the participants consent.

Data Availability Statement: Not applicable.

Conflicts of Interest: The authors declare no conflict of interest.

References

1. Tricio, J.; Laohapand, P.; Van Steenberghe, D.; Quirynen, M.; Naert, I. Mechanical state assessment of the implant-bone continuum: A better understanding of the Periotest method. *Int. J. Oral Maxillofac. Implant.* **1995**, *10*, 43–49.
2. Wright, W.E.; Davis, M.L.; Geffen, D.B.; Martin, S.E.; Nelson, M.J.; Straus, S.E. Alveolar bone necrosis and tooth loss: A rare complication associated with herpes zoster infection of the fifth cranial nerve. *Oral Surg. Oral Med. Oral Pathol.* **1983**, *56*, 39–46. [CrossRef] [PubMed]
3. Eckerbom, M.; Magnusson, T.; Martinsson, T. Reasons for and incidence of tooth mortality in a Swedish population. *Dent. Traumatol.* **1992**, *8*, 230–234. [CrossRef] [PubMed]
4. Krall, E.A.; Garvey, A.J.; Garcia, R.I. Alveolar bone loss and tooth loss in male cigar and pipe smokers. *J. Am. Dent. Assoc.* **1999**, *130*, 57–64. [CrossRef] [PubMed]
5. Duong, H.; Roccuzzo, A.; Stähli, A.; Salvi, G.E.; Lang, N.P.; Sculean, A. Oral health-related quality of life of patients rehabilitated with fixed and removable implant-supported dental prostheses. *Periodontology 2000* **2022**, *88*, 201–237. [CrossRef]
6. Kanehira, Y.; Arai, K.; Kanehira, T.; Nagahisa, K.; Baba, S. Oral health-related quality of life in patients with implant treatment. *J. Adv. Prosthodont.* **2017**, *9*, 476–481. [CrossRef]
7. Dental Implants Market Size, Share & Growth Report. 2030. Available online: https://www.grandviewresearch.com/industry-analysis/dental-implants-market (accessed on 6 March 2023).
8. Fiorillo, L.; Meto, A.; Cicciù, M. Bioengineering Applied to Oral Implantology, a New Protocol: "Digital Guided Surgery". *Prosthesis* **2023**, *5*, 234–250. [CrossRef]
9. Abraham, C.M. A Brief Historical Perspective on Dental Implants, Their Surface Coatings and Treatments. *Open Dent. J.* **2014**, *8*, 50–55. [CrossRef]
10. Block, M.S. Dental Implants: The Last 100 Years. *J. Oral Maxillofac. Surg.* **2018**, *76*, 11–26. [CrossRef]
11. Alqahtani, N.D.; Alzahrani, B.; Ramzan, M.S. Deep Learning Applications for Dyslexia Prediction. *Appl. Sci.* **2023**, *13*, 2804. [CrossRef]
12. Sethi, Y.; Patel, N.; Kaka, N.; Desai, A.; Kaiwan, O.; Sheth, M.; Sharma, R.; Huang, H.; Chopra, H.; Khandaker, M.U.; et al. Artificial Intelligence in Pediatric Cardiology: A Scoping Review. *J. Clin. Med.* **2022**, *11*, 7072. [CrossRef] [PubMed]
13. Zhang, G.; Luo, L.; Zhang, L.; Liu, Z. Research Progress of Respiratory Disease and Idiopathic Pulmonary Fibrosis Based on Artificial Intelligence. *Diagnostics* **2023**, *13*, 357. [CrossRef] [PubMed]
14. Basu, K.; Sinha, R.; Ong, A.; Basu, T. Artificial intelligence: How is it changing medical sciences and its future? *Indian J. Dermatol.* **2020**, *65*, 365–370. [CrossRef]

15. Chen, S.-L.; Chen, T.-Y.; Huang, Y.-C.; Chen, C.-A.; Chou, H.-S.; Huang, Y.-Y.; Lin, W.-C.; Li, T.-C.; Yuan, J.-J.; Abu, P.A.R.; et al. Missing Teeth and Restoration Detection Using Dental Panoramic Radiography Based on Transfer Learning with CNNs. *IEEE Access* **2022**, *10*, 118654–118664. [CrossRef]
16. Mao, Y.-C.; Chen, T.-Y.; Chou, H.-S.; Lin, S.-Y.; Liu, S.-Y.; Chen, Y.-A.; Liu, Y.-L.; Chen, C.-A.; Huang, Y.-C.; Chen, S.-L.; et al. Caries and Restoration Detection Using Bitewing Film Based on Transfer Learning with CNNs. *Sensors* **2021**, *21*, 4613. [CrossRef]
17. Li, C.-W.; Lin, S.-Y.; Chou, H.-S.; Chen, T.-Y.; Chen, Y.-A.; Liu, S.-Y.; Liu, Y.-L.; Chen, C.-A.; Huang, Y.-C.; Chen, S.-L.; et al. Detection of Dental Apical Lesions Using CNNs on Periapical Radiograph. *Sensors* **2021**, *21*, 7049. [CrossRef]
18. Chuo, Y.; Lin, W.-M.; Chen, T.-Y.; Chan, M.-L.; Chang, Y.-S.; Lin, Y.-R.; Lin, Y.-J.; Shao, Y.-H.; Chen, C.-A.; Chen, S.-L.; et al. A High-Accuracy Detection System: Based on Transfer Learning for Apical Lesions on Periapical Radiograph. *Bioengineering* **2022**, *9*, 777. [CrossRef]
19. Geetha, V.; Aprameya, K.S.; Hinduja, D.M. Dental caries diagnosis in digital radiographs using back-propagation neural network. *Health Inf. Sci. Syst.* **2020**, *8*, 8. [CrossRef] [PubMed]
20. Muramatsu, C.; Morishita, T.; Takahashi, R.; Hayashi, T.; Nishiyama, W.; Ariji, Y.; Zhou, X.; Hara, T.; Katsumata, A.; Ariji, E.; et al. Tooth detection and classification on panoramic radiographs for automatic dental chart filing: Improved classification by multi-sized input data. *Oral Radiol.* **2021**, *37*, 13–19. [CrossRef]
21. Kohlakala, A.; Coetzer, J.; Bertels, J.; Vandermeulen, D. Deep learning-based dental implant recognition using synthetic X-ray images. *Med. Biol. Eng. Comput.* **2022**, *60*, 2951–2968. [CrossRef]
22. Chen, S.-L.; Chen, T.-Y.; Mao, Y.-C.; Lin, S.-Y.; Huang, Y.-Y.; Chen, C.-A.; Lin, Y.-J.; Hsu, Y.-M.; Li, C.-A.; Chiang, W.-Y.; et al. Automated Detection System Based on Convolution Neural Networks for Retained Root, Endodontic Treated Teeth, and Implant Recognition on Dental Panoramic Images. *IEEE Sens. J.* **2022**, *22*, 23293–23306. [CrossRef]
23. Lin, S.-Y.; Chang, H.-Y. Tooth Numbering and Condition Recognition on Dental Panoramic Radiograph Images Using CNNs. *IEEE Access* **2021**, *9*, 166008–166026. [CrossRef]
24. Widiasri, M.; Arifin, A.Z.; Suciati, N.; Fatichah, C.; Astuti, E.R.; Indraswari, R.; Putra, R.H.; Za'In, C. Dental-YOLO: Alveolar Bone and Mandibular Canal Detection on Cone Beam Computed Tomography Images for Dental Implant Planning. *IEEE Access* **2022**, *10*, 101483–101494. [CrossRef]
25. Yadalam, P.K.; Trivedi, S.S.; Krishnamurthi, I.; Anegundi, R.V.; Mathew, A.; Al Shayeb, M.; Narayanan, J.K.; Jaberi, M.A.; Rajkumar, R. Machine Learning Predicts Patient Tangible Outcomes After Dental Implant Surgery. *IEEE Access* **2022**, *10*, 131481–131488. [CrossRef]
26. Hashim, D.; Cionca, N.; Combescure, C.; Mombelli, A. The diagnosis of peri-implantitis: A systematic review on the predictive value of bleeding on probing. *Clin. Oral Implant. Res.* **2018**, *29* (Suppl. 16), 276–293. [CrossRef] [PubMed]
27. Prathapachandran, J.; Suresh, N. Management of peri-implantitis. *Dent. Res. J.* **2012**, *9*, 516–521. [CrossRef]
28. Isobe, T.; Feigelson, E.D.; Akritas, M.G.; Babu, G.J. Linear regression in astronomy. *Astrophys. J.* **1990**, *364*, 104–113. [CrossRef]
29. Lu, L.; Zhou, Y.; Panetta, K.; Agaian, S. Comparative study of histogram equalization algorithms for image enhancement. *Mob. Multimed. Image Process. Secur. Appl.* **2010**, *7708*, 770811. [CrossRef]
30. Zhu, Y.; Huang, C. An Adaptive Histogram Equalization Algorithm on the Image Gray Level Mapping. *Phys. Procedia* **2012**, *25*, 601–608. [CrossRef]
31. Chen, H.; Zhang, K.; Lyu, P.; Li, H.; Zhang, L.; Wu, J.; Lee, C.-H. A deep learning approach to automatic teeth detection and numbering based on object detection in dental periapical films. *Sci. Rep.* **2019**, *9*, 3840–3851. [CrossRef]
32. Jang, W.S.; Kim, S.; Yun, P.S.; Jang, H.S.; Seong, Y.W.; Yang, H.S.; Chang, J.-S. Accurate detection for dental implant and peri-implant tissue by transfer learning of faster R-CNN: A diagnostic accuracy study. *BMC Oral Health* **2022**, *22*, 591. [CrossRef]
33. Liu, M.; Wang, S.; Chen, H.; Liu, Y. A pilot study of a deep learning approach to detect marginal bone loss around implants. *BMC Oral Health* **2022**, *22*, 11. [CrossRef] [PubMed]
34. Lin, N.-H.; Lin, T.-L.; Wang, X.; Kao, W.-T.; Tseng, H.-W.; Chen, S.-L.; Chiou, Y.-S.; Lin, S.-Y.; Villaverde, J.F.; Kuo, Y.-F. Teeth Detection Algorithm and Teeth Condition Classification Based on Convolutional Neural Networks for Dental Panoramic Radiographs. *J. Med. Imaging Health Inform.* **2018**, *8*, 507–515. [CrossRef]
35. Takahashi, T.; Nozaki, K.; Gonda, T.; Mameno, T.; Wada, M.; Ikebe, K. Identification of dental implants using deep learning—Pilot study. *Int. J. Implant. Dent.* **2020**, *6*, 53. [CrossRef] [PubMed]

Disclaimer/Publisher's Note: The statements, opinions and data contained in all publications are solely those of the individual author(s) and contributor(s) and not of MDPI and/or the editor(s). MDPI and/or the editor(s) disclaim responsibility for any injury to people or property resulting from any ideas, methods, instructions or products referred to in the content.

Article

Surface Accumulation of Cerium, Self-Assembling Peptide, and Fluoride on Sound Bovine Enamel

Konstantin Johannes Scholz [1,*], Karl-Anton Hiller [1], Helga Ebensberger [1], Gerlinde Ferstl [1], Florian Pielnhofer [2], Tobias T. Tauböck [3], Klaus Becker [3] and Wolfgang Buchalla [1]

[1] Department of Conservative Dentistry and Periodontology, University Hospital Regensburg, Franz-Josef-Strauß-Allee 11, 93053 Regensburg, Germany
[2] Institute of Inorganic Chemistry, University of Regensburg, Universitätsstr. 31, 93047 Regensburg, Germany
[3] Department of Conservative and Preventive Dentistry, Center for Dental Medicine, University of Zurich, Plattenstrasse 11, 8032 Zurich, Switzerland
* Correspondence: konstantin.scholz@ukr.de

Abstract: The accumulation of caries-preventive compounds on sound enamel is crucial in order to improve the inhibition of carious lesion initiation. The aim of this research was to investigate the initial accumulation of cerium, oligopeptide p11-4, and fluoride from NaF or amine fluoride (AmF) on sound enamel in vitro by means of energy dispersive X-ray spectroscopy (EDX). Polished bovine enamel specimens (n = 120 from 60 teeth) were fabricated. Out of these, 12 specimens each were treated with $CeCl_3$ (cerium(III) chloride heptahydrate 25%), oligopeptide p11-4 (Curodont Repair, Credentis), NaF (10,000 ppm F^-), AmF (amine fluoride, Elmex Fluid, CP-GABA GmbH, 10,000 ppm F^-), or Aqua demin (control). After rinsing with water, the surface elemental composition (Ce, N, F, Ca, P, O, Na, Mg) was measured (EDX; EDAX Octane Elect detector, APEX v2.0), expressed in atomic percent (At%) and analyzed (non-parametric statistics, α = 0.05, error rates method). Another 12 specimens per treatment group were fabricated and used for analyzing accumulation in cross-sections with EDX linescans and two-dimensional EDX-mappings. The surface median atomic percent of cerium (At%Ce) was 0.8 for $CeCl_3$, but no Ce was found for any other group. N, specifically for oligopeptide p11-4, could not be detected. Fluorine could only be detected on fluoridated surfaces. The median atomic percent of fluorine (At%F) was 15.2 for NaF and 17.0 for AmF. The Ca/P ratio increased significantly compared to the control following the application of NaF and AmF ($p < 0.001$), but decreased significantly for $CeCl_3$ ($p < 0.001$). In cross-sectioned specimens of the $CeCl_3$-group, 12.5% of the linescans revealed cerium at the enamel surface, whereas 83.3% of the NaF linescans and 95.8% of the AmF linescans revealed fluorine at the enamel surface. Following the application of oligopeptide p11-4, no traces of N were detectable. In the depth of the samples, no signal was detected for any of the corresponding elements exceeding the background noise. Cerium and fluorine (from both NaF and AmF), but not the oligopeptide p11-4, precipitated on sound enamel.

Keywords: chemical composition; EDX; caries prevention

1. Introduction

Untreated caries of permanent teeth is a prevalent condition with an estimated 2 billion worldwide cases in 2019 [1]. Coronal carious lesions typically start with lesion initiation in sound enamel [2]. Hence, the approach to combat caries is twofold: to prevent demineralization of sound enamel and to promote the remineralization of previously demineralized areas [3,4]. For all cariostatic compounds that act in addition to the local presence of ionic calcium and phosphate, adherence or accumulation at the enamel surface is therefore a preferred quality in order to positively influence the balance between demineralization and remineralization during daily acidic challenges [5].

Fluorides, e.g., applied in form of dentifrices or varnishes, have been used for a long time in the prevention and treatment of initial carious lesions [6,7]. These act primarily via local effects, for example through the initial formation of calcium fluoride (CaF_2) on the enamel surface at acidic pH [8–10] or through accumulation within the hydration layer of enamel crystals and diffusion of 1–2 nm into these crystals [11]. In addition to fluoride, for which cariostatic effects are well documented, a number of novel, potentially cariostatic compounds have emerged.

Lanthanoid compounds such as cerium salts, although not yet used clinically, have recently shown anti-erosive and cariostatic potential [12–14]. Although not fully understood, the incorporation of cerium at the positions of calcium in the crystal lattice of hydroxyapatite may increase acid resistance. The lower solubility of cerium phosphate or cerium-substituted apatite, compared to corresponding naturally occurring calcium phosphates, may explain a potential caries-preventing effect of cerium in enamel [15]. The oligopeptide p11-4 ($C_{72}H_{98}N_{20}O_{22}$), designated as a *self-assembling peptide*, is described to bind calcium ions [16,17]. Nevertheless, oligopeptide p11-4 also may inhibit initiation of initial enamel caries by binding to sound enamel, due to its calcium-binding capacity [17].

In view of its potential properties to prevent enamel demineralization, it was the aim of this study to investigate the initial surface accumulation of cerium and oligopeptide p11-4 on sound enamel in vitro and compare these with fluoride from NaF or amine fluoride, both well-established compounds in caries prevention. The corresponding null-hypothesis of the study was that topical application of cariostatic agents based on cerium(III)-chloride, oligopeptide p11-4, amine fluoride, or sodium fluoride has no significant influence on the elemental composition of sound enamel.

2. Materials and Methods

For all in vitro experiments, permanent inferior incisors of freshly slaughtered bovine animals were extracted and stored at 4 °C for a maximum of 3 months in 0.5% chloramine solution before use.

2.1. Enamel Preparation and Treatment

The crowns from 60 bovine inferior incisors were hand-sectioned into 120 equally-sized labial enamel specimens with underlying dentin (10 × 10 × 3 mm; one incisal and one cervical specimen per tooth) using a cutting disc (Superdiaflex H 365F 190 Horico Dental, Berlin, Germany) under copious water cooling. Roots and pulpal tissue were removed. The central enamel region of each specimen was ground flat and polished under continuous water cooling with Si-Carbide paper (Metaserv Motopol 8, Buehler, Leinfelden-Echterdingen, Germany; 150 rpm, FEPA P1200, CarbiMet, 40 s, FEPA P4000, MicroCut, 60 s; both Buehler, Germany). After polishing, each specimen consisted of at least a layer of 1 mm of enamel and 1 mm of underlying dentin. The dentin on the pulpal side of the specimen and the unpolished marginal enamel areas were covered with nail varnish. The resulting 120 specimens (Figure 1) were randomly allocated to 5 treatment groups (n = 24): $CeCl_3$ (25% cerium(III)chloride heptahydrate in aqueous buffer-solution, pH = 4; Merck KGaA, Darmstadt, Germany), oligopeptide p11-4 (pH = 6.2; Curodont Repair, Credentis, Windisch, Switzerland), NaF (sodium fluoride, 10,000 ppm F^- in aqueous buffer-solution, pH = 4; Merck KgaA, Darmstadt, Germany), AmF (amine fluoride, 10,000 ppm F^-, pH = 4; Elmex Fluid, CP GABA GmbH, Hamburg, Germany), and Aqua demin (control). The solutions according to treatment groups were applied on the polished sound enamel. For $CeCl_3$, NaF and AmF, 0.1 mL of the solution was passively applied from a pipette, left for 60 s, and subsequently rinsed off for 30 s using demineralized water. For oligopeptide p11-4, one unit of approximately 60 µL of the solution was applied using the applicator from the Curodont system, left for 300 s, and subsequently rinsed off for 30 s using demineralized water. For Aqua demin (control), 30 s rinsing with demineralized water (1.82 × 10^7 µSv; TKA GenPure, TKA xCAD, TKA Wasseraufbereitungssysteme GmbH, Niederelbert, Germany) without further treatment was performed.

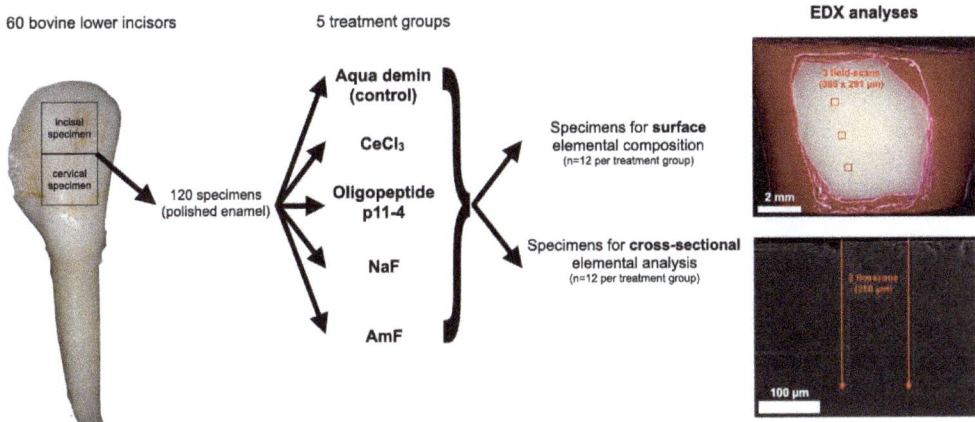

Figure 1. Flowchart of the experimental steps. From 60 bovine lower incisors, 120 polished enamel specimens were randomly allocated to 5 treatment groups: Aqua demin (control), cerium(III)-chloride ($CeCl_3$), oligopeptide p11-4, sodium fluoride (NaF), and amine fluoride (AmF). The surface elemental composition (Ce, N, F, Ca, P, O, Na, Mg) was measured in three fields of the treated enamel surface using energy dispersive X-ray spectroscopy (EDX). The accumulation on the surface was analyzed in cross-sections by EDX linescans and two-dimensional EDX element mappings.

2.2. Surface Visualization (LV-SEM)

All 12 specimens from every group were dried in an exsiccator using activated silica gel (Silica-Gel with indicator Orange-Gel, Merck, Germany) for 24 h. Within 4 h they were mounted onto aluminum stubs (Baltic Präparation, e.K., Wetter, Germany) using double-sided adhesive carbon discs and conductive adhesive paste (Leit-Tab and Leit-C-Plast, Baltic Präparation e.K.). Exemplary superficial SEM micrographs (FEI Quanta 400 FEG, Thermo Fisher Scientific, FEI Deutschland GmbH, Dreieich, Germany) were taken from the enamel surface in low vacuum mode (secondary electron mode, 1.5 Torr, accelerating voltage 10 kV, working distance 10 mm, horizontal field width 10.82 µm) without previous sputtering, using a large field detector (LFD) and pressure limiting aperture (PLA).

2.3. Surface Elemental Composition (EDX)

Using the same specimens, the surface elemental composition was measured in three fields (366 × 291 µm) at a distance of at least 500 µm from each other and at least 500 µm within the margin of the treated enamel surface (Figure 1), using EDX (EDAX Octane Elect detector, APEX v2.0, AMETEK EDAX GmbH, Weiterstadt, Germany) and calibration with standard customized coefficients (SCC). The EDX measurements were performed in low vacuum mode (PLA, 1.5 Torr, accelerating voltage 10 kV, working distance 10 mm, 50 µm aperture, 100 live seconds, amp time 3.84 µs, image resolution 1024 × 800 pixels). Atomic percent (At%) of the elements Ce, N, F, Ca, P, O, Na and Mg were calculated from every field. At%Ce, At%N, or At%F were the target parameters of the experiment being selective indicators for precipitation of $CeCl_3$, oligopeptide p11-4, or fluorides. C, Cl, and Si were not included in the analysis, because they were not within the scope of the study, and their concentration may be influenced by storage and polishing procedures.

2.4. Cross-sectional Elemental Analysis (EDX)

From the remaining 60 specimens (12 per group), cross sections through the specimen perpendicular to the enamel surface were made following treatment to analyze surface accumulation "from the side" and potential in-depth penetration (Figure 1). Before cutting, the enamel surface was gently air-dried, covered with Clearfil SE Bond (Kuraray, Chiyoda,

Japan) and low viscosity bulk-fill composite (SDR flow+, Dentsply Sirona, York, NY, USA), and light cured according to the manufacturer instructions (VALO curing light, up 5919-I, Ultradent Products, South Jordan, UT, USA) in order to mechanically stabilize the enamel surface during the following cutting procedure. Subsequently, the specimens were centrally cut perpendicular to the enamel surface using a saw microtome (Leitz 1600; Leica Microsystems, Wetzlar, Germany), dried and mounted as described for surface elemental composition specimens.

In order to verify the accumulation of the target elements Ce, N and F on the enamel surface, cross-sectional EDX linescans were taken perpendicular from the cut enamel surface, including the surface and deeper areas (FEI Quanta 400 FEG, EDAX Octane Elect detector, APEX v2.0), using low vacuum mode (1.5 Torr, PLA, accelerating voltage 10 kV, working distance 10 mm, aperture 50 µm). Within each scan, the counts of either Ce, N, or F were used as target elements. For each specimen, two parallel central EDX linescans with a distance of 100 µm from each other and perpendicular to the original enamel surface were recorded. Each line comprised a row of single measurements with 2 µm line width along a length of 250 µm with 0.9 µm intervals in between two single measurements (dwell time 20 ms; amplification time 7.68 µs; 50–80 frame iterations to collect necessary counts). For each element, the EDX counts were plotted against the sample depth, and a two-dimensional fit (TableCurve 2D, v5.01 S4STAT, Chicago, IL, USA) was applied. For every linescan, the counts of the target element in >100 µm depth from the enamel surface resembled a horizontal line and were therefore defined as background noise. From all fitted EDX linescans, the functions obtained by TableCurve 2D that showed a peak of EDX counts of Ce, N, or F at the enamel surface was counted and evaluated as an additional indicator of a consistent accumulation of the target elements.

2.5. Determination of Nitrogen in the Oligopeptide p11-4 Delivery-System (Curodont Repair)

No information on the concentration of oligopeptide p11-4 within Curodont Repair is provided by the manufacturer. Therefore, and because of the results of the above described experiments, the nitrogen content of Curodont Repair was determined by EDX. Hitherto the relative elemental composition of the manufacturer's applicator brush alone, the oligopeptide p11-4 fluid alone and oligopeptide p11-4 fluid applied according to manufacturer's instructions using the respective applicator brush were analyzed. The fluids were applied on aluminum stubs that were covered with adhesive carbon discs (Leit-Tab) and allowed to dry without rinsing off. The residue was analyzed for its elemental composition with respect to C, N, O, Na, and S using EDX (all measurements: low vacuum mode, 1.5 Torr, accelerating voltage 10 kV, horizontal field width 340 µm). Additionally, the Leit-Tab without test materials was examined.

2.6. Data Analysis

For surface EDX data, non-parametric statistical procedures were used to analyze At% of respective elements (SPSS version 25.0, IBM, Armonk, USA). The median of the three measured fields per specimen was used as the representative value of every specimen. Ca/P ratios were calculated. For all groups, medians and 25% and 75% percentiles were calculated from the specimens' representative values. The Mann–Whitney U Test was used to test for statistically significant differences between groups. The level of significance was set to $\alpha = 0.05$ and adjusted to $\alpha^*\left(k\right) = 1 - \sqrt[k]{1-\alpha}$ with k = number of pairwise tests to be considered in case of multiple comparisons according to the error rate method [18].

3. Results

Relative atomic percent [At%] composition at the enamel surface and the Ca/P ratio of the investigated groups are shown in Table 1 and Figures 2 and 3.

Table 1. Results of atomic percent [At%] and Ca/P ratio at the enamel surface following treatment according to group (n = 12). Since data are not symmetrically distributed, and some of the sums of the medians may differ from 100%. Asterisks indicate significant difference between the respective group and the control (Aqua demin). Data are also depicted in Figures 2 and 3.

	Aqua Demin (Control)		$CeCl_3$		Oligopeptide p11-4		NaF		AmF	
	Median	25–75%	Median	25–75%	Median	25–75%	Median	25–75%	Median	25–75%
At%Ce	0.00	0.00–0.00	0.75 *	0.60–1.43	0.00	0.00–0.00	0.00	0.00–0.00	0.00	0.00–0.00
At%N	0.00	0.00–0.00	0.00	0.00–0.00	0.00	0.00–0.00	0.00	0.00–0.00	0.00	0.00–0.00
At%F	0.00	0.00–0.00	0.00	0.00–0.00	0.00	0.00–0.10	15.20 *	12.88–16.85	17.04 *	8.85–21.23
At%Ca	21.85	20.35–22.63	20.90	19.85–22.08	20.80	20.25–22.08	22.35	21.53–23.15	24.55 *	23.58–25.48
At%P	13.40	12.63–13.77	13.20	12.85–13.60	13.00	12.58–13.51	11.00 *	10.43–11.18	11.22 *	10.38–12.90
At%O	63.60	62.62–65.78	64.10	62.50–64.98	65.00	63.19–66.18	50.70 *	48.93–52.18	47.55 *	40.41–52.38
At%Na	0.40	0.40–0.50	0.40	0.40–0.40	0.40	0.40–0.50	0.60 *	0.53–0.60	0.45	0.40–0.50
At%Mg	0.50	0.40–0.60	0.43	0.40–0.58	0.40	0.40–0.50	0.60	0.43–0.70	0.50	0.40–0.64
Ca/P ratio	1.63	1.62–1.65	1.60 *	1.55–1.62	1.62	1.60–1.63	2.03 *	1.96–2.12	2.17 *	1.92–2.40

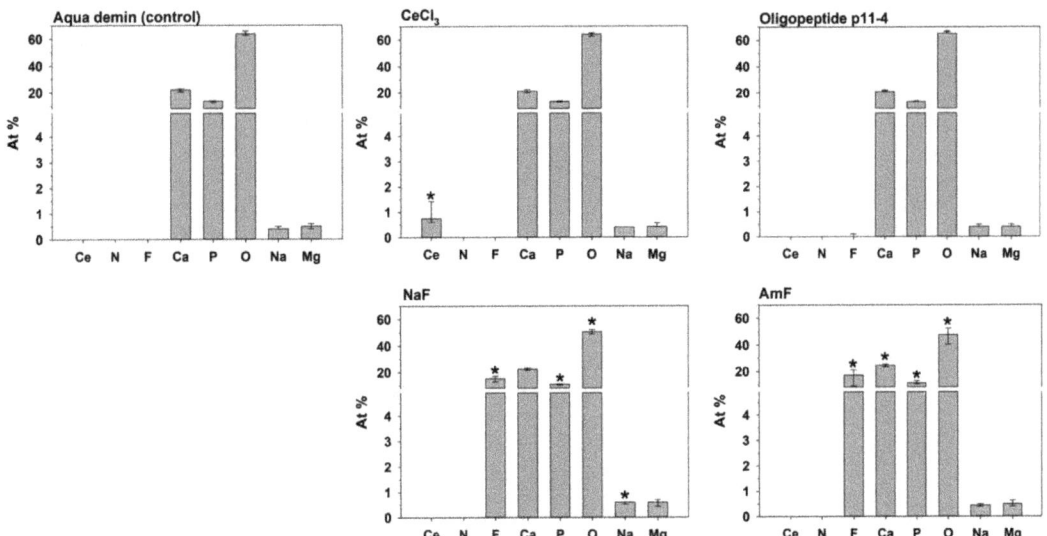

Figure 2. Median and 25–75% percentiles of the elemental composition [At%] at the enamel surface displayed in a separate diagram for each group (n = 12). For a single element, an asterisk indicates a significant difference between the respective group and the control (Aqua demin).

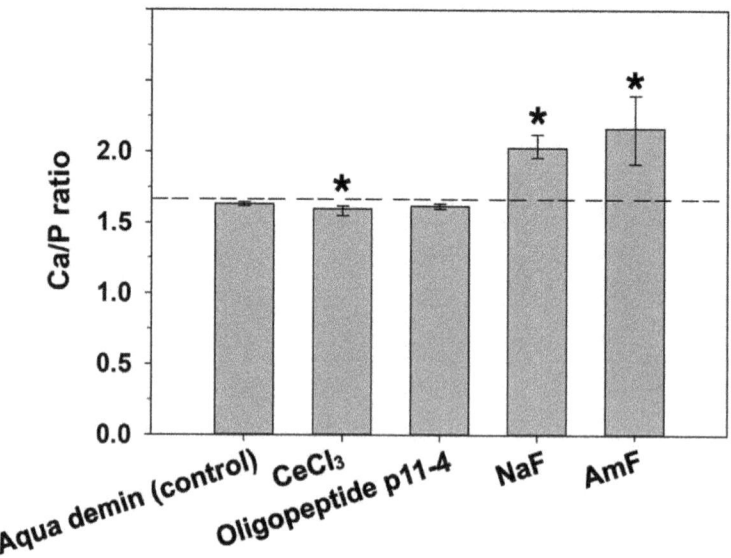

Figure 3. Ca/P ratio of the respective groups (median and 25–75% percentiles; n = 12) at the enamel surface. Asterisks indicate significant differences compared to the control (Aqua demin). Dashed line shows stoichiometric ratio (1.667) of hydroxyapatite.

Control enamel surfaces (Aqua demin, treatment with deionized water only) comprised Ca, P, O, and, to a lesser degree, Na and Mg. The Ca/P ratio in the control group was near the ratio of stoichiometric hydroxyapatite of 10:6 = 1.667. None of the target elements Ce, N, or F were found. Cerium was found on enamel surfaces after cerium(III)-chloride application (group $CeCl_3$) only. Nitrogen could neither be detected after application of oligopeptide p11-4 that contains nitrogen, nor in any other group. Fluorine was always found after application of NaF or AmF, but not in any other group. According to the error rate method (k = 8), $CeCl_3$, NaF, and AmF differed significantly from control (Aqua demin) regarding their elemental compositions, but oligopeptide p11-4 did not.

In detail, NaF application also led to significantly more At%Na ($p \leq 0.001$) compared to Aqua demin, but less At%O and At%P ($p \leq 0.001$). Treatment with amine fluoride (AmF) also exhibited significantly more At%Ca ($p \leq 0.001$) compared to Aqua demin, but significantly less At%O ($p \leq 0.001$), and At%P ($P = 0.003$). A significant increase of the Ca/P ratio (Figure 3) compared to the control treatment (Aqua demin) was found for NaF ($p \leq 0.001$) and AmF ($p \leq 0.001$), in contrast to $CeCl_3$, which showed significant decreased Ca/P ratio ($p \leq 0.001$) compared to the control treatment (Aqua demin). Oligopeptide p11-4 did not show a difference compared to control (Aqua demin) in the Ca/P ratio. Furthermore, regarding the both fluorine-containing test materials, application of NaF led to significantly more At%Na ($p \leq 0.001$) and significantly less At%Ca ($p \leq 0.001$) as compared to application of AmF, but there were no significant differences in At%F.

Low vacuum micrographs (Figure 4) revealed superficial, net-like deposits after application of $CeCl_3$. Enamel surfaces of group Oligopeptide p11-4 did not show any deposits and were not discernable from the control (Aqua demin). In group NaF and AmF, globular precipitates on the enamel surface similar to CaF_2 deposits can be seen.

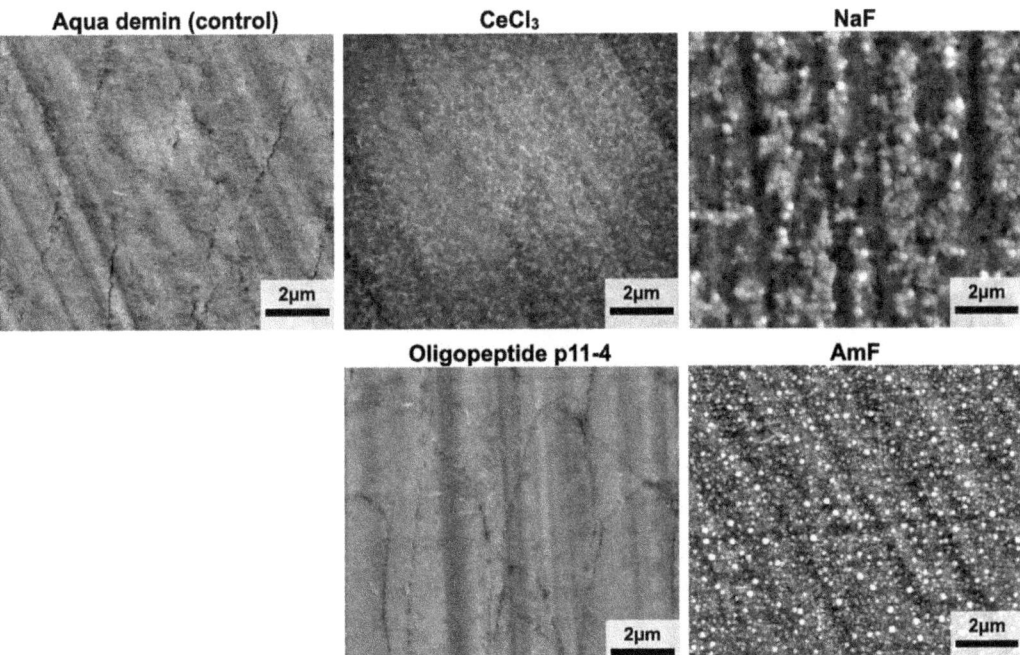

Figure 4. Low vacuum (secondary electron mode) SEM images. Globular precipitates comparable with CaF_2 deposits were visible for groups NaF and AmF. The surfaces of specimens from group $CeCl_3$ showed net-like superficial deposits. The images from the oligopeptide p11-4 group and Aqua demin (control) are visually indistinguishable.

In the cross-sectioned specimens (Figure 5), distinct surface accumulations appeared in the form of peak functions for $CeCl_3$ based on the cerium counts in 3 out of 24 (12.5%) linescans, for NaF based on the fluorine counts in 20 out of 24 (83.3%) linescans, for AmF based on the fluorine counts in 23 out of 24 (95.8%) linescans, but not in oligopeptide p11-4 groups based on the nitrogen counts and not for Aqua demin (control) for any of the target elements. Notably, the peaks for $CeCl_3$ and NaF are only about twice the background noise, while for AmF it is about 15 times higher.

$$y = a + \frac{b}{d+e}\left[1 - e^{-c(x-f)} - \frac{d}{d+e-c}\left(1 + ce^{-(d+e)(x-f)} - (d+e)e^{-c(x-f)}\right)\right] \quad (1)$$

$$y = a + b\,\text{erfc}\left[\left(\frac{x-c}{d}\right)^2\right], \text{ with } \text{erfc}(x) = 2\int_x^\infty \frac{1}{\sqrt{\pi}}e^{-u^2}du\,; x \geq 0. \quad (2)$$

The fits showed a clear superficial accumulation of fluorine-containing deposits in all specimens in which NaF (b) or AmF (c) were applied. In some CeCl3 (a) samples, cerium-containing accumulations were detected at the surface, but with a much smaller difference between peak and background compared to the fluoride accumulations. None of the target elements Ce, N, or F were found following treatment with oligopeptide p11-4 or control (Aqua demin). A different scale (y-axis) was used for better visibility.

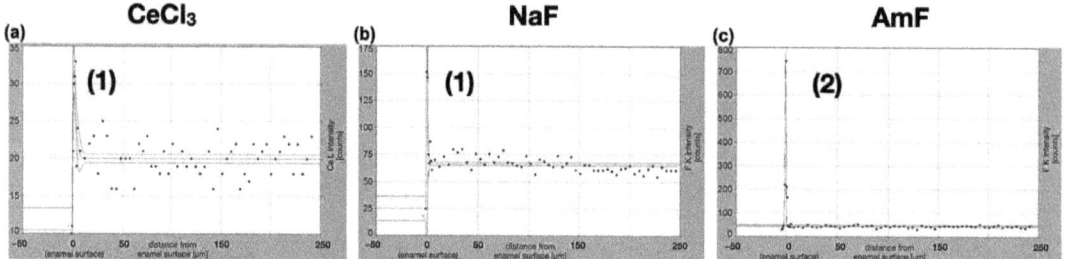

Figure 5. Visualization of linescans from the surface to a depth of 250 µm from the surface. For every linescan, the counts of the target element in >100 µm depth from the enamel surface resembled a horizontal line and were therefore defined as background noise. Counts (y-axis) of respective elements were plotted as a function of depth into enamel (x-axis). Two-dimensional fits were calculated (green lines) with corresponding 95% confidence limits (purple lines). Best fits were an *Equilibrium Peak function*(1) for CeCl$_3$ (r^2 = 0.62; (**a**)) and NaF (r^2 = 0.86; (**b**)) and a *Complementary Error Peak function* (2) for AmF (r^2 = 0.97; (**c**)).

The elemental composition of the product containing oligopeptide p11-4 used in this study (Curodont Repair) is depicted in Table 2. The caked solution of Curodont Repair applied with the applicator brush provided by the manufacturer comprised 2.3 At%N, the solution not in contact with the respective brush 1.5 At%N, and the specific brush itself 5.6 At%N. The Curodont system contains nitrogen, indicating the presence of oligopeptide p11-4.

Table 2. Relative elemental composition of the manufacturer's applicator brush, the test material Oligopeptide p11-4 applied according to manufacturer's instructions on a Leit-Tab, the oligopeptide p11-4 fluid on a Leit-Tab, and the Leit-Tab without test material application.

Element [Atom%]	C	N	O	Na	S
Oligopeptide p11-4 manufacturer's applicator brush	63.4	5.6	31	0	0
Oligopeptide p11-4 applied on Leit-Tab according to manufacturer	54.3	2.3	43.3	0	0.1
Oligopeptide p11-4 fluid on Leit-Tab	66.1	1.5	30.9	0.7	0.8
Leit-Tab without test material application	87.5	0	12.1	0.1	0.3

4. Discussion

In the present study, test materials with cariostatic potential were applied to sound bovine enamel. As the controls (treated with Aqua demin) always contained 0 At% of the target elements cerium (At%Ce), nitrogen (At%N), and fluorine (At%F) by median, the necessary condition to detect and analyze the cariostatic test materials used in this experimental setup was established. Moreover, the target element N proved to be reliably detectable with the EDX setup used.

For a locally applied cariostatic to actually achieve the intended preventive effects in a clinical situation, e.g., positively influencing the balance between demineralization and remineralization or inhibiting bacterial biofilm formation, it is a basic prerequisite that it can adequately attach to the enamel [5]. Despite the widespread use of fluorides, with an estimated 1.5 billion daily users of fluoridated toothpaste in 2015, dental caries is prevalent worldwide [1,19,20]. Therefore, a deeper understanding of the mechanisms of action of fluorides in the context of their cations and alternative cariostatic compounds is essential.

In a previous study, we established energy dispersive X-ray spectroscopy (EDX) as a method to detect and analyze CaF$_2$-like precipitations after fluoride gel application on sound human enamel under high vacuum conditions [10]. In contrast to this former study, here we used SEM imaging and EDX, both under low vacuum conditions, to allow us to study sample surfaces without any experimental modifications, especially without a surface metal coating [21,22]. Generally, elements with larger atomic numbers ($Z > 10$) can be analyzed with high accuracy using EDX [23]. However, we were able to reliably measure elements with an atomic number ≤ 10, in the case of the present study, mainly F, O, and N, by system calibration with customized coefficient-standards (SCC) and using an EDX system with a Si_3N_4 window, which has higher transmittance compared to generally used polymer windows, especially for low keV X-rays emitted by elements of lower atomic numbers [24]. To date, there are no other studies directly aiming for detection of oligopeptides on dental hard tissues by targeting the nitrogen atoms using energy dispersive X-ray spectroscopy. However, measuring peptide nitrogen with EDX has already been applied in other fields such as the detection of peptides on nanofibers for peripheral nerve regeneration [25,26] or the detection of oligopeptide integrated into polymeric fibers [27].

Among the test materials applied in this study, two of the treatment solutions are marketed, clinically applicable compounds (oligopeptide p11-4: Curodont Repair; AmF: Elmex Fluid). NaF was used in the same fluoride concentration and pH-value as AmF. $CeCl_3$ was prepared as an experimental solution.

At%Ce > 0 were found for all areas treated with cerium(III)-chloride without significant influence on the other elements. When applied to sound enamel, cerium might have a cariostatic effect inhibiting the onset of a carious lesion by replacing single calcium ions in the hydroxyapatite lattice, leading to a more stable substituted apatite [14,15]. Another in vitro study showed a positive effect of 10% cerium chloride application on the reduction in quantitative light-induced fluorescence loss during demineralization and remineralization cycles compared to a placebo solution [28]. Our study showed that cerium can adhere to sound enamel areas with a median of 0.8 At%Ce. Since cerium could possibly act as a substituent for calcium within the hydroxyapatite lattice, this could explain the lower Ca/P ratio of specimens treated with $CeCl_3$ compared to control specimens.

After the application of the two different fluoride-containing test materials, although identical in fluoride content and pH, elemental composition differed between those two for some elements. Despite different cations, both fluoride preparations in the present study had a pH of 4, leading to precipitation of CaF_2-like globular structures that can be seen on SEM images (Figure 4) and were confirmed by the high surface At%F. This is in accordance with other in vitro studies that showed fluoride precipitation after the application of acidic fluoride compounds [8,10,29,30]. Surface fluoride accumulation was also observed in most of the cross sectioned samples for NaF and AmF. Following application of $CeCl_3$, cerium was detectable in some cross-sectioned samples, but less frequently as compared to fluorine at fluoridated samples. This can be explained by a presumably thicker layer of the precipitates containing fluoride compared to the precipitates containing cerium, which is also supported by the higher At% for the fluoride preparations compared to the At%Ce for $CeCl_3$ in surface elemental composition analysis. On the other hand, two randomly located linescans were performed per sample, which is why especially thin accumulations were not detectable in all linescans, although they were revealed to be present in all surface elemental composition analyses. Oligopeptide p11-4 could neither be detected in cross sectional specimens nor by direct elemental analysis of the treated surface.

In the present study, nitrogen from oligopeptide p11-4 was found in the liquid and the applicator of the test material as depicted in Table 2, but not after application on enamel and rinsing with demineralized water, as performed for all test materials. Within the test material oligopeptide p11-4, the measurements indicate an uneven distribution of the oligopeptide over the applicator and the liquid, whereas a stable adherence of the peptide on sound enamel was not achievable. The Ca-binding capacity reported for oligopeptide p11-4 seems not to be sufficiently strong to establish its bond to the sound enamel surface.

A limitation of the study might be that we investigated the direct interaction of the applied test materials with sound polished enamel. Presence of a pellicle or pH-cycling might influence outcomes regarding superficial elemental composition. While this study shed light on the potential of novel anti-cariogenic compounds in order to prevent the onset of carious lesions starting with sound enamel, future research may focus on the persistence and efficacy of surface precipitations and in-depth penetration of such anti-cariogenic compounds to promote remineralization of previously demineralized areas varying in mineral content and porosity, in order to fully comprehend their potential during demineralization and remineralization.

5. Conclusions

Cerium and fluorine could be detected significantly on all bovine enamel surfaces after application of $CeCl_3$ and NaF or AmF, respectively, which were found to be significantly different to the untreated control. In contrast, nitrogen was not detected after application of oligopeptide p11-4 and did not lead to any significant difference in superficial elemental composition compared to untreated control specimens.

Author Contributions: Conceptualization K.J.S., K.-A.H., W.B.; methodology H.E., G.F., K.B., F.P.; validation T.T.T., F.P., W.B.; formal analysis K.-A.H., K.J.S.; investigation K.J.S., H.E., G.F., K.-A.H.; data curation K.-A.H., K.J.S.; writing—original draft preparation K.J.S.; writing—review and editing W.B., K.-A.H., T.T.T., F.P., K.B.; visualization K.-A.H., H.E., G.F; supervision W.B., K.J.S.; project administration K.J.S., K.-A.H., H.E., G.F. All authors have read and agreed to the published version of the manuscript.

Funding: Konstantin J. Scholz and Florian Pielnhofer received funding from the University of Regensburg (UR Fellows program). Konstantin J. Scholz received funding from the Medical Faculty of the University of Regensburg (ReForM A program) and the DGZMK (German Society of Dental, Oral and Craniomandibular Sciences; Deutsche Gesellschaft für Zahn-, Mund- und Kieferheilkunde; science funding).

Institutional Review Board Statement: No human material and only tooth samples from dead cattle were used for this study. No separate ethical approval was required for this study as stated by the Ethics Committee of the Faculty of Medicine, University of Regensburg (Regensburg, Germany). All experiments were performed in accordance with relevant guidelines and regulations.

Informed Consent Statement: Not applicable.

Data Availability Statement: All relevant data generated or analyzed during this study are included in this article. Further enquiries can be directed to the corresponding author.

Acknowledgments: Rainer Müller (Institute of Physical and Theoretical Chemistry, University of Regensburg, Regensburg, Germany) is acknowledged for valuable discussions in the initial phase of this study. Felix Bressmer (Department of Conservative Dentistry and Periodontology, University Medical Center Regensburg, Germany), Andrea Gubler, and My-Lien Lai (Department of Conservative and Preventive Dentistry, University of Zurich, Switzerland) are acknowledged for support in specimen preparation.

Conflicts of Interest: The authors declare no conflict of interest.

References

1. Wen, P.Y.F.; Chen, M.X.; Zhong, Y.J.; Dong, Q.Q.; Wong, H.M. Global Burden and Inequality of Dental Caries, 1990 to 2019. *J. Dent. Res.* **2022**, *101*, 392–399. [CrossRef] [PubMed]
2. Arends, J.; Christoffersen, J. Invited Review Article: The Nature of Early Caries Lesions in Enamel. *J. Dent. Res.* **1986**, *65*, 2–11. [CrossRef] [PubMed]
3. Philip, N. State of the Art Enamel Remineralization Systems: The Next Frontier in Caries Management. *Caries Res.* **2018**, *53*, 284–295. [CrossRef]
4. Pitts, N.B. Are We Ready to Move from Operative to Non-Operative/Preventive Treatment of Dental Caries in Clinical Practice? *Caries Res.* **2004**, *38*, 294–304. [CrossRef] [PubMed]
5. Twetman, S. Prevention of Dental Caries as a Non-communicable Disease. *Eur. J. Oral. Sci.* **2018**, *126*, 19–25. [CrossRef]
6. Walsh, T.; Worthington, H.V.; Glenny, A.M.; Appelbe, P.; Marinho, V.C.; Shi, X. Fluoride Toothpastes of Different Concentrations for Preventing Dental Caries in Children and Adolescents. *Cochrane Database Syst. Rev.* **2010**, *2*, 22. [CrossRef] [PubMed]

7. Lenzi, T.L.; Montagner, A.F.; Soares, F.Z.M.; de Oliveira Rocha, R. Are Topical Fluorides Effective for Treating Incipient Carious Lesions? A Systematic Review and Meta-Analysis. *J. Am. Dent. Assoc.* **2016**, *147*, 84–91.e1. [CrossRef]
8. Dijkman, T.G.; Arenas, L. The Role of 'CaF2-like' Material in Topical Fluoridation of Enamel in Situ. *Acta Odontol. Scand.* **2009**, *46*, 391–397. [CrossRef]
9. Hellwig, E.; Lennon, Á.M. Systemic versus Topical Fluoride. *Caries Res.* **2004**, *38*, 258–262. [CrossRef]
10. Scholz, K.J.; Federlin, M.; Hiller, K.; Ebensberger, H.; Ferstl, G.; Buchalla, W. EDX-Analysis of Fluoride Precipitation on Human Enamel. *Sci. Rep.* **2019**, *9*, 7. [CrossRef]
11. De Leeuw, N.H. Resisting the Onset of Hydroxyapatite Dissolution through the Incorporation of Fluoride. *J. Phys. Chem. B* **2004**, *108*, 1809–1811. [CrossRef]
12. Wegehaupt, F.J.; Sener, B.; Attin, T.; Schmidlin, P.R. Anti-Erosive Potential of Amine Fluoride, Cerium Chloride and Laser Irradiation Application on Dentine. *Arch. Oral Biol.* **2011**, *56*, 1541–1547. [CrossRef] [PubMed]
13. Wegehaupt, F.J.; Sener, B.; Attin, T.; Schmidlin, P.R. Application of Cerium Chloride to Improve the Acid Resistance of Dentine. *Arch. Oral Biol.* **2010**, *55*, 441–446. [CrossRef] [PubMed]
14. Wegehaupt, F.J.; Buchalla, W.; Sener, B.; Attin, T.; Schmidlin, P.R. Cerium Chloride Reduces Enamel Lesion Initiation and Progression in Vitro. *Caries Res.* **2014**, *48*, 45–50. [CrossRef]
15. Feng, Z.; Liao, Y.; Ye, M. Synthesis and Structure of Cerium-Substituted Hydroxyapatite. *J. Mater. Sci. Mater. Med.* **2005**, *16*, 417–421. [CrossRef]
16. Aggeli, A.; Fytas, G.; Vlassopoulos, D.; McLeish, T.C.B.; Mawer, P.J.; Boden, N. Structure and Dynamics of Self-Assembling β-Sheet Peptide Tapes by Dynamic Light Scattering. *Biomacromolecules* **2001**, *2*, 378–388. [CrossRef]
17. Kind, L.; Stevanovic, S.; Wuttig, S.; Wimberger, S.; Hofer, J.; Müller, B.; Pieles, U. Biomimetic Remineralization of Carious Lesions by Self-Assembling Peptide. *J. Dent. Res.* **2017**, *96*, 790–797. [CrossRef]
18. Miller, R.G., Jr. *Simultaneous Statistical Inference*; Springer Series in Statistics: Berlin/Heidelberg, Germany, 2011; Volume 2, ISBN 9781461381242.
19. Gkekas, A.; Varenne, B.; Stauf, N.; Benzian, H.; Listl, S. Affordability of Essential Medicines: The Case of Fluoride Toothpaste in 78 Countries. *PLoS ONE* **2022**, *17*, e0275111. [CrossRef]
20. FDI World Dental Federation. *The Oral Health Atlas—The Challenge of Oral Disease*; Myriad Editions: Brighton, UK, 2015; Volume 2, ISBN 978-2-9700934-8-0.
21. Scholz, K.J.; Bittner, A.; Cieplik, F.; Hiller, K.; Schmalz, G.; Buchalla, W.; Federlin, M. Micromorphology of the Adhesive Interface of Self-Adhesive Resin Cements to Enamel and Dentin. *Materials* **2021**, *14*, 492. [CrossRef]
22. Sato, S.; Matsui, H.; Sasaki, Y.; Oharazawa, H.; Nishimura, A.; Adachi, A.; Nakazawa, E.; Takahashi, H. The Efficiency of X-Ray Microanalysis in Low-Vacuum Scanning Electron Microscope: Deposition of Calcium on the Surface of Implanted Hydrogel Intraocular Lens (IOL). *J. Submicr. Cytol. Path.* **2006**, *38*, 1–4.
23. Scimeca, M.; Bischetti, S.; Lamsira, H.K.; Bonfiglio, R.; Bonanno, E. Energy Dispersive X-ray (EDX) Microanalysis: A Powerful Tool in Biomedical Research and Diagnosis. *Eur. J. Histochem.* **2018**, *62*, 2841. [CrossRef] [PubMed]
24. Rafaelsen, J.; Nylese, T.; Bolorizadeh, M.; Carlino, V. Windowless, Silicon Nitride Window and Polymer Window EDS Detectors: Changes in Sensitivity and Detectable Limits. *Microsc. Microanal.* **2015**, *21*, 1645–1646. [CrossRef]
25. Nune, M.; Subramanian, A.; Krishnan, U.M.; Sethuraman, S. Peptide Nanostructures on Nanofibers for Peripheral Nerve Regeneration. *J. Tissue Eng. Regen. M* **2019**, *13*, 1059–1070. [CrossRef] [PubMed]
26. Nune, M.; Krishnan, U.M.; Sethuraman, S. PLGA Nanofibers Blended with Designer Self-Assembling Peptides for Peripheral Neural Regeneration. *Mater. Sci. Eng. C* **2016**, *62*, 329–337. [CrossRef] [PubMed]
27. Gharaei, R.; Tronci, G.; Davies, R.P.W.; Gough, C.; Alazragi, R.; Goswami, P.; Russell, S.J. A Structurally Self-Assembled Peptide Nano-Architecture by One-Step Electrospinning. *J. Mater. Chem. B* **2016**, *4*, 5475–5485. [CrossRef]
28. Jaisingh, R.; Shanbhog, R.; Nandlal, B.; Thippeswamy, M. Effect of 10% Cerium Chloride on Artificial Caries Lesions of Human Enamel Evaluated Using Quantitative Light-Induced Fluorescence: An in Vitro Study. *Eur. Arch. Paediatr. Dent.* **2017**, *18*, 163–169. [CrossRef]
29. Comar, L.P.; Souza, B.M.; Al-Ahj, L.P.; Martins, J.; Grizzo, L.T.; Piasentim, I.S.; Rios, D.; Buzalaf, M.A.R.; Magalhães, A.C. Mechanism of Action of TiF4 on Dental Enamel Surface: SEM/EDX, KOH-Soluble F, and X-Ray Diffraction Analysis. *Caries Res.* **2017**, *51*, 554–567. [CrossRef] [PubMed]
30. Petzold, M. The Influence of Different Fluoride Compounds and Treatment Conditions on Dental Enamel: A Descriptive in Vitro Study of the CaF2 Precipitation and Microstructure. *Caries Res.* **2001**, *35*, 45–51. [CrossRef]

MDPI
St. Alban-Anlage 66
4052 Basel
Switzerland
www.mdpi.com

Bioengineering Editorial Office
E-mail: bioengineering@mdpi.com
www.mdpi.com/journal/bioengineering

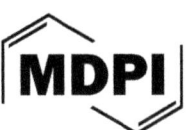

Disclaimer/Publisher's Note: The statements, opinions and data contained in all publications are solely those of the individual author(s) and contributor(s) and not of MDPI and/or the editor(s). MDPI and/or the editor(s) disclaim responsibility for any injury to people or property resulting from any ideas, methods, instructions or products referred to in the content.

www.ingramcontent.com/pod-product-compliance
Lightning Source LLC
LaVergne TN
LVHW070629100526
838202LV00012B/763